Struik Lifestyle
(a imprint of Random House Stru
Company Reg. No. 1699/003153/(
80 McKenzie Street
Cape Town 8001
South Africa
www.randomstruik.co.za

First published in 1994 by Viking, a division of the Penguin Group
Second edition published in 2009 by Random House Struik (Pty) Ltd

PUBLISHER: Linda de Villiers
MANAGING EDITOR: Cecilia Barfield
EDITOR: Gill Gordon
DESIGNER: Ilze van der Westhuizen
ILLUSTRATOR: James Berrangé
PROOFREADER: Glynne Newlands

Reproduction by Hirt & Carter Cape (Pty) Ltd
Printed and bound by Kyodo Nation Printing Services Co., Ltd, Thailand

ISBN 978 1 77007 753 9

Over 40 000 unique African images are available to purchase from our
image bank at **www.imagesofafrica.co.za**

AUTHOR'S DEDICATION

This book is dedicated to my daughter Alexandra who, like me, is a dreamer; to my wife Jean Anne who manages to keep my feet on the ground even when my head is under water; to all those divers whose ingenuity and courage from the time of Alexander the Great have made the sport possible; and to all modern scuba divers who delight in the underwater world.

CONTENTS

FOREWORD TO THE FIRST EDITION

Some books for divers seem to be written for instructors, others for research specialists or book reviewers, and a few for all three. This one is really written for committed and serious divers from Openwater I to Instructor level, diving medical technicians, and even diving physicians who have just recently entered the field of diving medicine. The text presents all areas of diving medicine from early history to recent scientific developments.

Approximately one-third of the text is devoted to the important issue of fitness to dive. Today's divers are considerably more knowledgeable than those of thirty years ago about the physiology and medicine of diving, as evidenced by their regular attendance at diving symposia and their ever-increasing demand for educational materials. Those medical conditions that militate against pursuing diving as a recreational or professional activity are cleary discussed and, for some conditions, excellent examples are used, often with pleasant humour to stress the issue.

The classification of decompression disorders has been the subject of considerable discussion and review by diving physicians recently, and a descriptive approach was proposed by Francis and Smth ('Describing Decompression Illness') which does not need formal acceptance of a mechanism or site. It utilises a description of symptoms, their rate of progression and their response to treatment, rather than the older classification of Type I or Type II decompression sickness. The author uses this classification of decompression disorders in his sections on treatment. The system is simple and it works.

The understanding of safe and efficient diving is greatly aided by this exceptionally complete and well-written book. *Safe Diving* is thoroughly recommended to all divers from student level to instructor – and to those physicians or diving medical technicians who may be required to provide medical treatment to those who venture under the sea.

Leon J. Greenbaum, Jr., PhD
Executive director: Undersea and Hyperbaric Medical Society
Bethesda, Maryland
United States of America

FOREWORD TO THIS EDITION

The beauty and mystery of the sea have always fascinated man. Fired by a desire to embrace its charm and challenge its fury we have engaged in various pursuits, from sailing its surface to delving its depths. In respect of the latter, scuba diving holds a particular intrigue, being a remarkable tale of the triumph of human ingenuity over environmental adversity, one that has demanded huge investments from science and medicine over several centuries.

Allan Kayle has been able to capture the essence and culmination of this quest in a book spanning less than 400 pages. With his exceptional gifts of language, imagination and understanding, Allan takes the reader by the hand, and reveals this fascinating world in a practical and completely accessible way. All who engage the underwater realm will benefit from his work – from the ardent researcher to the novice recreational diver.

Safe Diving first appeared in 1994. What impressed me immediately was the grace and deceptive simplicity with which complex terms as well as scientific and medical controversies were reduced to the level of advanced common sense. In this edition, Allan follows the tried and tested approach of introducing history and physics, followed by the importance of diving medicals and how the various parts and systems within the body may affect diving safety and enjoyment. Next he tackles the operational areas of diving maladies and accidents and how to manage them. His flow-diagrams, charts and decision-trees not only offer a logical approach to many diverse problems, they also illuminate the priorities of care in pragmatic, chronological order. The illustrations are superb, while the updated, expanded and enriched text is a sheer joy.

As executive director of DAN Southern Africa, I endorse this work fully and recommend it to all who seek excellence, safety and enjoyment in their respective underwater pursuits.

Frans J Cronje
MBChB, MSc
President and executive director: Divers Alert Network Southern Africa
Past-president: Southern African Undersea & Hyperbaric Medical Association
17th President of the International Congress of Hyperbaric Medicine

INTRODUCTION

Over the past 25 years I have seen and chatted to thousands of divers. We've spoken about bends and arterial gas embolism, bone necrosis and oxygen toxicity, nitrogen narcosis and middle ear problems. Over a sea of beer we've sailed through the hazards of squeezes and squalls, swum through kelp, and coughed through lung injuries and carbon monoxide.

Although sport diving has now become hugely popular worldwide and vast amounts of diving information are just a click away on the internet, there is still a lot of confusion, misinformation and even mystery about diving. Most divers know of the dangers, but not so many really know what to do when they occur. This book is for the diver who has enough knowledge to feel insecure when faced by a diving emergency. It is a look at diving from a casualty's point of view. It explains basic medical fitness to dive and explores the advisability of diving with, or after, an underlying illness.

Attention is devoted to the hundreds of illnesses common to everyone, such as influenza, diarrhoea, stomach acid reflux, high cholesterol levels and high blood pressure. Heart disease, including heart valve problems, coronary artery disease, coronary artery stenting and bypass surgery, and their effects on diving are considered, as well as the host of diseases particular only to divers. A no-nonsense approach is provided to diving accidents and ailments – how to help and get help when a potential disaster threatens.

The growth of DAN worldwide, and the advantages of becoming a member of this international diver-orientated rescue service, cannot be overstressed. For the sake of completeness, diving laws, altitude tables, and the latest approach to therapeutic oxygen and mixed gas recompression tables are included.

Asthma and diabetes mellitus have long been the subject of intense controversy in diving circles. The requirements and advisability of diving with these conditions is provided. Nitrox diving has become immensely popular and the benefits and dangers of breathing an oxygen-enriched mix are included, as well as an assessment of diving with semi-closed and closed breathing sets using helium. Factors predisposing to bubble formation after diving, as well as recent work indicating the possibility of reducing bubble formation in sport divers, are given.

The term Acute Decompression Illness – as approved at the Undersea and Hyperbaric Medical Society in 1990 and the European Undersea Biomedical Society in 1991 – has been used throughout this book. It includes both decompression injuries as well as pulmonary barotrauma resulting in arterial gas embolism.

Hundreds of medicines and drugs are mentioned in these pages. Their generic names have been used instead of the more popular trade names. There were three reasons for doing this. The first was the fact that various pharmaceutical companies make the same generic compound but market it under different names. Secondly, many drug companies change the trade name of their product in different countries. The third, and most important, reason was to force the diver to obtain professional medical advice in identifying and obtaining a particular generic drug, and to seek help about the wisdom of using that drug in his or her particular case.

None of the drugs or medications named in this book should be used without consulting your doctor in advance for a prescription and proper consideration of any allergic or untoward side effect in your individual case. The same applies to all members of any diving group. Divers are sociable creatures and are frequently more than willing to share their resources with less-fortunate members of their diving group. This may include medications for buddy or other divers suffering from ailments such as seasickness, a coral scratch or an equalising problem. It is imperative to understand that non-qualified help is then being given and, should anything untoward or life-threatening occur, responsibility for any potential disaster shifts squarely on to the well-meaning diver. It is essential that qualified confirmation about the safety of any medicine or drug incorporated in a medical kit be obtained individually by each and every diver.

AIDS has been given special attention because of the escalating spread of the epidemic and the potential danger of assisting a bleeding victim who may be HIV-positive. The awful consequences of contracting the disease while saving a life have made safety precautions necessary in handling wounds and administering CPR.

The recommendations for the provision of effective CPR have changed radically in the last few years. The previous formula for one or two rescuers, and their rates of providing artificial respiration and cardiac massage, has been supplanted by a faster, more effective, but more energy-demanding input for either one or two rescuers. In non-diving cases, the total elimination of the need for artificial respiration (mouth to mouth) in CPR was recommended in 2008.

If you are a diver, this book belongs in your kit bag, the cubby hole of your 4x4, or the waterproof compartment of your dive boat. Keep it handy, refer to it whenever you have a medical question or problem, and use it to guide you if things get rough. I hope you never really need it.

Dr Allan Kayle, Johannesburg, 2009.

AUTHOR'S ACKNOWLEDGEMENTS

The author wishes to thank the following people and organisations: the Royal Navy and US Navy for giving permission to reproduce the Therapeutic Oxygen Tables in chapter 44; DAN Southern Africa for providing details of the relevant contacts for emergency diver assistance worldwide; Dr Leon Greenbaum, past executive director of the Undersea and Hyperbaric Medical Society for writing the Foreword to the first edition; Dr Frans Cronje, president of DAN Southern Africa, for contributing the Foreword to this edition; Gill Gordon, who edited this edition, and whose additional research and input added immeasurably to the quality of the text; and James Berrangé, who created the numerous illustrations provided in this edition.

ABOUT THE AUTHOR

Allan Kayle graduated from the Medical School of the University of the Witwatersrand, Johannesburg, in 1965. He joined the full-time staff of the Department of Physiological Chemistry and was awarded the PhD degree in 1972.

In 1981 he completed his advanced sport diving training under the auspices of the National Association of Underwater Instructors (NAUI) and attended a South African Navy course in submarine medicine in Simon's Town.

In 1983 he was granted a permit by the National Monuments Council to salvage the historical wreck of HMS *Birkenhead* which sank off the Cape coast in 1852. His book about this, *Salvage of the Birkenhead*, was published in 1990. Over the years, he has written regular feature articles on the technical and medical aspects of diving for *Divestyle* magazine and was a contributor to the *South African Second Underwater Handbook* published in 1989.

In 1993, he was nominated by Scuba Schools International (SSI) for their highest award – the Platinum Pro 5000. In the same year, **Safe Diving** was first published; with a second edition released in 1996. Also in 1996, his book, *How to Manage Diving Problems*, was published, with revised editions in 2004 and 2005. In 2001, he contributed the chapter dealing with diving health hazards and their management in South African commercial divers, for the *Handbook of Occupational Health Practice in the South African Mining Industry* published by SIMRAC (Safety in Mines Research Advisory Committee).

In April 1994 he was officially certified by the British Health and Safety Executive and the British Department of Transport as a diving physician for internationally operative commercial divers. This certification was reaffirmed in May 1998. In 2001 he was medical adviser for Stott-Comex Offshore, an international commercial diving company working in the Mossel Bay offshore oil fields.

Dr Kayle is a founder member of the Southern African Undersea and Hyperbaric Medical Association (SAUHMA). He became president of the association in September 1994 and was re-elected for a second term of office in October 1999. He served on the board of DAN Southern Africa from 2001 to 2008.

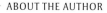

01

HISTORY OF DIVING

Man has always dived. Starting with simple plunges for fish, breathhold diving was used by pearl, shell and seafood divers from about 4500 BC. Free diving for sponges began during ancient Greek times and continued for many centuries. The ancient Greeks even incorporated the legal rights of divers – the deeper the dive, the greater their share of profits.

BREATHHOLD DIVING

The navies of Greece and Rome dominated early recorded diving history. During the Trojan wars, around 1190 BC, breathhold divers were used to sabotage wooden enemy ships by drilling holes in their hulls, cutting anchor lines and constructing submerged wooden port defences against assailing ships. Philo of Byzantium, an engineer and architect to Alexander the Great, recommended replacing anchor ropes with chains to foil enemy divers.

Using divers, Pompey's son, Gnaeus, refloated ships sunk by the Romans to obstruct the entrance to the harbour of Oricus in Greece, and then captured the port. Mark Antony attempted to impress Cleopatra during a fishing competition by having his divers secretly load his hook with a steady supply of fish. Cleopatra reacted by ordering one of her divers to attach a salted fish to his hook!

Between the 16th and 18th centuries, the native coral divers of Margarita Island in the Caribbean were reportedly able to dive up to 30 metres depth for 15 minutes, all day and every day. They claimed their stamina was due to the use of tobacco! For centuries, the pearl diving industry used the basic technique of breathholding, notably among the *Ama*, or 'sea women', of Japan where the technique was employed for over 2000 years. This is dying out, although *Ama* divers perform for show at the Mikimoto company's Pearl Island in the Bay of Toba, Japan, and pearl divers of the Tuamoto Archipelago in the South Pacific still use the breathhold method.

SNORKELS

The first major technical advance in diving was the use of a length of bamboo or hollow reed as a snorkel when hunting in water. This allowed the diver to replenish his air requirements while stealthily approaching his prey, but restricted depth to just below the surface. Artistotle recorded this method being used in ancient Greece, while Christopher Columbus wrote of North American Indians using it to hunt for wild fowl. Across the globe, Australian aborigines used it to trap wild duck.

In the late 15th century, Leonardo da Vinci made drawings of breathing tubes. The breathing device amounted to a snorkel but, as the dead space was large, carbon dioxide would have accumulated. He also designed a diver's fin and suggested that divers could breathe from 'a wine skin to contain the breath'; initiating, perhaps, the first scuba design? In 1680, Borelli in Italy examined Da Vinci's designs and disagreed with them. He felt that exhaled air would have to be cleansed before rebreathing and proposed that cooling it through a copper tube would be effective. He was not too far off the mark. Modern rebreathing sets use breathing gases stored in ultra-cold liquid form, with the exhaled carbon dioxide and water vapour being frozen out.

OPEN DIVING BELLS

After snorkels, the next advance in boosting underwater endurance was the development of open diving bells. Alexander the Great is rumoured by Ethicus to have built one in 332 BC, but the stories relating to it are surely the antecedents of modern fishing tales. Alexander apparently entered a 'glass barrel' and was 'swallowed by the sea'. On his return he proclaimed, 'Sir Barons, I have just seen that this whole world is lost, and the great fish mercilessly devour the lesser.' Allegedly, one fish was so big that it took three days to swim past the appalled Alexander in his submerged bell!

During the 1530s, Guglielmo de Loreno built weighted wooden chambers that were filled with air, but open at the bottom. In 1620, Sir Francis Bacon described one as: 'A sort of metal barrel lowered into the water, open end downward. The diver can put his head in and so recover his breath.' The air could not be purified or replaced, and it was not until 1691 that Edmund Halley, the British astronomer of comet fame, extended the scope of these open bells (damaging an eardrum in doing so). He patented an open diving bell that could be replenished with air. Efficient pumps had yet to be invented, but his bell was supplied from weighted barrels of air which the divers hauled down from the surface. Keeping the barrels well below the bell allowed the barrel air to escape through the hoses and up into the bell. Halley also freed divers of the need to breathhold when away from the bell by designing hose systems to supply the diver with air from the bell. Primitive, but they managed dives to 20 metres of sea water (msw) for one and a half hours. Using Halley's diving bells, 50 bronze cannons, each weighing half a tonne, were recovered from the *Wasa*, a Swedish warship that sank in 30 msw.

SURFACE AIR SUPPLY

Although Otto von Guericke developed the first air pump in 1650, dependable hand-operated air pumps only became available during the late 1700s and it then became possible to supply a submerged diver with air from the surface. This is the first record of helmets being used. The early ones were really miniature open bells – in effect, an inverted bucket over the head. Excess air pumped into these helmets escaped through the open bottom and created a flushing system. The diver could breathe as long as he stood upright. If he stooped or stumbled, the helmet simply flooded.

Next came the idea of tailoring the diving bell to the shape of a man, thereby providing him with a watertight cover and an air supply. The first diving suit comprised a copper helmet with glass viewpoints, firmly attached to a full rubber suit. It was designed in 1837 by Augustus Siebe who called it a 'closed dress'. Now more commonly known as the standard diving suit or standard rig, it enabled a diver to move freely without water entering his helmet. Incoming air was pumped down a hose into the helmet and surplus air escaped through an outlet valve. Using these rigs, the first diving school was established by the Royal Navy in 1843. Siebe's design has since evolved into the modern surface-supplied dry suit and hard hat.

But with the advent of the closed dress (standard diving suit) and the resultant longer dives came 'the bends', a phenomenon previously described in caisson workers – bridge builders who worked in fixed underwater pressurised chambers and tunnels. The bends were first noted by Robert Boyle in 1667, when he observed gas bubbles in the eye of a snake after experimental decompression, but the cause was unknown.

In the late 19th century, the great French physicist, Paul Bert, suggested that nitrogen bubbles were the cause, and he showed that a gradual ascent from depth could prevent the onset of the condition, while recompression could relieve the pain. A British physiologist, John Scott Haldane, was appointed to investigate the problem and continue Bert's work. Haldane noted that a diver could be lifted from 10 msw to the surface without suffering decompression pain, and he postulated staged decompression stops, allowing enough time at progressively shallower stages for excess gas to be exhaled. The idea was tested on goats, then on men in pressurised chambers and, finally, in 1906, on sea dives to 64 msw. Haldane published the first dive tables in 1910 and, in 1915, a team of US Navy divers, breathing air, located a submarine sunk to a depth of 93 msw and and raised it to the surface.

It is extremely doubtful whether a modern diver would dream of diving to, let alone working at, 93 msw with only air as a breathing source. But it was accomplished, despite extreme narcosis, an oxygen partial pressure of over two atmospheres which should have caused underwater convulsions, and an enormous risk of acute decompression illness.

THE ORIGIN OF SCUBA

The next step was to liberate the diver from a the constraints of a surface air hose and a heavily weighted suit. In the 19th century, compressors could achieve a maximum pressure of only 40 atmospheres (see page 20), which meant a very limited time under water. Modern scuba divers now return to the surface when their cylinder pressure is 50 atmospheres because they are running out of air! But, at the time, 40 atmospheres was all they had and they worked with it.

In the early 1800s, an American engineer, Charles Condert, carried air compressed in a copper tube coiled around his body. The air was released into a hood covering the upper part of his body. A small hole was supposed to allow exhaled carbon dioxide to escape, but in 1831 Condert died while using his system. Then, in 1865, two French technicians, Benoit Rouquayrol and Auguste Denayrouze, invented an aerophore: a full-face mask supplied from the surface, but fitted with an air receiver carried on the back so that the diver could uncouple himself from his hosing for a few minutes. This was the first Self-Contained Underwater Breathing Apparatus, or SCUBA.

At the same time, work was proceeding to develop oxygen rebreathing sets and the first practical one was built by an Englishman, Henry Fleuss, in 1878. It was a closed circuit set that supplied pure oxygen to the diver and removed exhaled carbon dioxide via a rope soaked in potassium hydroxide. The system was dangerous, as the effects of oxygen toxicity were largely unknown, but it was the forerunner of military oxygen sets, submarine escape sets, fire-fighting sets and mine rescue equipment.

In 1918, the Japanese Ogushi Peerless Respirator was patented. It was a scuba system using a cylinder carried on the back and it passed field tests to 324 ft. The diver controlled his air supply by using his teeth to trigger air flow into his mask. Then, in 1933, a Frenchman, Yves le Prieur, designed a system whereby the diver carried the cylinder on his chest and released air into his mask by manually opening a tap. Le Prieur's system was adopted by the French Navy. In 1930, rubber goggles with glass lenses were developed by Guy Gilpatric, and face masks and snorkels soon became commonplace. Three years later, the first swim fins were patented by another Frenchman, Louis de Corlieu.

DEVELOPMENT OF SCUBA TECHNOLOGY

What we now know as scuba was developed in 1943. French engineer, Emile Gagnan, devised a reducing valve for use in gas-powered cars. With oceanographer Jacques-Yves Cousteau, he modified this valve to construct the first underwater demand valve, which was triggered by the diver's breathing and automatically compensated for changes in depth and pressure. It was simple and reliable and, in the years following World War II, the 'Aqua Lung' heralded the beginning of sport scuba diving.

From here, things developed rapidly, with advances in equipment, technology and training, and the establishment of organisations to meet the needs of the new recreational diving community. The University of California introduced the first wet suit in 1956, and the first buoyancy compensator, called the Stabilization Jacket, was introduced by Scubapro in 1971. The first commercially available dive computer, the Orca Edge, was introduced in 1983. In 1980, the Divers Alert Network (DAN) was founded at Duke University, North Carolina, as a non-profit organisation with the aim of promoting safe diving (see page 350).

Complex, self-monitoring closed circuit scuba sets were first developed during the 1950s. Over the years, these were upgraded into ultra-sophisticated electronically controlled systems that accurately regulated the required gas and volume flow from oxygen and diluent helium cylinders.

With the development of mixed gas diving came technical diving, enabling divers to dive rapidly to great depths using mixed-gas scuba and then decompress under water for many hours during the subsequent ascent. In 2001, the UK's John Bennett reached

Boyle's Law, Charles's Law and the Pressure Law can all be combined into one formula, known as the UNIVERSAL GAS EQUATION.

$$\frac{P1V1}{T1} = \frac{P2V2}{T2}$$

Examples

Mike Hood goes to his local dive shop to have his scuba cylinder filled. He wants the cylinder filled to 200 ATA. The ever-lazy Pete Muckitt does not bother to put the cylinder in a tub of water to keep it cool. As the pressure in the cylinder increases, so does the temperature, up to 47°C. Mike then heads for his favourite dive site at Flounder-on-Sea, where the water temperature is 7°C and begins to holler and curse. What is the pressure in his cylinder? Which law are we using?

P1 = 200 ATA
V1 = K (constant) (for practical purposes, the volume of his cylinder does not change)
T1 = 47°C = 320°A
P2 = ?
V2 = K
T2 = 7°C = 280°A

$$\frac{200 \times K}{320} = \frac{P2 \times K}{280}$$

$$P2 = \frac{200 \times K \times 280}{320 \times K}$$

P2 = 175 ATA (Pressure Law: V is K)

Dr Parrotfish taps one litre of gas from a decompression chamber into a balloon for analysis. The chamber is baking in the midday sun, which has raised the temperature inside the chamber to 37°C. When he gets back to the laboratory, the temperature is a refreshing 17°C. What is the volume of the sample, and which law are we using?

P1 = K
V1 = 1 litre
T1 = 37°C = 273 + 37 = 310°A
P2 = K
V2 = ?
T2 = 17°C = 273 + 17 = 290°A

$$\frac{K \times 1}{310} = \frac{K \times V2}{290}$$

$$V2 = \frac{290 \times K \times 1}{310 \times K} = \frac{290}{310} = 0.935 \text{ litre} \ (= \text{Charles's Law})$$

4. DALTON'S LAW

John Dalton was a Quaker who lived in 18th-century England and played bowls on Thursday afternoons. He was the first person to describe colour-blindness and the atomic theory. He was also very interested in gas mixtures and, since laws were in vogue, he invented Dalton's Law.

In a mixture of gases, the total pressure is equal to the sum of the partial pressures of the individual gases in the mixture.

In a sample of air at sea level, the total pressure is 1 ATA. This consists of approximately 80% nitrogen and 20% oxygen (ignoring traces of carbon dioxide, water and argon).

> Total pressure = 1 ATA
> Nitrogen = 80% = 0.8 ATA
> Oxygen = 20% = 0.2 ATA
> Total of nitrogen and oxygen = 0.8 + 0.2 = 1.0 ATA

Simple enough, but it can become tricky. For instance: A diver breathes a mixture of helium, nitrogen and oxygen. At 90 metres, the helium flowing through his demand valve has a partial pressure of 8 ATA. At the surface, the partial pressure of the nitrogen in his purged gas is 0.15 ATA.

PROBLEM: What is the percentage oxygen in the mix?

ANSWER: At 90 metres, the total pressure is: 9 ATA + 1 ATA = 10 ATA. His helium exerts a pressure of 8 ATA in his demand valve, i.e. 8/10 of the total **ambient** pressure or 80% of the mix is helium. At the surface, nitrogen exerts a partial pressure (pp) of 0.15 ATA or 15% of 1 ATA. So 15% of the mix is nitrogen.

According to Dalton's Law:

$$ppHe + ppN_2 + ppO_2 = \text{total pressure}$$
$$80\% + 15\% + x = 100\%$$
$$x = 5\% \text{ oxygen}$$

Dalton's Law is important in:
1. calculating the proportions of various gases in a breathing mixture to avoid nitrogen narcosis or oxygen toxicity, and
2. calculating the depth at which trace contaminants, such as carbon monoxide, become significant as toxic gases.

Example

> Nitrox Albert wants to dive to 140 metres. He knows that helium is expensive, so he wants to add some nitrogen to the mixture, equivalent to the nitrogen partial pressure at 30 metres breathing air. He also does not want the partial pressure of oxygen to be greater than 0.5 ATA at the bottom. What is his mix?

ANSWER: We must calculate the proportions of oxygen and nitrogen required. The rest is helium.

Oxygen:

> The pressure at 140 metres is 14 ATA + 1 ATA = 15 ATA.
> This is his **ambient** 'atmospheric' pressure.
> His oxygen partial pressure at this depth must be 0.5 ATA.
> Expressed as a percentage: $\dfrac{0.5 \times 100}{15}$ = 3.33% oxygen

Nitrogen:

> We want the ppN_2 to be the same as the ppN_2 at 30 metres on air,
>> i.e. the **equivalent nitrogen partial pressure.**
> In air, N_2 = 80%
> At the surface its pp is 0.8 ATA
> At 30 metres, its pp is 0.8 x 4 (3 ATA + 1 ATA) = 3.2 ATA
> So we want 3.2 ATA of N_2 at 140 metres (15 ATA)
> As a percentage: $\dfrac{3.2}{15}$ x 100 = 21.33% nitrogen

> Therefore, the mix is:
> Oxygen: 3.33% + Nitrogen: 21.33% = 24.66%
> Helium: 100 – 24.66 = 75.34%

PROBLEM: If the minimum ppO_2 safe to breathe is taken as 0.15 ATA, could Nitrox Albert breathe this mix at the surface? Oxygen = 3.33%.
At 1 ATA, the partial pressure of oxygen would be 0.033 ATA, and the mix would be fatal, as gross oxygen starvation (hypoxia) would occur. Up to what ascent from bottom depth could he breathe the mixture?

ANSWER: The percentage oxygen in the mixture is 3.33%
This would exert a ppO_2 of 0.15 ATA

$$\text{At} \quad \frac{0.15}{x} = \frac{3.33}{100}$$

$$x = \frac{15 \text{ ATA}}{3.33}$$

$$= 4.5 - 1 \text{ ATA} = 3.5 \text{ ATA}$$

$$= 35 \text{ msw}$$

NOTE: Although the partial pressure of a gas varies with changes in depth, the percentage does not. Percentage is constant. Dalton's Law also explains the blackout of ascent in breathhold divers after hyperventilation.

5. HENRY'S LAW

William Henry was a melancholic chap who committed suicide at Pendlebury, UK, in 1836. However, he did leave a legacy in the form of Henry's Law.

At a constant temperature, the amount of gas that will dissolve in a liquid is proportional to the partial pressure of the gas over the liquid.

This law involves gases and liquids and refers to the dissolving of gases into liquids. In the diving sense, the liquid would be body tissues, and the gas would be the gas breathed i.e. air or a mixture.

At 1 ATA, Martin, a diver at Crankshaft Bay, has about one litre of gaseous nitrogen dissolved in his body. (He is said to be saturated with air-nitrogen at 1 ATA.) If he was hunting for abalone and scuba-dived to 20 metres (3 ATA), he would eventually reach equilibrium again and have three litres of nitrogen dissolved in his body (if he were not arrested first for pilfering marine resources without a permit!).

Time is needed for the absorption of nitrogen. The longer the dive, the more nitrogen is dissolved. When Martin surfaces, the air he breathes is again at 1 ATA. The nitrogen dissolved in his body will then reverse its direction, i.e. out of his tissues and into the air via his lungs. If the pressure drop is too rapid, his tissues may have more nitrogen than they can hold in solution, leading to the formation of bubbles, which can cause acute decompression illness.

The science behind Henry's Law is also directly responsible for:
- nitrogen narcosis,
- oxygen toxicity, and
- high pressure nervous syndrome.

During diving, the partial pressures of any gas increase with descent, and decrease on ascent. At depth, the gradient is gas to lungs to blood to tissues. On return to the surface, the gradient is tissues to blood to lungs to air.

ARCHIMEDES' PRINCIPLE

In times long past, when the earth was flat and magicians and monsters prevailed, a fat man weighed a lot and a thin man didn't. Nowadays, with man standing on the moon, even weight is not what it used to be. As the moon's gravity is less than that of the earth, a fat man standing on its surface would weigh less, even though the total amount of blubber on his well-covered bones was the same. To put it another way, his mass is constant but his weight is dependent on gravity.

The Germans introduced the term 'weight-force' to distinguish between mass and weight. Weight-force is the product of mass and gravity and is expressed in newtons.

Weight-force (G) = m x g newtons (N)
When m = mass in kilograms
g = local acceleration due to gravity in m/sec/sec.

Example

Skinny Sam decides to step on to the scales at his local laundromat. He gets a reading of 65 kg. This is his mass. The local acceleration due to gravity is 9.812523 m/sec/sec. This means that if Sam were falling in this particular area, he would accelerate by 9.812523 metres per second per second, that is, for every second he fell, he would travel 9.812523 metres per second faster than the previous second.

As G = mg
Sam's weight-force would be 65 x 9.812523
or 637.814 N

In English-speaking countries, there is no word for 'weight-force' and the word 'weight' is loosely used to mean both mass or weight-force. So, Sam would say he weighs 65 kg or that his 'weight' is 65 kg. To distinguish between mass and weight-force one looks at the units.

If the units are in kilograms, mass is meant.

If the units are in newtons, force is meant.

If Sam were on Jupiter with a gravity 12 times that of the earth, he would have a weight of 637.814 x 12 or 7653.77 N, but his mass would still be 65 kg. On the moon, his weight would be 106.30 N and his mass would again be 65 kg.

Now, back in time to Archimedes, where 'weight' is expressed in kilograms so mass is the order of the day. Around 250 BC, Archimedes invented the water screw. One day he displaced his mass in his bathtub and ran naked through the streets of Syracuse screaming '*Eureka! Eureka!*' King Hieron II had just received a nice new golden crown and he wanted to know whether it was pure gold or mixed with silver. He handed the problem to Archimedes, whose bath gave him the answer. Archimedes first weighed the crown, then, immersing it in water, he noted the amount of water it displaced. He then weighed an identical mass of pure gold, and immersed that in water. If the two amounts of water that were displaced were the same, then the crown would be pure gold.

I don't know the end of the story, so the crown's purity remains a secret forever. But Archimedes' principle states:

Any object, wholly or partially immersed in liquid, is buoyed up by a force equal to the mass of liquid displaced.

Example

Supposing a diver weighing 70 kg fully geared up steps off his boat into the water. If he displaces 75 kg of water, he will float, being 5 kg lighter than the mass of water displaced. He is **positively buoyant**. This makes descent difficult, but ascent easy. If he displaces 65 kg of water, he will sink, being 5 kg heavier than the mass of water displaced. He is **negatively buoyant**. This makes descent easy, but ascent difficult. If he displaces exactly 70 kg of water, he is **neutrally buoyant** and will neither sink nor float. He experiences a sense of weightlessness similar to an astronaut in zero gravity. He can descend or ascend with ease.

Now suppose he decides to descend. As he does so, Boyle's Law comes into operation. His neoprene sponge wet suit contains thousands of tiny gas bubbles which become compressed with the increasing pressure. This reduces his suit's volume and so decreases the mass of water he displaces. The deeper he goes, the more negatively buoyant he becomes, and his descent becomes easier and faster. Sport divers use a buoyancy compensator, which can be partially inflated at depth to counter this negative buoyancy, and to assist ascent if required.

PROBLEM: Long-suffering Charlie takes his mother-in-law diving. He helps her tog up, and carefully attaches 16 kg of lead weights to her weight belt. When she enters the water, her weight is 80 kg. She displaces 80 litres of sea water. Is he, finally, rid of her? (The density of sea water is 1.025 and density = mass : volume.)

ANSWER: No. She is 2 kg buoyant. He should have used more weight!

03

DIVING MEDICALS AND SCUBA DIVING

All around the world, qualified scuba divers receive their training at clubs affiliated to their relevant national union, such as SAUU in South Africa, BS-AC in Britain or CMAS in France, or at private dive schools operating under the auspices of US-based institutions such as NAUI, SSI, YMCA, NASDC or PADI.

Diver training courses on offer cover everything from the basics to instructor certification. In most cases, divers emerge from their basic courses with an adequate understanding and only need additional diving time and experience to complete their metamorphosis into *Homo scubiens*.

But are novice divers safe under water? Most of the national unions compel their trainee divers to undergo a medical examination before starting training to ensure that their state of health meets the particular, and often peculiar, demands of diving. Reputable private dive schools do the same. Medicals should be repeated every two years if the diver is under the age of 40, and annually if older. But there is always the law of the 'buck'. It costs money to have a medical and a chest X-ray; these raise the price of the diving course and many divers are on a tight budget to pay for tuition, buy a wet suit, a BC, scuba cylinder, demand valve and so on. They investigate the diving school market: 'Hey,' they say, 'here's a school that doesn't need a medical unless you're over 40. We're only 19, and we run marathons – hell, we're fit enough! Why waste money on a medical? We'd rather use the bucks to buy a mask!'

Here's why you need that medical. These stories are all true.

Joe had just returned from Israel where he did a one-day 'resort diving course' and had fallen in love with the sport. He approached a diving school and was told to have a medical. He said he had recently had one in Israel and passed A1. The dive school believed him. During the openwater diver training, Joe completed his bottom time and ascended normally with his instructor. At the surface, he suddenly started choking and gasping and lost consciousness. All attempts at resuscitation were futile. The post-mortem examination revealed air bubbles in the arteries of his brain and heart. Joe had suffered an arterial gas embolus from a ruptured lung on a controlled ascent. Discussion with his family revealed that he had had a previous spontaneous pneumothorax (see page 65). Joe had lied, and he died for his ambition to dive.

Mike (23) was an athlete, a long-distance runner and a league squash player. At his medical he appeared a perfect physical specimen – muscular, lean and powerful. He was asked to pass a specimen of urine. 'I can't,' he replied. 'I went just before I came here. I'll bring one later.' 'No,' he was told. 'Have some water and read a magazine.' Mike passed his specimen after further argument. It was loaded with sugar plus ketones. 'I didn't want to tell because I knew I would fail,' he said ruefully. 'I am an uncontrolled diabetic on insulin.' (See page 141.)

Nineteen-year-old Tim had completed his openwater one course and was keen to advance his training. When he changed diving schools, he was told to have a medical. Due to his youth, his first dive school had decided he 'did not need an examination.' At his medical he was tense and reticent, revealing his history only with persuasion. Eventually the dam broke. He had been diagnosed with multiple sclerosis and had been admitted to hospital twice in the previous year. His breathing muscles and his limbs had been paralysed, necessitating an artificial ventilator. He had also been on huge doses of cortisone. He could not face the horror of his illness and on both occasions had attempted suicide by alcohol overdose. As a result, Tim was on antidepressants and was seeing a psychiatrist. He had completed his openwater one course between his admissions to hospital.

Unbelievable? Here is another. Pete arrived for his medical with his form filled out and his X-rays in his hand. Like all would-be divers, he was excited at the prospect of getting underwater and impatient to have his medical behind him. On closer scrutiny, the X-rays showed a tumour at the root of his left lung. The 26-year-old was referred to his doctor as an emergency.

All diving schools require their students to sign an indemnity form, releasing the school from any financial or legal obligation should a diving accident occur. But there is nevertheless an unwritten inescapable moral obligation – ensuring that their students are medically fit to dive. Potential divers have families, fiancées, wives, husbands and children who need them and care for them. It is a woeful and terrible task to inform these people that their loved one is dead. Does a diving instructor actually have to see the uncomprehending anguish on the face of a four-year-old and her weeping mother before accepting and implementing this moral responsibility?

As the number of sport divers increases, accidents and deaths will continue to happen. All newcomers to the sport are just dying to dive. They have no idea of the hazards. They are thinking of beaches and palm trees and beautiful coral in crystal-clear water. They look to qualified divers for informed advice. If someone asks, tell them to have a medical. Don't let them dive to die.

04

IMPLICATIONS OF AGE, GENDER AND BODY BUILD

The basic health demands of diving are simple, but a diver's mind and body must be able to safely handle the physical loads of pressurised gases in and out of solution, as well as the inherent demands and dangers of the sea.

AGE LIMITS

Who is too old to dive? Who is too young to dive? The truth is that no one really knows and only common sense can dictate a practical policy. The risks involved in being too young or too old relate primarily to the potential for drowning or developing the bends. Either can kill, so the issue of age is relevant.

MATURITY The question of when one is too old to dive is relatively easy to answer. Forty is generally considered the age at which one becomes an 'older' diver. Even in the absence of any underlying disorder such as high blood pressure, lung disease or coronary artery disease, vital nitrogen parameters invariably become less efficient due to the ageing process (these include tissue nitrogen-load tolerance and degassing, venous transport of post-dive gas and bubbles, and lung degassing of nitrogen). The 40-plus diver is invariably less fit than his or her younger counterpart, or has to expend more time in intensive training to achieve comparable fitness. But this degree of precious training time is rarely available to people who, by now, are usually peaking in their chosen careers.

All of this means that older divers are more prone to drown under challenging water conditions. Standard dive tables are no longer ideal, as they are designed for people half an older diver's age. 'Middle-age spread' with its increased fatty reservoir for fat-soluble nitrogen compounds the problem.

To ensure safety under water, older divers should follow very conservative depth/ dive durations, making a mandatory 5-minute stop at 5 msw after any dive. For older divers using standard sport diving tables, this author recommends a 'five per cent shortening' of the no-decompression-stop dive time for each decade after 40, and avoiding all obligatory decompression-stop dives.

All divers over the age of 40 should have an annual diving medical conducted by a certified dive doctor.

YOUTH Children younger than 12 should probably not dive. If they do, it should certainly be no deeper than 9 msw and always with perceptive parental supervision. There are several reasons for this. Bone growth and lengthening occurs at the growth cartilage (epiphyseal cartilage) near the ends of each limb bone. These growth cartilages are responsible for the deposition of new bone and normal lengthening with growth of the limbs.

A limb bend, presenting, for example, with an aching elbow or knee in an adult, while certainly requiring chamber recompression therapy, is generally a relatively minor incident without long-term complications. But bubble injury in sensitive juvenile limb growth plates could lead to stunting or even deformation of further limb growth. These growth plates eventually disappear normally, becoming incorporated into the bone of a limb. At this point bone growth stops permanently.

Final bony fusion of limb epiphyseal cartilage usually occurs between the ages of 13 and 16 years in girls, and 15 and 18 in boys. This makes age 12, which is generally accepted as the minimum age for entry into a scuba diving course, purely arbitrary, as active growth plates are still present. It also puts the responsibility for ensuring that tissue nitrogen loading is never excessive squarely into the dive instructor's hands, as well as those of the parents.

As children are inherently adventurous and liable to dive without consideration of risks, perhaps venturing beyond safe time, depth and sea condition limits, it is essential that these dangers are carefully explained to them during their scuba courses, and that a parent always dives with them. If neither parent dives, the child must not dive until at least 16 years of age.

Buoyancy control can be a real problem in children and even in small adults. At the beginning of a dive, the scuba cylinder is full of compressed air, making it negatively buoyant, so the child sinks easily. However, at the end of the dive the near-empty and now-buoyant cylinder can either initiate an uncontrollable ascent or one that is too fast, or it can make the mandatory 5-minute stop at 5 metres of sea water (msw) a difficult exercise without surfacing.

The size problems associated with juvenile divers are usually easily circumvented by ensuring that two children do not form a buddy pair, or even dive with a single adult. Each child should team up with a competent buddy pair of adult divers (at least one of them a parent). This trio diving is recommended because it ensures that each adult also has back-up buddy support in the event that something should go wrong under water. Expecting a juvenile diver to render active physical support and rescue a diver twice his or her mass from the water in an emergency is stretching things a little far. Should the adult then require CPR, juvenile lungs simply do not have the volume capacity to effect efficient ventilation in an adult, while the muscle power required to achieve proper chest and heart compression may not be present either.

PHYSICAL FACTORS AFFECTING WOMEN

There are specific differences particular to women divers, not because of any lack of ability or understanding, but simply because women are women. These differences are due to both physical and psychological factors. Some are advantageous, some disadvantageous, and others are myths.

FAT DISTRIBUTION   In general, women have a greater natural distribution of fatty tissue underlying the skin than men. Their relative lean body mass (their mass minus that of fat) is less than that of males. As a result, women tend to tolerate cold conditions better than men do and hypothermia often takes longer to develop in women. However, their relatively increased amount of fatty tissue provides a potentially greater store for nitrogen retention, and the risk of the bends is therefore theoretically higher in women than in men. In practical terms, though, this difference is rarely encountered, provided standard diving tables are followed.

MENSTRUATION   Let's explode a myth. Many female divers refrain from diving during their periods, believing that sharks will detect bleeding and eat them up. This is untrue. The use of internal tampons provides a convenient method of controlling flow, while the incidence of shark attacks on menstruating women is actually lower than on non-menstruating women. But what happens to tampons when women dive? Will pressure force a tampon beyond ready recovery by the user? Will the little string disappear, making an embarrassing visit to a doctor necessary? No. Tampons are porous and therefore unaffected by water depth, making them safe for diving.

Heavy periods can cause problems, however. Regular blood loss with inadequate dietary replacement of iron may cause iron deficiency and anaemia. This can place a female diver at risk at times when strength and stamina are demanded, such as when swimming against powerful currents, because the oxygen-carrying capacity of blood is reduced. Women with heavy flows should seek medical advice to confirm that their iron stores and haemoglobin are adequate.

Some women experience severe abdominal pain, irritability, nausea and vomiting with or just before their periods. These are a potential source of danger under water – inability to swim properly due to cramps, hasty and unwise responses, and inhalation of vomit may occur. The decision to dive must allow for these. If drugs are required to control these symptoms, the answer is easy: do not dive at period time.

BREAST IMPLANTS   Here is another myth. Some divers still believe that breast implants will burst as a result of pressure changes incurred while diving (or flying in aeroplanes!). They won't. Implants are filled with saline or silica gel, and it is only gas spaces that obey Boyle's Law and undergo substantial pressure-volume changes (see page 21). Implants are not inflatable pneumatic bladders! However, they will absorb some inert gas during a dive, resulting in the formation of inconsequential small bubbles inside an implant. Allow six weeks after implant surgery before resuming diving.

ORAL CONTRACEPTION The majority of oral contraceptives contain combined derivatives of the female hormones oestrogen and progesterone. The basic idea of the pill is to stop cyclical ovulation and the release of a viable egg or ovum from an ovary each month. Without ovulation, no fertilisation can occur. Considering the number of females worldwide actively enjoying sport diving, it is obvious that hundreds of thousands, even millions, must be taking oral contraceptives.

For safety, however, remember that one of the side-effects of the pill is an increased tendency for platelets to clump, leading to abnormal blood clotting, especially inside calf veins where blood flow is slower and more sluggish than anywhere else in the body. Venous nitrogen bubbles that can form after a dive also stimulate platelet aggregation around them so the risk of venous thrombosis in female divers does increase with the pill. A few precautions will help to avoid the problem: practise safe diving techniques, taking care to avoid excessive bubble loading; ensure the calf muscles are not compressed; and sit or lie with the knees extended after diving to allow easy venous return from the calves.

PREGNANCY The majority of female divers are of child-bearing age and so, not unexpectedly, many of them fall pregnant. Naturally, they want to know whether they should dive with their descendents under their wet suits. A negative reply causes indignation: 'But my friend dived right through her pregnancy and even while she was breastfeeding her twins!'

So, aside from being unaffected by the nitrogen equivalent of carbonated milk, who is this initially smaller-than-a-kiwi-fruit-sized result of parental genetic fusion to dictate maternal exposure to the hyperbaric environment? Why should foetal needs be any different from the mother's? Why shouldn't a pregnant woman dive until her bulk threatens to rip her double-lined two-tone lycra suit? And what if she promises to do only shallow dives and never, ever, any decompression-stop dives?

The answer has to do with the foetal lungs. Unborn babies float in amniotic fluid, a protective liquid that suspends them within the muscular wall of their mother's uterus. Their lungs are non-functional in their liquid environment and all of their oxygen, carbon dioxide and nitrogen needs are handled via the umbilical cord and placenta. The placenta is not just a lump of inconvenient flesh that is discarded after a delivery. It is an amazing union of mother and child, a unique organ comprising half of mother's tissue and half of child's, with maternal capillaries looping to touch, but never joining, the baby's matching capillary loops. It is an intimate network of totally separate blood supplies, providing sustenance and oxygen to the baby, and removing metabolic end-products and carbon dioxide for excretion via the maternal kidneys and lungs. A mother and child's circulations do not mix; they are the blood supplies of two different people – the mother's capillaries providing and nurturing, and the child's taking and excreting.

The giving and taking includes the gases of diving. During a dive, the mother gives her child hyperbaric oxygen plus a hefty nitrogen load. The child offloads carbon dioxide and then tries to degas nitrogen after the dive. But junior hasn't got functional lungs, and depends on the placenta to return nitrogen to the mother's blood. This is the first snag.

Nitrogen decompression requires a gradient. It's fine for mom – she's got a gradient to 0.79 atmospheres at the beach. Junior has a gradient from himself to mom's already nitrogen-loaded venous system and, for the first few minutes of decompression, mom may even continue to supply nitrogen to junior. In other words, there is a delay. Junior has to join the queue to degas. This means he has a higher residual nitrogen time than his mother, who is already putting on her wet suit for a repetitive dive because her tables or dive computer say it's fine. Baby bubbles loom! But things are even more dangerous. Junior also has normal shunts between the right and left sides of his heart (foramen ovale), and between the pulmonary artery and aorta (ductus arteriosus). Any foetal venous bubbles can easily embolise into the child's arterial system.

The next snag is nausea. During the first three months of pregnancy, many women develop nausea and vomiting. If this occurs on land or on a boat, fluid loss results in relative or absolute dehydration. A decrease in total body water means a faster rate of tissue nitrogen loading during diving – and this naturally includes junior. Then, if mom decides to retch under water, inhalation of vomit and sea water may follow, progressing to hypoxia, near-drowning, or worse.

Saturation divers breathing oxygen at a partial pressure of higher than 0.5 ATA for prolonged periods are prone to develop acute pulmonary oxygen toxicity, with coughing, burning chest pain, breathlessness and eventually respiratory failure.

Unborn babies live under conditions of relatively low oxygen partial pressure. Nature has supplied them with a special oxygen carrier, foetal haemoglobin, which has a very high affinity for oxygen. After birth, foetal haemoglobin is rapidly replaced by adult haemoglobin, which is maintained for life. Foetuses and newborn babies don't do well with high oxygen partial pressures. Cataracts in the lens of the eye can occur, as well as acute respiratory distress that is very similar to the acute pulmonary oxygen toxicity found in saturation diving.

When a pregnant woman dives to 20 metres, she receives oxygen at a partial pressure of 0.63 ATA. Her baby gets a little less, but the threat of oxygen toxicity is there. Congenital abnormalities in the newborn occur nearly six times more frequently in females who continue to dive regularly when compared with non-divers. The risk increases should the pregnant (and invariably fatter) mother suffer a bend or arterial gas embolism and require pure oxygen therapy under pressurised conditions in a chamber.

Later in pregnancy, other problems arise. The expectant mother becomes clumsy and may trip over her fins, lose her balance while hefting a heavy cylinder, or injure herself in a rocking ski-boat. The presence of a large belly makes breathing difficult, and an agile physical response to underwater stress is a doubtful prospect.

A normal baby and healthy mother warrant a nine-month lay-off from diving.

BREASTFEEDING Pregnant divers sometimes ask: 'Is it safe to dive while breast-feeding?' The answer is 'Yes'. Diving will not affect breast milk production, nor predispose the mother to milk retention or mastitis. Although diving will cause a temporary increase in nitrogen partial pressure in unreleased breast milk, feeding is done at ambient surface pressure and any excess gas load to the baby will be minimal, or be relieved with a good burp.

MISCARRIAGE If loss of the foetus occurs within the first six weeks of pregnancy and the abortion is complete, diving may resume after one week. However, later abortions usually require a dilatation and curettage (D&C), and six weeks should be allowed to pass before returning to diving.

MENOPAUSE With the onset of menopause, at around age 50, female divers are exposed to an increased risk of osteoporosis – the decalcification of bone that renders them more liable to bony injury after even relatively minor trauma. Additionally, the skin and other tissues become more fragile, with easy bruising and skin bleeding. It has become common for women near the onset of menopause to take calcium supplements, vitamins and female hormone replacement therapy. Remember to take care to avoid venous thrombosis.

HYSTERECTOMY Diving may recommence six weeks after a hysterectomy, provided the reason for having the hysterectomy is now absent too.

PHYSICAL MISMATCHING A large part of sport diver training is devoted to diver rescue and resuscitation. The novice diver learns how to share an air supply, and how assist an unconscious diver to the surface and get him or her aboard a boat. But what happens if she weighs 57 kg and he tips the scales at 126 kg? Such buddy pairs do occur, and it then becomes necessary to ensure that they always dive with another pair. Three divers should easily manage what a slightly built buddy would struggle or fail to accomplish.

PSYCHOLOGICAL FACTORS Women divers usually fall into one of two groups. Most are extremely safe divers who dive efficiently, intelligently and well. They take few risks and are very considerate buddy partners. However, some women fall into the 'fragile league'. They encourage or request their male partners to prepare their equipment, fill their air cylinder from the compressor, carry their gear to the boat, and plan the dive schedule from the tables. With time, they forget how to fill a scuba cylinder, calculate air depth-time durations, or plan a dive. If problems arise, they are then incapable of providing an intelligent solution. These ladies become a liability to their buddies and incompetent in an emergency.

There is no place for sloppiness in diving – a member of a buddy pair may one day have to rely on the other for his or her life.

BODY BUILD

There are three basic human body builds: the skinny ectomorphs, the muscular mesomorphs and the tubby endomorphs – with varying combinations of each.

Ectomorphs have very little body fat for insulation and their diving Achilles' heel is hypothermia. Skinny divers should always wear a wet suit.

Tubby endomorphs, on the other hand, are amply insulated. They also have the further advantage of buoyancy – their shape approximates that of a sphere and, in accordance with Archimedes' Principle, they displace the maximum volume of water per given mass. This means that compression of their wet suit at depth will have less effect in creating negative buoyancy. Unfortunately, the disadvantages of fatty insulation outweigh inherent warmth and floating power. A large fat reserve means a large potential nitrogen storage capacity, as nitrogen is about five times more soluble in fat than in blood or muscle tissue. So, fat divers are more prone to the bends. They are also more prone to high blood pressure, heart disease and diabetes, which could disqualify them from diving altogether. In addition, being less agile, they are more liable to injury in a boating accident or to a mishap in a diving emergency that requires a rapid physical response.

Lucky mesomorphs are intermediate, with reasonable insulation, easy buoyancy, and good physical power and agility when needed.

It is extremely difficult, and requires great dedication, to change one's body build. Few have this determination and even fewer are blessed with a naturally pure mesomorphic body. But, like any sport, efficient diving does place demands on one's habits. Good eating habits with minimal intake of animal fats, regular exercise, minimal alcohol and no smoking will help keep an average sport diving enthusiast in good condition for safe diving, even if the belt buckle is a notch or two too wide.

PHYSICAL FITNESS AND VO2

A reasonable degree of fitness is needed to dive. But what is reasonable? In fitness tests, the laboratory standard measures aerobic capacity. This is the volume of oxygen used at maximal exercise capacity, known as VO2 max. A staged exercise, such as running on a treadmill, is performed until the subject is exhausted. Exhaled breath is analysed for oxygen and carbon dioxide and compared to air. This analysis measures the metabolic capacity of the entire body and is expressed as millilitres of oxygen (O_2) per kilogram body mass per minute (ml/kg/min). Normal VO2 max values are 17–85 or more ml/kg/min.

As multiple units may be difficult to understand, the term MET was introduced. It means 'metabolic equivalents' and is a ratio. The resting VO2 in men is taken as 3.5 ml/kg/min. Maximal aerobic capacity in MET is VO2 max divided by 3.5.

A diver with a VO2 max of 50 ml/kg/min will exercise to 14.29 MET. As women generally have a higher percentage body fat, their MET value would be disadvantaged, so a resting standard of 3.2 ml/kg/min is used for females. The normal MET max figures are 5–25 in men and women. As fat is metabolically inert during exercise, thin people are advantaged and will have higher MET max readings. A fat-free or lean body mass can be used for more accurate MET max levels (ml/kg/min/LBM).

One generally does not use one's MET max capacity. Swimming hard requires about 13 MET. Sport divers swimming gently in coral waters need about 3 MET of exertion but they should be capable of 10 MET at least.

BODY MASS INDEX

The body mass index, or BMI, is a scale that is used to predict body composition in large groups. BMI is unreliable in single predictions. A fat diver will have a greater BMI than a lean one. A very muscular diver with the same height and mass as a fat diver will have the same BMI. So significant limitations in the value of BMI do exist.

The formula comprises the body's mass in kilograms, divided by the square of the height in metres. It has no units, so rounded-up figures are used.

$$\text{BMI} = \frac{\textbf{Body mass (kg)}}{\textbf{Height (m)}^2}$$

The normal BMI range is 18.5–24.9; underweight is less than 18.5, overweight is considered to be in the 25–29.9 range and obese over 30. A BMI over 30 would usually disqualify a person from diving for reasons including obesity, unfitness, diabetes, blood fat abnormalities, high blood pressure and coronary artery disease – the so-called metabolic syndrome. Fat people are generally unfit and become exhausted easily. Abdominal fat restricts breathing, resulting in CO_2 build-up, a higher risk of decompression illness and a reduced ability to respond to physical challenges. Having a heart attack underwater is usually lethal.

MYOCARDIAL INFARCTION (HEART ATTACK) Branches of the left and right coronary arteries supply the heart muscle with blood. As blood cannot adequately flow into powerfully contracting ventricular muscles, the coronary arteries are the only arteries in the body that supply their end-organ (heart muscle) with blood during ventricular relaxation. The elastic recoil of the aorta is the driving force for blood to flow into the coronary arteries. Gradual obstruction of these arteries by fatty deposits on their walls, followed by a sudden blockage due to the formation of a blood clot on the roughened surface, leads to a heart attack.

Deprived of essential oxygen, the portion of heart muscle beyond the block dies. If a major branch is involved, the person dies. Death is usually due to the sudden onset of abnormal heart rhythms, especially ventricular fibrillation, resulting in ineffectual pumping and cessation of the blood supply to the brain. Resuscitation must commence within four minutes of the onset of ventricular fibrillation or brain death will begin. (See cardiopulmonary resuscitation, page 230.)

Sport divers should wait for one year after a heart attack before resuming diving, provided chest pain or irregular rhythms do not occur at maximal treadmill exercise testing, a stress ECG shows no strain pattern, and the diver is examined by a cardiologist twice a year and by a diving physician once a year. In addition, the diver must always wear a full wet suit and hood to protect against cold exposure. Avoid swimming against a current, or surf entries into powerful waves; and avoid staged decompression stops (except for a mandatory 5-minute stop at 5 msw with all dives). The maximum suggested diving depth is 18 msw.

CORONARY ANGIOPLASTY Advances in medical technology have revolutionised the management of coronary artery disease and nowadays, surgery is the treatment of choice. A diagnosis of angina pectoris, the chest pain felt when coronary artery blood supply is inadequate, is followed by coronary angiography, where radio-opaque dye is injected into the coronary arteries. If a significant block is found and the arteries are amenable to surgery, there are two possible treatments: coronary angioplasty and coronary bypass surgery. If surgery is technically impractical because of extensive coronary artery disease, palliative oral therapy becomes the treatment of choice.

Coronary angioplasty dilates and opens narrowed coronary arteries by means of a small inflatable balloon at the tip of a long catheter that is introduced through a femoral artery in a groin and pushed via the aorta into the coronary arteries. A stent is then often inserted. This is a metal coil or tube that holds and maintains the artery open. In the early stages of a heart attack it is also often possible to inject streptokinase, an enzyme that dissolves blood clots, into the affected coronary artery and so abort the attack. New developments involve high-energy lasers and arterial shaving techniques to vaporise or remove obstructing fatty plaques and clots, and restore coronary artery patency.

Diving after an angioplasty **may** be permitted by a diving physician, provided the restrictions described above for diving after a heart attack are adhered to.

CORONARY BYPASS SURGERY Recircuiting coronary artery blood flow is being performed routinely in many centres around the world. The operation involves the initial removal of lengths of superficial veins from the legs. These vein segments are then grafted to the coronary arteries, one end above and the other below the site of arterial obstruction. The area of disease is left alone and simply bypassed through the transplanted veins. In most cases, the operation is virtually curative, in that the need for oral medication stops and the patient can resume a fully active lifestyle with minimal restrictions.

Sport divers can consider returning to diving provided the conditions outlined above for diving after a heart attack are met. The issue of pleural scarring after open chest surgery, which can lead to pulmonary barotrauma with diving, must be discussed by the diver and his physician.

DISORDERS OF RHYTHM AND RATE (ARRHYTHMIAS)

There are many disorders of heart rhythm and rate, the commonest being a too-fast or too-slow heart rate. A normal heart rate is between 60 and 90 beats a minute. The majority of arrhythmias are not indicative of underlying disease, and merely reflect excesses in lifestyle. Immoderate use of alcohol, nicotine, caffeine or decongestants, as well as fatigue, anxiety or stress, all cause a rapid resting heart rate, often with occasional extra abnormal beats. These extra beats disappear with effort. A very slow heart rate often occurs in super-fit athletes, but increases normally during exercise.

Any other unusualness in heart rhythm or rate requires investigation to exclude underlying disease such as an overactive thyroid gland, anaemia, high blood pressure or coronary artery disease. The nature and severity of the cause will determine further fitness to dive. Uncontrolled abnormalities of rhythm and rate, or those due to or requiring drug therapy, usually exclude diving.

VALVULAR DISEASE

Abnormalities of the valves of the heart are invariably first detected because of characteristic murmurs heard on clinical examination.

A pulmonary flow murmur, which is very common in young people, is of no clinical significance, merely reflecting vigorous blood flow through the pulmonary valve of the heart. It is not a contraindication to diving. Another common murmur that usually poses no threat to divers is that of the billowing mitral leaflet syndrome (also called click-murmur syndrome or Barlow's syndrome). The murmur is due to a rather floppy leaflet of the mitral valve between the left atrium and ventricle. It is detected by hearing a classic murmur and click when listening to the heart through a stethoscope. In some cases palpitations occur, with runs of rapid heart beats and, if beta-blockers are needed, the person may be unfit to dive.

Some congenital valve abnormalities do not necessarily exclude diving. A bicuspid aortic valve, where the aortic valve guarding against reflux of blood back into the left ventricle has two cusps instead of three, is an example. If not incompetent or heavily calcified on assessment by a cardiologist, the person may dive. The most common pathological murmurs are due to valvular scarring and distortion by rheumatic heart disease in young people; and, in older divers, to the hardening and calcification of the aortic and mitral valves. If narrowing or leaking of the affected valves is considered significant by a physician, diving is prohibited. Bubble initiation is a real risk on actively moving valves that have lost their smooth surfaces.

Cardiac surgery incorporating the implantation of artificial heart valves also bars diving in most cases. People who have had such surgery commonly use anticoagulants to prevent clotting on the valves, and the risk of massive haemorrhage with any barotrauma, plus the effects of cold water stress, exercise, and the demands of nitrogen loading and degassing, make diving unacceptable.

PACEMAKERS

Electronic pacemakers, inserted under the skin and taking control of the heart rate, are used when cardiac or coronary artery disease presents with abnormal rhythms, causing fainting episodes or are possibly life-threatening. The problems of diving with a pacemaker are the original reasons for inserting it; the effects of pressure on a possibly non-pressure-resistant electronic instrument, and the need for the pacemaker to accelerate heart rate during exercise. Variable rate pacemakers are available, but before making any decision to dive with a pacemaker, detailed discussion between the manufacturer, cardiologist, diving physician and the patient is essential.

BLEEDING DISORDERS

Any disorder that predisposes to a bleeding tendency usually means total disqualification from diving. Whether due to the use of anticoagulant drugs such as Warfarin or heparin, liver disease, bone marrow problems, leukaemia or inherited disorders such as haemophilia, a tendency to haemorrhage could be fatal when diving.

Associated chronic anaemia may be present. Any pressure-volume changes with depth could result in uncontrolled bleeding in the lungs, middle ears, sinuses and gut. The regular infusion of fresh-frozen plasma into the blood of haemophiliacs and allied bleeders can only offer some protection under normal surface circumstances. It can never handle the potential catastrophe of pulmonary barotrauma or trauma due to injuries from boat propellers or marine animal bites. But there are divers who dive while on anticoagulant treatment. Their rationale is that they always dive carefully and safely. It cannot be medically condoned and the risk is entirely in their own hands. No one can guarantee that an emergency under water will not occur.

BLOOD DONORS

A donor should wait for 24 hours after donating blood before diving again, provided he or she is not anaemic. The reason is a lower total oxygen-carrying capacity by haemoglobin plus the loss of blood volume. Under diving conditions, the available oxygen is at a higher partial pressure than at the surface and a significant amount can dissolve in plasma. The main reason is related to the loss of about one-sixth of the total **fluid** volume of blood, the **only** route for inert gas carriage from the tissues to the alveoli. After 24 hours it is safe to recommence diving as the blood fluid volume balance will have been restored, even though the cellular and protein elements still have to be replaced. Replacement of red cells takes about two months.

PERIPHERAL VASCULAR DISEASE

A number of diseases, such as arteriosclerosis and diabetes, affect the small peripheral vessels of the body. This reduces the blood supply to the tissues of the arms and legs, especially the lower legs, feet and hands, which become permanently cold, with decreased hair and nail growth. Under exercise conditions, the oxygen supply becomes very inadequate and muscle cramping occurs, classically in the calf muscles while walking. This is called claudication. The affected person has to stand and wait until the acidic products of metabolism, such as lactic acid, can be removed from the area and the oxygen debt repaid. Diving aggravates this because cold water causes spasm of already inadequate blood vessels, worsening of the blood supply and easy cramping. Tissue degassing is also affected and diving is dangerous.

CHILBLAINS (Raynaud's Phenomenon) is a minor and temporary form of peripheral vascular disease. Spasm of the blood supply to the fingers and toes occurs in cold weather. These digits become cold, white and numb, the skin becomes painful and itchy and then rebound flushing occurs. In severe cases, blistering or even sores can develop. Diving in cold water intensifies this and the fingers can become very pallid, totally numb and difficult to move. Restoration of the blood supply after the dive is accompanied by intense burning and itching plus red flaring of the skin as spastic vessels dilate. Wearing gloves and bootees while diving often helps, while taking vitamin B6 assists in improving peripheral blood supply.

VARICOSE VEINS

Varicose veins generally cause no problem with diving, as the surrounding water pressure provides even support to dilated and tortuous veins. Severe cases should be treated surgically as the veins may bleed profusely with accidental trauma. Coral cuts on the legs, and bumping and scraping on boats are common injuries among divers.

CAROTID SINUS SYNDROME

The carotid sinuses, dilations of the carotid arteries, are located at the main branching of the arteries in the hollows of the neck just below the angles of the jaw. They function as blood pressure sensors and monitors. If an increase in blood pressure is sensed, nerve reflexes are initiated in the carotid sinuses which then cause slowing of the heart rate and a drop in blood pressure.

Problems can occur if the wet suit (or dry suit) is too tight around the neck. This occurs most commonly with pullover non-zippered wet suits or tight-fitting hoods.

The pressure of a too tightly fitting suit or hood stimulates the carotid sinuses and results in a profound slowing of heart rate and a steep drop in blood pressure to well below normal levels. This leads to sudden faintness or giddiness, even loss of consciousness or a seizure. Carotid sinus syndrome is possibly involved in cases of sudden death occurring in scuba divers, and is more prevalent and grave in older divers.

Prevention Ensure that dive suits are not too tight-fitting around the neck; slit tight pullover wet suits to avoid any neck constriction.

Management If a diver presents with sudden giddiness or loss of consciousness, whatever the possible cause, it is essential to ensure that the neck is free of constriction. If the casualty's upper neck is encased in tight rubber, cut free the rubber with your dive knife to ensure that no suit pressure exists, or peel off the hood. This also allows free access to the carotid pulses, which are the primary pulse monitors in CPR.

ANAEMIA

Anaemia is a reduction in the amount of haemoglobin, the oxygen-carrying iron-protein in red blood cells. It may be acute, following a sudden haemorrhage, and can lead to shock and even death; or chronic, being associated with simple iron deficiency, inherited anaemias such as thalassaemia and spherocytosis, or many other diseases, including cancer. Anaemia presents with fatigue, weakness, pallor, low blood pressure and breathlessness. As it reduces the oxygen-carrying capacity of blood, diving should be avoided until it is corrected. If an enlarged spleen is present, diving is barred, as there is a high risk of rupturing the spleen.

One type of anaemia, sickle-cell anaemia, is an inherited condition in which normal adult haemoglobin (haemoglobin A) is replaced by haemoglobin S. Red cells cluster together within blood vessels under low oxygen partial pressures. This results in so-called crises, with tissue death beyond the red cell mass. Carriers have both types of haemoglobin and they don't have crises, but they do sickle with hypoxia (a deficiency in the amount of oxygen delivered to the body tissues). As hypoxia is rare in sport diving, selected carriers may dive. However, people with full sickle-cell anaemia must not dive, as their decompression risks are high.

LEUKAEMIA

Leukaemia, which is a cancer of the white blood cells, is the leading cause of death in young adults. It may be acute or chronic; myelogenous or lymphoblastic leukaemia. Treatment involves chemotherapy and/or bone marrow transplants. Diving with leukaemia depends on several things:
- Being in full remission with no associated anaemia or enlarged spleen. The danger of rupturing the spleen with diving activity is very real.
- Being off all chemotherapy, fully recovered from any side-effects of treatment and having good immune resistance.
- Having good general fitness.

If all these parameters are present, diving may be considered.

07

PULMONARY REQUIREMENTS OF SCUBA DIVING

In contrast to the hydraulically operated cardiovascular system, the respiratory system is a pneumatic system. There are two lungs, each surrounded by a tough but flexible double sheath, the pleura. The lungs are encased by the rib cage and the diaphragm, a powerful flat sheet of muscle dividing the chest, or thorax, from the abdomen below. Although the lungs and heart actually fill the thorax, the pleural cavity is a potential space between the lungs and the ribs.

The Pulmonary System

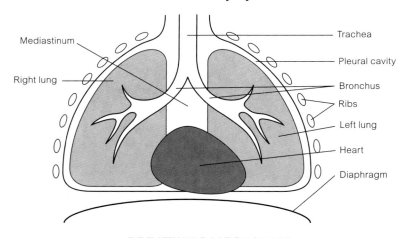

Mediastinum
Right lung

Trachea
Pleural cavity
Bronchus
Ribs
Left lung
Heart
Diaphragm

BREATHING MECHANICS

The lung bellows work as follows: the intercostal muscles between the ribs contract and pull the ribs outwards. At the same time, the diaphragm contracts downwards. This means that the volume of the chest increases. A vacuum forms in the potential space between the lungs and the rib cage. The lungs expand to fill this space and air is sucked into the lungs – this is **inspiration**. The muscles of the chest wall and diaphragm then relax and the rib cage springs back to its resting position. Air is squeezed out of the lungs – this is **expiration**. Inspiration is active, and expiration passive, under resting conditions. During exercise, additional chest muscles assist with the need for rapid inhalation, and exhalation becomes active too.

RESPIRATORY TREE

Like the arterial network, the respiratory system is a branching system. Inhaled air passes into the trachea, the rigid air pipe in the front of the throat below the larynx. In the chest, the trachea divides into two bronchi. Each bronchus passes into a lung. Within the lung, bronchi subdivide until the terminal bronchioles. Each of the millions of terminal bronchioles ends in a grape-like cluster of alveoli.

ALVEOLI

It is important to understand the physical scope of the lungs. Alveoli are not just air-filled sacs dangling from bronchioles. The number of alveoli has been estimated at 750 million, with a total surface area for gas exchange equal to that of the playing surface of eight full-size snooker tables, or 25 times the total surface area of the skin. Surrounding the alveoli is a capillary network processing the venous (right) side of the heart's entire blood output per minute.

To achieve this prodigious surface area in the relatively paltry volume of the chest, alveoli have to be very small and thin-walled. This means that bronchioles have to be small, too. They are: each semiglobular alveolus in a particular cluster is about 0.1 mm in diameter and one cell thick, and each bronchiole about 0.3 mm wide. And, from a diving point of view, therein lies their weakness.

A scuba diver risks exposing alveoli that are mere fractions of a millimetre in diameter and just one cell thick to several atmospheres of pressure change. At only 10 msw the air pressure in a human chest is two atmospheres, in other words, it equals the pressure inside a motor car tyre!

To tolerate this, the pressure inside and outside the lungs must be equal at all times. A pressure difference of only 0.1 ATA may be enough to rupture the lungs, meaning that if a scuba diver lying at the bottom of the shallow end of a swimming pool inhales fully and then stands up, his or her lungs may burst.

GAS EXCHANGE

Lungs have a huge thin-walled surface area that is exposed to air on one side and a massive network of blood on the other. This allows for very rapid gas exchange. The ultimate function of the lungs is to absorb oxygen and eliminate carbon dioxide. Both absorption and elimination are fluid-gas operations, transferring oxygen from air to blood, and carbon dioxide from blood to air.

The exchange occurs across a single layer of cells that line millions of air-filled alveoli and a single layer of cells that line the giant network of blood-filled pulmonary capillaries. So blood and air are both necessary for breathing. This may be obvious, but it is not that simple.

An efficient blood supply is essential – this is called **perfusion**. A good air supply is needed – this is called **ventilation**. And a rapid transfer of gas between air and blood is required – this is called **diffusion** (see illustration on next page).

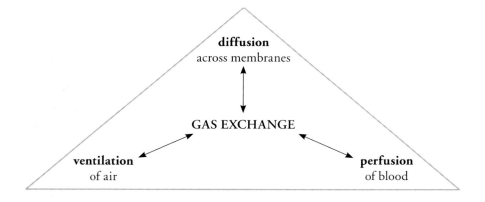

diffusion
across membranes

GAS EXCHANGE

ventilation
of air

perfusion
of blood

Perfusion, ventilation and diffusion are what lungs are about and they must all be normal and balanced for efficient gas exchange to occur. If any one of them fails, gas exchange is impaired. A failure of perfusion of normally ventilating lungs will achieve no gas exchange. Good perfusion of non-ventilating alveoli will achieve no gas exchange. Good perfusion and ventilating of non-diffusing alveoli will achieve no gas exchange. Balance is essential.

PULMONARY ASSESSMENT IN SCUBA DIVERS

A full assessment of lung function entails measuring all three aspects of pulmonary activity – ventilation, perfusion and diffusion. However, as avoiding pulmonary barotrauma is the only reason for doing lung function testing in an apparently normal scuba diver, only ventilation is directly assessed.

There are three aspects to assessing ventilation:
 – clinical assessment by a doctor,
 – chest X-ray, and
 – lung function test.

The clinical assessment forms part of any routine check-up and confirms the absence of any obvious disease. The diver's health history is investigated and the presence of normal air entry and exhalation listened for.

An X-ray gives an idea of the gross anatomy of the chest, and demonstrates heart size and shape, the major vessels and bronchi, the presence of overinflation or under-inflation of lungs, scarring and tumours, diaphragm movement on inhalation and exhalation and, very importantly, air-trapping in the bullae (pathological blister-like areas in the lung or on its surface). These are usually totally asymptomatic on land and the person is completely unaware of their presence unless they suddenly burst and a spontaneous pneumothorax occurs. But, under diving conditions, and filled with air under pressure at depth, bullae can easily burst on ascent with potential collapse of the lung, tearing of lung tissue, haemorrhage into the chest, and arterial gas embolism. Air-trapping, unless enormous, is not detectable clinically or on lung function testing.

An X-ray is essential and should comprise both inspiratory and immediate expiratory chest views to assess diaphragm movement and detect bullae.

A lung function test assesses all lung volumes and flow rates. It directly measures air volumes moving into and out of the lungs, rates of flow achieved, and rates of change of flow. It computes residual volumes of airways, and detects any restriction to inspiration and any obstruction to exhalation under resting and forced respiratory conditions. Changes in the elasticity of the lungs, their compliance in moving readily with inspiration and expiration, and resistance to flow in airways are assessed. Conditions such as asthma and emphysema are readily detected.

Pulmonary barotrauma is a result of failure of exhalation of compressed air. In order to reduce the costs of evaluating a sport diver, a minimum basic assessment of lung function measures volumes and flow rates during exhalation only.

At least three parameters must be measured:

1. FVC – **Forced Vital Capacity** is the volume of air exhaled between a full inhalation and a maximal forced exhalation. It is the maximum volume of air a diver can move into or out of the lungs. It varies with age, gender, height, weight and population group. Standard tables or computerised machines are used to predict the volume in each person tested. The FVC normally lies between 3.0 and 7.0 litres in adults. Asthmatics often have a normal FVC. The minimal FVC acceptable for diving is 75 per cent of predicted FVC.

2. FEV1 – **Forced Expiratory Volume in one second** is the volume of air exhaled in the first second of a maximal exhalation. It is the first second of the FVC and indicates any airway resistance. The higher the resistance to exhalation, the lower will be the volume of air exhaled in the first second. The FEV1 is always reduced with any obstructive airways disease, including asthma.

3. FEV1% – As both the FVC and FEV1 vary with height, weight, age, gender and population group, their volumes in litres mean little unless a standard table or computer are at hand. So a ratio is used which is independent of all the variables. The volume of air exhaled in the first second is calculated as a percentage of total air exhaled:

$$\text{FEV1/FVC} \times 100 = \text{FEV1\%}$$

A diver with normal lung function will be able to exhale about 80 per cent of his FVC in one second. The minimum FEV1% acceptable varies between authorities; in the UK the lowest accepted is 70–75 per cent. As asthmatics always have a low FEV1, they will also have a low FEV1%.

Many doctors still use peak flow meters to measure the peak flow rate (PFR) as a test for respiratory efficiency in divers. However, the peak flow meter has no place in diving medicine. Even people with severe obstructive airways disease can sustain a very high flow rate for a fraction of a second. The peak flow meter will provide a favourable reading, while the person completes their expiration with a six-second-long wheeze. Spitting or tonguing the mouthpiece will also provide normal results. The peak flow meter is useful only in assessing an individual's response to treatment for obstructive pulmonary disease.

There is one lung volume people cannot use or change – the air volume remaining after maximal exhalation. Called the **residual volume (RV)**, it is the volume of the tubular airways inside the lungs – the bronchi and bronchioles. Its importance relates to the maximum depth that can safely be reached by a breathhold diver. An average total lung volume (TLV) is about 6 litres. This is the sum of FVC and RV (TLV = FVC + RV). An average residual volume is about 1.2 litres. One can now ask, how deep can one go on a breathhold dive, assuming average lung volumes?

On descent, the surrounding water pressure compresses the air in one's chest. One can therefore descend until total lung air has been compressed to equal the surface residual volume. With a TLV of 6 litres and a RV of 1.2 litres (one fifth), one can therefore dive to 5 ATA or 40 msw. At this point, lung air volume will be one fifth of that at the surface (see Boyle's Law, page 21). Descending below this depth results in blood pooling in the great veins of the chest to further equalise the decreasing air volume. What follows is a crushing of the chest wall and rupture of internal tissues and veins, along with massive intrathoracic haemorrhage.

Despite the theoretical safe average maximum of 40 msw, free dives have been made to below 100 msw. These divers require extraordinarily flexible chest walls, lung volumes with relatively very small RVs, and immense venous pooling capability. It is doubtful whether breathhold dives to these depths can be done without causing some pathology.

Divers who have a breathing source under water do not undergo these volume changes, as the pressure of the inhaled air is set to the ambient surrounding pressure at all times. The total lung volume is the same at the surface and at depth. What does vary is the density of the gas mix with pressure, as well as the partial pressures of the components in the mix (see Dalton's Law, page 24).

BREATHHOLD DIVING

A breathhold diver is deliberately risking asphyxiation. During breathholding, the body continues to use oxygen and produce carbon dioxide. So the partial pressure of oxygen in the blood will drop (hypoxia) and the partial pressure of the carbon dioxide will rise (hypercapnia – eventually leading to carbon dioxide narcosis). Either effect can cause unconsciousness, commonly at 5 msw during the ascent, and together they form a very dangerous pair.

Breathhold diving, especially with prior hyperventilation, is a classic exercise in diving physics. At the surface of the water, hyperventilating flushes out alveolar carbon dioxide. Following Henry's Law (see page 26), arterial blood carbon dioxide levels also drop (hypocapnia). Obeying Dalton's Law, alveolar oxygen and nitrogen pressures increase to compensate for the low level of carbon dioxide. During descent, water pressure increases and Boyle's Law reduces lung air volume. Dalton's Law continues to operate with a proportional rise in the partial pressure of alveolar oxygen. Henry's Law now drives this oxygen into pulmonary capillary blood and pulmonary arterial carbon dioxide into alveolar gas. Alveolar oxygen drops and carbon dioxide rises[1]. The high arterial partial pressure of carbon dioxide is the stimulus for the overwhelming desire to breathe that ends a breathhold dive and forces a diver to surface. This will normally occur while the partial pressure of oxygen is still sufficient for body requirements. However, should the arterial oxygen level drop below a critical level of 4 kilopascals (kPa), unconsciousness under water may occur without any warning. The same may happen if the carbon dioxide level rises above 6 kPa.

At the same time, other profound physiological changes are occurring in the diver. Lung ventilation stops, but diffusion and perfusion continue. At a depth of 10 msw the early effects of chest squeeze occur. Lung air volume has halved, lung tissue is compressed and alveolar architecture is distorted. Interference with normal perfusion threatens as the lungs become 'stiff' and engorged with blood.

Spear fishermen are breathhold divers. They are often very competitive and want to stay under water for as long as possible, so:
– they train in order to increase their circulatory efficiency
– they acclimatise to a raised level of carbon dioxide in the blood; regular divers may find their 'carbon dioxide threshold' or stimulus to breathe is set higher than non-divers,
– they move as little as possible under water to conserve oxygen and reduce carbon dioxide production, and
– they **hyperventilate** before the dive. This is the dangerous one. Let's look at two examples:
    • Nick promised his wife some fresh crayfish. Using a snorkel, he dives to 10 msw (2 ATA). At this depth, his lung air volume has halved (Boyle's Law), and the partial pressure of oxygen in his alveoli has doubled (Dalton's Law). This is beneficial in that more oxygen is now available. After 45 seconds, the high partial pressure of carbon dioxide forces him to surface, waving a crayfish. All is well, as his oxygen level is still adequate.
    • Jeff is a competitive spear fisherman. He hyperventilates at the surface, breathing in and out as deeply as possible, until he feels dizzy. What he has done is to flush out his lungs and alveoli so that the partial pressure of carbon dioxide in his alveoli has dropped to 2.7 kPa (normal alveolar carbon dioxide at sea level is just over 5 kPa). This gives him a 'start', as the time required to build up the carbon dioxide to trigger levels will be longer. He has also increases his alveolar oxygen, the lost carbon dioxide being replaced by air. He now dives to 20 msw (3 ATA). The oxygen concentration in his lungs triples, giving him even more duration.

---

1   A South African doctor, Pieter Landsberg, found that after vigorous hyperventilating, these alveolar changes are not invariable and do not reliably reflect the blood gas status. At the end of the dive, alveolar carbon dioxide may be very high or low, with low or moderate oxygen.

Jeff waits and waits for his fish and, just when he feels he must ascend, he gets his chance and spends a further 10 seconds spearing it. The desire to breathe is now very strong and he ascends rapidly. As he does so, the water pressure drops, but so does the partial pressure of oxygen in his alveoli. At 5 msw his blood oxygen drops so much that he suddenly loses consciousness. Luckily, a buddy is at hand to bring him to the surface and resuscitate him.

This is the classic description of **blackout of ascent** – the cause of death by drowning in many healthy breathhold divers. It is caused by a deadly sequence of events. The increased ambient pressure at depth decreases the lung air volume and increases alveolar partial pressure of oxygen, so causing a higher gradient of oxygen into the blood from the lungs. Hyperventilating before the dive drops the baseline carbon dioxide level in the lungs and arterial blood, and increases the time before a high arterial blood carbon dioxide stimulus forces the diver to surface. If excessive, it also raises blood alkalinity, causing a drop in available blood calcium – this, then, can cause tetany (intense limb-muscle cramps).

Oxygen is steadily removed from alveolar air during the dive but, at the bottom, the level is adequate, even at the end of the dive. Ascent, especially fast ascent, causes the oxygen level in the lungs to fall sharply with a rapid drop or even a reversal in the gradient of oxygen into the blood, resulting in a severe arterial hypoxia of ascent, (especially in the last 5 msw) and sudden blackout.

The safety of the dive depends on:

1. **Ventilation** A large FVC with relatively small RV will provide a greater oxygen reserve. This ratio is reduced with any respiratory ailment. Hyperventilation should be limited to four breaths.

2. **Diffusion** An efficient alveolar/capillary junction is needed for rapid transfer of oxygen and carbon dioxide. This is reduced by factors such as smoking or respiratory infections.

3. **Perfusion** A good alveolar blood supply is needed for efficient degassing and upgassing. Any illness affecting blood supply to the lungs will reduce perfusion.

4. **Fitness** This improves muscle oxygen utilisation for a given exercise load. Oxygen consumption and carbon dioxide production during hyperventilation will affect the safe duration of the dive. So will oxygen consumption and carbon dioxide production during the dive.

5. **Blood carbon dioxide load between dives** Inadequate time for breathing, and carbon dioxide unloading at the surface between breathhold dives, will cause rapid hypercapnia (an excess of carbon dioxide in the blood) and even carbon dioxide narcosis and syncope (fainting) at the bottom with the next dive.

6. **Dive depth** The deeper the dive, the greater the chances of chest squeeze, the higher the oxygen gradient into blood at the bottom, and the steeper the hypoxia (deficiency in the amount of oxygen delivered to body tissues).

7. **Dive duration** Breathhold dives of longer than 80 or 90 seconds place the diver in extreme jeopardy.

8. **Rate of ascent** Very rapid ascents cause a rapid drop in the delivery of alveolar oxygen and result in hypoxia on ascent.

9. **Patent foramen ovale** A flap-valve between the right and left upper chambers of the heart is present in up to 25–37 per cent of people. If right-to-left shunts, such as a PFO (see page 44), are present, this author believes they may operate with the increased water pressure on the chest in breathhold diving and be an important cause of death in breathhold diving.

As the breathhold diver descends, water pressure around him or her increases. The chest and lungs become compressed and 'stiff', lung capillaries are flattened, and the right side of the heart, a very low pressure system, meets increased resistance to its attempts to pump blood into lung blood vessels. The pressure in the right atrium rises and the PFO opens. Venous blood, high in carbon dioxide and very low in oxygen, is shunted into the left side of the heart and back into the general circulation. Less blood reaches the lungs. This results in a decreased transfer of blood carbon dioxide into alveoli, plus a reduced draw on available alveolar oxygen during the dive. Arterial blood oxygen drops dramatically and carbon dioxide rises sharply. Analysing the gas in the alveoli at this point would show a relatively low carbon dioxide level and ample oxygen! Bottom syncope may then occur, due to profound arterial hypoxia and carbon dioxide narcosis. Or a rapid ascent could beat diffusion of oxygen from, and carbon dioxide into, expanding alveoli and result in blackout of ascent.

NOTES:

- Deep dives to below 30 msw without hyperventilating may cause blackout of ascent as the alveolar oxygen partial pressure will increase at least four times, with very rapid absorption, followed by an equivalently rapid drop on ascent.

- The same laws also apply to nitrogen. At depth, the nitrogen partial pressure in the alveoli will also increase. This is equivalent to breathing air at depth. Repetitive deep dives on a snorkel may cause excessive amounts of nitrogen to be absorbed, resulting in bends occuring on breathhold dives.

- Oxygen utilisation by the tissues does not increase with depth. It increases with work. A diver at 10 msw and a diver at 100 msw will use the same amount of oxygen (when expressed in surface volumes) for the same work, ignoring the work of breathing a denser mix. This is why a two per cent oxygen mix is safe at 90 msw but 20 per cent is required at the surface. Their partial pressures are the same (0.2 ATA) under the different conditions.

- Similarly, the body does not produce more carbon dioxide at depth than at the surface. Metabolic requirements do not change – only pressures do.

METABOLISM

The gases oxygen and carbon dioxide have been mentioned again and again. The following questions arise:
- Why do we need oxygen?
- What is oxygen used for?
- Where does carbon dioxide come from?

The fine details are very complex and totally out of the scope of diving. However, the basic essentials are easily explained with an analogy. Take a petrol engine. The fuel is octane, which consists of 8 atoms of carbon and 18 atoms of hydrogen linked in a straight chain (C_8H_{18}).

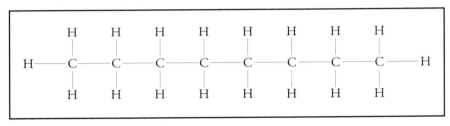

Inside the cylinders, the octane is mixed with air (i.e. oxygen), pressurised and sparked. The octane combines with the oxygen and explodes. If conditions were perfect, the end products would be carbon dioxide (CO_2) and water (H_2O).

Octane + oxygen = carbon dioxide + water + energy + heat

As conditions are never perfect, some of the octane is incompletely combusted and forms carbon monoxide (CO). Complete combustion yields carbon dioxide only. The tissue cells are our engines, billions of them. Our fuel is glucose from our diet. Glucose combines with oxygen to produce carbon dioxide, water, energy and heat.

Glucose + oxygen = carbon dioxide + water + energy + heat

Obviously, we do not explode oxygen and glucose under pressure. The overall reaction is broken down by steps into many smaller reactions, each controlled by enzymes and releasing some of the energy and heat, and all strictly controlled. Our body heat is the result of this process. The carbon dioxide we breathe out is the end-product, together with some water vapour. The rest of the water formed is handled by the kidneys. For every molecule of oxygen used, a molecule of carbon dioxide is formed.

At **rest**, we use about 0.25 litres of oxygen per minute. With **hard swimming**, we use up to four litres of oxygen per minute. Note that this is only oxygen used, not total air consumption. Not all the oxygen we breathe in is used. Inspired air contains about 21 per cent oxygen and exhaled air approximately 16 per cent oxygen.

How is oxygen carried to the tissues?

Within the blood are trillions of red blood cells, or erythrocytes. Within these cells is an iron-containing pigment called haemoglobin, which gives blood its red colour. (In plants, the equivalent pigment is chlorophyll, which gives them a green colour.) Haemoglobin traps oxygen under conditions of high oxygen partial pressure (i.e. in the lung capillaries) and releases it under conditions of low oxygen partial pressure and high carbon dioxide partial pressure (i.e. in the tissues).

Most of the body's oxygen is carried bound to haemoglobin. Only a small percentage is dissolved free in plasma, the straw-coloured liquid portion of blood that remains when all the blood cells are removed.

What controls breathing?

Since breathing is an automatic process that does not require any conscious attention, there obviously must be a control mechanism. The respiratory centre that controls breathing is located in the brain. It receives its information regarding breathing rate and depth from the following (among others):

1. **Carbon dioxide partial pressure** The partial pressure of carbon dioxide in the blood is the most powerful stimulus to breathe. A rise in the carbon dioxide level in the blood stimulates ventilation.
2. **Oxygen partial pressure** This is a much weaker stimulus to breathe, however, a low partial pressure of oxygen does stimulate inspiration.
3. **Heat** A rise in body temperature stimulates inspiration, while a fall in body temperature depresses breathing.
4. **Acidity** Lactic acid is formed when the oxygen supply of actively exercising muscles falls. This increase in acidity stimulates ventilation in order to increase oxygen uptake.
5. **Joint movement** An active movement of a joint triggers nerve reflexes to the respiratory centre in the brain and stimulates ventilation.

Under normal conditions, the circulating level of carbon dioxide is the main controlling force. But the body is beautifully coordinated. An increase in ventilation is linked to an increase in perfusion in order to maintain balance. All of the above respiratory-stimulating factors also stimulate heart output, with increased perfusion of the lungs with blood in order to take full advantage of the increased ventilation.

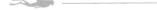

08

IMPLICATIONS OF RESPIRATORY DISEASE ON DIVING

Normal breathing is essential for safe diving. During a dive, the lungs are exposed to more potential danger than any other organ. It is imperative that a diver with a history of any significant respiratory problem has a comprehensive medical, incorporating a chest X-ray with inspiratory and expiratory views and a full lung-function test. Conditions that can affect the efficiency of the bellows system – its ventilation, perfusion or diffusion – must, temporarily or permanently, bar a diver from the sport.

VENTILATION ABNORMALITIES

Ventilation of the lungs requires efficient inspiration (breathing in) and expiration (breathing out). There are a number of conditions that can impair either one or the other, or both of these actions. Some, such as bronchitis and pneumonia, are acute and temporary, and diving may resume after full recovery and clinical reassessment. Others, such as a spontaneous pneumothorax, are acute and require permanent suspension from diving. Many are ongoing and therefore automatically preclude diving – emphysema or lung damage caused by chronic dust inhalation (pneumoconiosis) fall into this category.

Disorders of inspiration (restrictive pulmonary disease)

Failure of easy inspiration occurs when the normal compliance of the lungs is lost, that is, they lose their elasticity and can no longer inflate normally to follow the expansion of the chest wall during inspiration. This occurs most commonly in quarry and mine workers and, depending on the type of dust involved (coal, asbestos, silicon or cement), leads to intense scarring of the lungs. Pulmonary fibrosis may follow congenital cystic disease of the lung, a lung infection, or abnormalities of the immune system of the body. The diagnosis is readily made via a chest X-ray, while lung function testing will reveal impaired respiratory results. The risk of pulmonary barotrauma while diving is enormous and diving is therefore prohibited.

Both inspiration and expiration are impaired by emphysema, which is most commonly caused by smoking. Overinflation of the lungs occurs due to the breakdown of alveoli, with a drastic reduction of alveolar surface area. The chest becomes barrel-shaped and the movement of the chest wall between full inspiration and expiration is greatly reduced. Emphysema sufferers often purse their lips and blow during expiration, unconsciously increasing the partial pressure in their lungs to drive oxygen from the alveoli into the blood. Obviously, they may not dive.

A short-term reduction in inspiration occurs commonly with rib injuries, and illnesses such as pleurisy and chest shingles, where pain limits adequate inhalation. All lung-function tests should be normal on recovery.

Disorders of expiration (obstructive pulmonary disease)

Expiration disorders cause airway obstruction and increased resistance to exhalation. Those disorders listed above that cause ongoing inspiratory impairment usually have an obstructive element too, with significantly increased bronchiolar resistance. The most common chronic disorders of expiration are asthma, chronic bronchitis and chronic obstructive pulmonary disease (COPD).

The most dangerous acute combined inspiratory and expiratory condition is a spontaneous pneumothorax, where the lung can neither fill nor empty normally. Benign and malignant tumours, tuberculosis and fungal infections of the lung may be both obstructive and restrictive, and all prohibit one from diving.

ABNORMALITIES OF PERFUSION AND DIFFUSION

Interference with the normal blood supply of the lungs impairs diffusion of oxygen, carbon dioxide and nitrogen. This occurs with pulmonary embolism, which occurs when a deep vein thrombosis (blood clot) in the calf muscle loosens and is carried as an embolus to the main venous return to the heart, and then pumped into the pulmonary arteries.

It can also happen following thrombosis of the superficial leg veins. Sarcoidosis, a condition characterised by the formation of granulomatous lesions in the lung, affects the alveolar membranes and interferes with diffusion. All perfusion and diffusion abnormalities must preclude diving.

SPONTANEOUS PNEUMOTHORAX

If air is allowed to enter the pleural cavity – the space between the surface of a lung and the chest wall – the lung bellows system instantly fails. The vacuum that exists in the pleural space on inspiration, forcing the lung to inflate, is eliminated. The lung collapses and ventilation and diffusion cease. This is called a pneumothorax.

Factors that predispose to a spontaneous pneumothorax under non-diving conditions are lung blisters and bullae, lung cysts, and cavities resulting from diseases such as tuberculosis (TB). In most cases the lung collapses without any warning, often when the person is straining to lift a heavy object, sneezing or vomiting.

These actions suddenly increase the pressure inside the lungs, resulting in tearing through the area of weakness on the surface of the lung. Sudden one-sided chest pain occurs, plus difficulty in breathing. If the torn area allows air flow in one direction only by acting as a flap valve, each successive breath pumps more air into the pleural cavity and progressively compresses the affected lung.

Pneumothorax (collapsed lung)

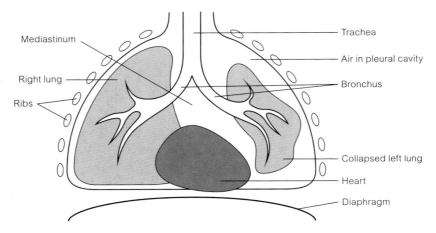

This is a **tension pneumothorax.** If it is allowed to proceed, it will steadily pressurise the chest, compressing the heart, mediastinum (the centre of the chest cavity containing the heart, major blood vessels and the division of the trachea into its two main bronchi) and the other lung into the opposite side of the thorax. If left untreated, the person will die of cardiopulmonary failure.

The incidence of recurrence of a spontaneous pneumothorax is high, with one-third of cases having another episode within three to five years.

Under scuba diving conditions, a pneumothorax may be precipitated by breath-holding during ascent, coughing or vomiting under water, or blowing very hard while performing a Valsalva manoeuvre (see page 115).

Unless the leak is extremely small, the consequences are very grave. Air expanding inside the pleural cavity on ascent cannot escape, so it will pressurise the chest as with a tension pneumothorax and then drive the lungs up into the throat and beyond. If a tension pneumothorax develops at depth, the diver will die under water. Ascent becomes impossible because of gas expansion, and remaining under water is impossible because of air supply limitations and progressive cardiopulmonary failure. A history of spontaneous pneumothorax must permanently preclude diving.

But – and such is the enthusiasm of divers for their sport that there is always a 'but' – some divers have continued diving after a pneumothorax by subjecting themselves to surgical stripping of the pleura of both lungs (pleurectomy). The pleural cavity is eliminated, the lungs then healing by attaching themselves directly to the chest wall. This procedure would seem a drastic for an otherwise healthy individual to undertake in order to scuba dive, and both lungs must be treated because surface blisters and blebs, if present, are most commonly found on both lungs. The question of lung scarring then predisposing to lung tissue tearing during diving with resultant arterial gas embolism must also be considered.

A pneumothorax can also occur following injury to the chest wall due a stab wound, fractured ribs or open chest surgery for reasons such as coronary artery by-pass procedures. It is important to exclude air-trapping by scarring and adhesions after surgery. A normal lung function test, chest X-ray, possible computerised lung scan (spiral CT scan), helium loop test and uneventful chamber pressure test dive in an experienced diver could make requalification acceptable, provided that the underlying cause of the need for surgery does not persist.

ASTHMA

Asthma is a condition associated with increased resistance to easy air flow out of the small tubular airways within the lungs. Up to about ten years ago, no diver with asthma, however mild, was medically fit to dive. It was felt that the danger of fatal lung injury during a rapid, emergency or uncontrolled ascent was so great that the risk was unacceptable.

The majority of asthmatics who want to dive comprise a subtle medical group. Their total lung volumes are usually entirely normal, many are athletes who excel at long distance running, competitive sport and even mountain climbing. They have normal lungs on chest X-rays. So why can't they dive? Because they take longer than normal to breathe out fully on volume/flow electronic lung function testing.

Divers breathe compressed air. On descent, their second stage regulators ensure that the gas pressure entering the lungs exactly equals surrounding water pressure. So far, asthmatics have no problem. During ascent, however, the picture changes. Their regulators will still ensure that they inhale air at the steadily-decreasing ambient water pressure, but any exhaled gases are simply vented into the water. Their lungs are left to cope on their own, however, to ensure that overpressurisation does not occur during ascent – a feature of all diving breathing systems.

As the surrounding water pressure falls, so compressed air already in the lungs expands in accordance with Boyle's Law. If expanding air cannot vent freely from the lungs and into the water through the mouth-held regulator, the diver will surface with compressed air trapped in the chest. Lung tearing and rupture can then occur. And this pressure does not have to be much. Less than one metre of sea water or one tenth of an atmosphere overpressurisation of the lungs is enough to cause fatal lung damage! An asthmatic diver surfacing rapidly from 10 msw because of breathing difficulty, an out-of-air situation, panic or an over-inflated buoyancy compensator could result in up to two atmospheres absolute of gas pressure in the lungs at the surface – more than ten times the required pressure for lung rupture. Death may be instant.

What causes asthma?

For hundreds of years, doctors have treated spasm of the small airway tubules, as this was thought to be the cause of asthma. Each of these tiny tubules, or bronchioles, is surrounded by a layer of muscle, and the spasm of this muscle layer causes narrowing of the tubule, obstructing easy air flow and resulting in wheezing and difficulty in breathing, especially with exhalation. But simple bronchiolar spasm does not cause asthma! Spasm is not the cause of asthma – it is the effect. Treating the spasm alone is like giving a painkiller to cure a dental abscess. It won't work; it is the tooth that must be treated and the pain will then disappear spontaneously. The same applies to asthma. Treat the cause and the spasm will go.

So what is the cause of asthma; what causes the spasm? Allergy is the root cause – to dusts, pollens, cats or dozens of other allergens. Allergy causes inflammation and swelling, and inflammation of the bronchioles is the bottom-line disease process.

Inflamed bronchioles are irritable and readily go into spasm, which causes airway obstruction. However, it is important to understand that inflammation also has three other major effects: inflamed bronchioles are swollen and secrete mucus; swelling and mucous plugs in the tubules add to obstruction; in addition, ongoing inflammation causes progressive scarring of the bronchioles. Scar tissue cannot be removed and the resultant additional narrowing due to scarring is then permanent and breathlessness becomes irreversible. This is part of the development of emphysema.

Once it was realised that managing bronchial inflammation was the key to treating asthma, the focus shifted to developing anti-inflammatory sprays that could be inhaled, thereby providing medication directly where it was needed, at the bronchioles, without having to swallow tablets which would expose the entire body to medication and possible side effects.

Asthma treatment and diving

It is now universally accepted that the primary treatment for asthma is the ongoing use of inhaled cortisone in tiny microgram doses. This is neither controversial or arguable. There is absolutely no demonstrably effective equivalent in any form of alternative medicine. Any asthmatic who is not on a maintenance regime of twice daily inhaled cortisone sprays, such as Budesonide or Fluticasone is, quite simply being treated poorly and inadequately.

There is no place for the use of bronchodilators in the primary treatment of asthma. Bronchodilator drugs, such as salbutamol, do not treat the cause. They treat the spasm secondary to inflammation and have no effect on swelling, mucus production or the inevitable bronchiolar scarring that will occur. Inhaled cortisone does prevent the inflammatory cascade to scarring. For those who are scared of using cortisone, the tiny microgram doses inhaled are far too little to have significant generalised side-effects such as osteoporosis, weight gain, tissue thinning and other damage that occurs with prolonged ingestion of oral cortisone in milligram doses (1000 times more). The effects of not using inhaled cortisone are far more dire.

Bronchodilators are the secondary line of treatment in asthma and are used only for episodes of spasm that may occur despite the use of inhaled cortisone. Long-acting bronchodilators, such as salmeterol, are now available and, in combination with microgram doses of cortisone, are currently the optimal method of primary treatment.

In some cases, combination sprays of salmeterol and corticoids are still not enough.

Leukotriene receptor antagonists, such as montelukast and zafirlukast, have been developed which act on eosinophils, the white blood cells involved in the initiation of the inflammatory allergic cascade, and add a powerful new arm to asthma management.

With this new approach to the effective management of asthma, it has become possible for selected asthmatics to dive; this means asthmatics who are well-controlled, meticulous with their therapy, physically fit and with absent airway obstruction on medical assessment. Diving physicians have the responsibility of recognising asthma, assessing its severity and ensuring effective treatment, especially the need for scrupulous attention to inhaled cortisone treatment. **This does not mean that all asthmatics may dive.** Without demonstrably normal lung functions maintained by daily cortisone sprays, they are assuredly not controlled and uncontrolled asthma does kill divers.

Assessing asthma requires an annual full medical examination, including an electronic lung function test. This test must be normal at rest and remain normal after very strenuous exercise in the doctor's examination room. A reduced expiratory flow rate, especially mid-expiratory flow, means that control is inadequate and the danger of pulmonary barotrauma very real. Diving is not permitted. There is no place for a puff of Ventolin or other bronchodilator just before a dive. The spray cannot reach every single bronchiole in spasm whereas inhaled air pressure surely does. Compressed air trapped by swelling, spasm or mucous plugs will cause lung damage or death on ascent. DCI occurs about four times more commonly in asthmatics. CAUTION: Any diver who has asthma, however mild, must consult a diving doctor regularly and ensure that his or her physical health, fitness and asthma control are excellent before taking to the water.

SMOKING AND DIVING

Smoking is a disease that was introduced into Europe by Christopher Columbus, who caught the habit from a North American Indian. The weed *Nicotiana tabacum*, a relative of deadly nightshade, was then named after the French ambassador to Lisbon, Jean Nicot, who sent the seeds to the queen of France, Catherine de Médici. She subsequently died at Blois on 5 January 1589.

Smoking and diving don't mix. Tobacco smoke contains a number of chemicals including nicotine, carbon monoxide, assorted tars and sulphur cyanides. The harmful effects of smoking are both short-term and long-term, local and general.

LOCAL EFFECTS OF SMOKING

1. Irritation of the lining of the nose, mouth, throat, bronchi and alveoli occurs. This leads to chronic swelling of these membranes with catarrhal mucus production and mucous plugs. These cause obstruction of Eustachian tube function and difficulty in equalising the middle ears on descent, plus reverse squeeze on ascent; obstruction of sinus outlets leading to sinus squeeze and reverse squeeze; obstruction of bronchioles predisposing to chronic cough, air-trapping and pulmonary barotrauma of ascent.

2. Decreased permeability of alveolar walls reduces gas diffusion with inefficient oxygen uptake and carbon dioxide and nitrogen degassing.
3. Decreased elasticity and compliance of the lungs to chest wall movement occurs. Lung function tests show increased airway resistance to breathing. With time, breakdown of alveoli occurs, resulting in progressive and irreversible lung damage and emphysema.
4. Reduced resistance to infection of the nose, sinuses, throat, bronchi and lungs predisposes to rhinitis, sinusitis, pharyngitis, bronchitis and pneumonia.
5. Chronic irritation disposes to malignant change and cancer of the respiratory tree anywhere from mouth and nose to lungs.

GENERAL EFFECTS OF SMOKING

1. Smoking increases blood viscosity and stimulates spasm of arterioles, both of which cause increased resistance to blood flow and high blood pressure. This then predisposes to cerebral haemorrhage or thrombosis of the cerebral arteries and stroke.
2. Stimulation of heart rate occurs with irregular beats and rhythms. Simultaneous spasm of the coronary arteries may lead to a heart attack.
3. Absorption of cancer-producing chemicals occurs, with an increased incidence of cancer of the stomach, bowel, bladder, prostate, thyroid and liver.
4. Smoking causes a reduction in oxygen saturation and an increase in carbon dioxide and carbon monoxide retention.
5. Damage to the cardiovascular and respiratory systems causes irreversible loss of general health, physical fitness and endurance.

CORYZA AND INFLUENZA

Coryza (a common cold) and influenza (flu) occur very commonly, especially in the winter months. They are viral infections that can affect the nose, throat and lungs. In a diving situation, it may be difficult to equalise the middle ears and sinuses when you have a blocked and stuffy nose due to a cold.

A viral pulmonary infection due to influenza can result in coughing, swelling of the bronchioles, inflammation of the lungs and the formation of a mucus plug, all of which may predispose the diver to air trapping and barotrauma of ascent. Hampered diffusion may also cause hypoxia and the retention of carbon dioxide.

An additional complication is the possibility of developing a bacterial infection after exercising or diving with a cold or flu. This can lead to the development of bacterial pneumonia, with all its hazards. There is usually a fever and the phlegm becomes thick and yellow or green.

If you have a cold or flu, the best option is to avoid diving until the condition passes. A two to three week layoff is usually required.

09

NEUROLOGICAL REQUIREMENTS OF SCUBA DIVING

The ultimate reason for venturing under water is to provide sensory input to the brain. A scuba diver trains, spends money and risks life and limb to satisfy the demands of the large grey-white organ in his or her skull. Whether your objective is to study marine life, salvage a wreck, engage in underwater photography, or simply admire the sheer wonder of Nature, it is the brain that motivates and appreciates it all.

THE BRAIN

The brain serves and dominates everything in the body. It has millions of nerve fibres that extend to every single organ and tissue. It constantly receives masses of incoming sensory information regarding both the external environment and the internal operation of every organ and system in the body, then simultaneously and continuously transmits millions of motor impulses to coordinate and react to all this information. But, important as they are, sensory and motor activity are just the homework the brain does to enable it to bring to bear the highest faculties, such as understanding, appreciation, ambition, creativity, humour, hope and passion.

In the diving situation, a healthy brain and nervous system comprise the third great medical requirement. (Healthy cardiovascular and respiratory systems are the other two prime demands that together handle the gas needs that make it possible for the brain to appreciate the underwater environment.) A heavy nitrogen overload in or out of solution, failure of oxygen supply or a build-up of carbon dioxide will rapidly and fatally affect the extremely vulnerable brain.

The highest brain faculties, such as self-awareness, thought, speech, reading and writing, are centred in the grey matter of the two large convoluted hemispheres of the cerebral cortex. Here, too, are based primary control of voluntary movement and the ultimate awareness of sensation – sight, sound, taste, smell, fine and coarse touch, pressure, hot and cold appreciation, body position, vibration sense and pain sensitivity. The cerebral cortex correlates all these higher faculties and sensory inputs and then directs appropriate movements in response.

Below the base of the back of the brain lies a large motor subcentre, the cerebellum, which automatically coordinates and fine-tunes all the body's requirements for movement and proper balance.

The control centres of unconscious vital bodily functions, such as breathing, heart rate, blood pressure and temperature regulation, are found in the brain stem, the most primitive part of the brain, which is situated between the cerebral cortex and the spinal cord.

THE SPINAL CORD

At the joint between the skull and the first cervical vertebra of the neck, the brain stem emerges as the spinal cord and descends into the spinal canal of the vertebral column. Between each vertebra, spinal nerves emerge and, level by level, systematically supply the entire body with sensory fibres to detect every modality of sensation and motor fibres to control every voluntary and involuntary movement.

PERIPHERAL NERVES

The peripheral nerves are composed of both sensory and motor fibres that carry information to and from the brain via the spinal cord. This information is transmitted very rapidly, because nerve conduction is electrical.

In addition to the sensory and motor fibres that control voluntary movement, involuntary nerves belonging to the **autonomic nervous system** also exist. These relay the information that controls unconscious vital functions, such as digestion, circulatory control and breathing.

NEUROLOGICAL ASSESSMENT IN SCUBA DIVERS

Confirmation of the normal working of the nervous system is essential before diving. The highest brain faculties, together with the motor and sensory systems, are the three major aspects required for normal brain function. All three must be assessed.

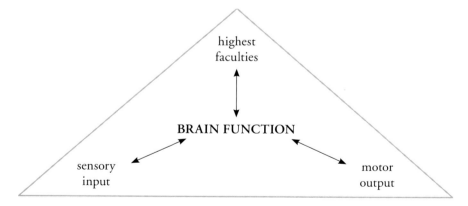

Any condition that predisposes to the failure or impairment of any of the highest faculties of the brain (such as self-awareness and orientation to place and time) must be immediately disqualifying. If there is a history of previous unconsciousness, due to injury for example, even with no residual defects at all, special investigations such as an electroencephalogram (EEG) are essential to exclude latent problems that may be present under diving conditions. Hyperventilation and breathing hyperbaric oxygen can precipitate a seizure. The EEG must therefore include a tracing of the electrical activity of the brain during hyperventilation.

Conditions that affect the spinal cord and peripheral nerves may or may not preclude diving – depending on their type, severity, and the ability and willingness of the diver and his or her buddy or buddies to adapt safely.

On a one-on-one buddy system the diver must have normal vision (excluding minor short-sightedness, far-sightedness and colour-blindness), hearing, sensation, muscle power, gait, balance and coordination. Balance is often tested by asking the subject to stand with the feet together and eyes closed. Excessive swaying (positive Rhomberg test) indicates a cerebellar problem. Tendon reflexes (e.g. the knee jerk) should be normal. Scratching the sole of the foot with a blunt object should result in the toes curling downwards. Should the big toe extend upwards and the other toes fan out (Babinski response), serious neurological impairment may be inferred and diving must be prohibited.

10

DIVING IMPLICATIONS OF NEUROLOGICAL DISEASE

Normal higher faculties are the prime neurological essentials for safe diving. Compromise may be possible in sport divers with sensory defects such as blindness in one eye, deafness, or even defects of the motor system such as poliomyelitis or paraplegia, but conditions causing even momentary aberrations of diver awareness and insight must disqualify any diving. These include both physical and psychological impairments.

PHYSICAL CONDITIONS IMPAIRING HIGHER FACULTIES

EPILEPSY

Epilepsy is a condition characterised by sudden and unheralded loss of consciousness. There are several types, the most dramatic being grand mal epilepsy where unconsciousness is associated with breathholding, prolonged convulsive spasms of body muscles, and a period of confusion and memory loss after the attack. Petit mal epilepsy, while also striking without warning, causes only a momentary lapse of consciousness with none of the profound motor disturbances of major seizures. The conversation or activity continues after a few seconds as if nothing has happened. Modern medication usually provides excellent control of epilepsy, enabling people with the condition to live absolutely normal lives.

The cause is unknown in most sufferers, but epilepsy can be the presenting feature of a cyst or tumour inside the brain; or follow a head injury with bleeding under the skull or scar tissue formation in injured brain tissue. However, whatever the cause, and no matter how effective treatment may be in controlling episodes, persons with epilepsy must not dive. The risk of even momentary unconsciousness underwater is unacceptable as diving, in itself, is a causative factor for epilepsy due to sensory deprivation, hyperventilation or breathholding and rising oxygen partial pressures in the inhaled gas with depth. This ban may be reconsidered in people who have been off all treatment for five years with no recurrence of epilepsy in that time and a normal EEG with hyperventilation and flickering light stimulation.

CONVULSIONS

Non-epileptic seizures or convulsions fall into a different category. Their cause is usually known and can generally be avoided. This includes low blood pressure, low blood sugar, alcohol and drug abuse etc. Diving is not necessarily prohibited, but prior medical approval is essential.

Fever convulsions during infancy are not included in the diving ban, provided they do not recur after the age of three.

FAINTING ATTACK (SYNCOPE)

The term **fainting attack** or **syncope** covers a number of conditions that can cause short-lived partial or complete loss of consciousness. It is very important not to be lulled into a false sense of security by assuming that the episodes are due to 'heat', 'low blood sugar' or 'low blood pressure' and are therefore insignificant from a diving point of view. All cases of syncope must be investigated before any further diving can be considered.

Once illnesses such as epilepsy, cerebral tumour, diabetes, heart problems and stroke have been excluded, the possibilities of heat aesthenia (see below), low blood pressure, low blood sugar and anxiety can be assessed. If these can be reasonably explained, they will not generally exclude further diving unless they are severe, as syncope under water is invariably fatal. In severe cases, diving is definitely out.

HEAT AESTHENIA This occurs in stuffy, crowded and poorly ventilated places. Although the body temperature usually remains normal, people sensitive to these environmental conditions may faint. Unlike epilepsy, heat aesthenia does not occur without warning. The victim feels faint and dizzy, and is often sweaty and very pale. He or she generally feels ill before losing consciousness. Lying down or sitting with the head between the knees in a well-ventilated or cool place usually relieves the episode before syncope occurs. It passes rapidly in any event and no confusional state occurs afterwards.

LOW BLOOD PRESSURE (HYPOTENSION) Many young people, especially young women, have blood pressures ranging around the 100/60 mark. After standing for some time, especially in hot conditions, or during their menses or when pregnant, gravity-pooling of blood in the veins of the lower body may occur. This reduces blood pressure even further and the supply of blood to the head may become inadequate. This can also happen when standing suddenly after sitting or lying down, and is especially common when getting up from a hot bath. The features are similar to those of heat aesthenia, ranging from dizziness to temporary unconsciousness, but pass quickly after lying down for a while.

Syncope due to heat aesthenia or low blood pressure is extremely unlikely under sport scuba diving conditions. The water is invariably much cooler than body temperature and gravity-pooling of blood cannot occur under the gravity-free conditions of total submersion with neutral buoyancy.

LOW BLOOD SUGAR (HYPOGLYCAEMIA) A drop in blood glucose is potentially hazardous underwater. In the absence of other disorders affecting glucose levels, such as diabetes mellitus, hypoglycaemia is usually the result of an excessively restricted diet, or anorexia or bulimia. It is far more common in females than males, probably because women are more figure-conscious than men, especially when they are going to expose their bodies on a beach or a boat on a diving holiday.

People on very restricted or crash diets must ensure they have a reasonable intake of carbohydrates a few hours before diving. This enables both liver and muscle tissue to recharge their reserves of glycogen, the storage form of glucose in the body. Under exercise conditions, this glycogen is broken down into glucose and provides the extra energy source needed for increased metabolic demands while ensuring that blood glucose is adequate for brain needs. The normal blood glucose level a few hours after eating is about 4–6 mmols/litre. Should the blood glucose level drop much below 3 mmols/litre, the picture closely resembles heat aesthenia and low blood pressure, with faintness, dizziness, pallor and profound sweating. The danger is that hypoglycaemic syncope may persist until sugar is administered. Underwater, this is patently impossible and, furthermore, pallor and sweating will not be noticed. Sudden unconsciousness may be the first sign.

ANOREXICS AND BULIMICS must not dive. They are pathologically reticent about telling the truth about their eating habits and are unable to control their obsession about being fat, even when clearly emaciated. Their carbohydrate energy reserves are very limited and their strength is greatly reduced. This makes them more liable to develop a severe drop in blood sugar with exercise underwater. In bulimics this is compounded by induced vomiting, with its resultant fluid loss, relative dehydration and an increased likelihood of bends.

ANXIETY AND LOW BLOOD CALCIUM (HYPOCALCAEMIA) Although in itself not a physical impairment, acute anxiety can result in grossly impaired changes in body chemistry. Aside from the increased tendency of very anxious people to panic given a stress challenge under water, hyperventilation is an additional risk. (This is very different to the controlled, deep hyperventilation of breathhold divers intent on reducing their arterial carbon dioxide levels.)

Anxiety-induced hyperventilation is rapid, shallow and ongoing, and can achieve profound hypocapnia (low blood carbon dioxide) with a sharp rise in the alkalinity of blood, a steep fall in ionised calcium, intense spasm of the hands and feet (tetany), and syncope. On land, syncope is curative for intensely agitated hyperventilators, as they stop their rapid breathing while unconscious and spontaneously recover when blood chemistry restores itself. Underwater, however, uncontrolled anxiety is dangerous.

CEREBROVASCULAR ACCIDENT (STROKE)

Sudden unconsciousness can occur with interruption of the normal circulation to the brain. This may be due to **thrombosis** with a clot obstructing a cerebral artery, **haemorrhage** due to the rupture of a blood vessel or an aneurysm in the brain, or

embolism of a blood clot to the brain. Whether there is full recovery or residual paralysis, weakness, numbness, loss of speech, etc., will depend on the exact site and the extent of the damage, but any history of cerebral vascular disease (even if the unconsciousness is very transient with full recovery) must permanently disqualify diving in the vast majority of cases.

ACUTE CEREBRAL DECOMPRESSION SICKNESS

A history of previous cerebral injury due to arterial gas embolism (AGE) or brain tissue nitrogen bubbling must be very carefully assessed. Any residual deficit must exclude further diving. This can be very difficult to detect as it may involve only subtle changes in dexterity, mental acuity or personality. British Naval policy requires confirmation by an approved doctor with a minimum of seven days off diving. The US Navy stipulates a four-week lay-off from diving. Many diving physicians will not permit any further diving, even with apparent full recovery. The situation therefore depends on the details of the diver's hyperbaric incident, the extent of recovery and the opinion of his or her medical advisor.

HEAD INJURY

Head injury at any time in the past, resulting in even brief unconsciousness and no residual brain damage, requires a full neurological assessment, including an EEG with a hyperventilation tracing. Any abnormality may exclude diving.

MIGRAINE

Migraine can be very problematic in sport diving and is a source of headaches to the diving physician as well as the subject. Among commercial and navy divers, migraine is usually grounds for disqualification from further diving. The difficulty relates to the time of onset and treatment. If a diver experiences a migraine before entering the water, the dive obviously must be aborted. Once underwater, the diver is subjected to cold, vascular changes and the demands of exercise. In addition, stress, nitrogen narcosis and skip breathing with carbon dioxide build-up may occur. Any one of these may precipitate or aggravate a migraine, leading to nausea, vomiting and vertigo under water in addition to the difficulty of coping with a violent head-ache. To complicate things, most cases of migraine have an aura before the headache starts. This may present as blurred or tunnel vision, flashing lights, ringing in the ears, etc. If these symptoms occur after a dive, it can be a problem distinguishing them from acute cerebral decompression illness, including AGE. When the diver then develops a blinding headache and begins to vomit, the dilemma worsens.

Painfully dilated blood vessels inside the confines of the skull bones, the under-lying membranes and the overlying scalp are thought to be the cause of migraine. Treatment is directed at narrowing these dilated blood vessels, but giving medication aimed at constricting blood vessels can have unpredictable effects on blood pressure, heart rate and heart rhythm when coupled with the vascular changes of diving.

Estimating the safety of scuba diving in known migraine sufferers must depend on the frequency, intensity and duration of past episodes. Diving must be forbidden if migraine episodes are severe, or while preventative treatments such as beta-blockers, clonidine, flunarizine or pizotifen are being used. Trying to abort an acute attack with ergotamine or sumatriptan before diving is exceedingly perilous. It is only if migraine episodes are infrequent, and the usual precipitating causes, such as caffeine, cheese amines, wine, etc., have been identified by experience and eliminated to the best of the diver's ability, that diving should be considered in migraine sufferers.

OTHER BRAIN CONDITIONS

Some illnesses primarily affect the brain tissue itself, causing compression of the brain inside the skull, interference with normal nerve pathways, or destruction of the fatty insulating myelin of nerve fibres. Impairment of the highest functions may be accompanied by changes in sensory and motor function. These illnesses include cysts and tumours, multiple sclerosis, brain syphilis and narcolepsy. In all instances, diving is forbidden. Scuba diving after acute inflammatory conditions of the brain, such as encephalitis and meningitis, depends on the completeness of recovery and the proven absence of any residual defects such as epilepsy.

PSYCHOLOGICAL CONDITIONS IMPAIRING HIGHER FACULTIES

DON'T JUST STAND THERE – PANIC!

Sign at the controls of Pentow Marine's salvage vessel, the *Reunion*.

PANIC

Panic is sudden, unreasoning and overpowering fear, which overrides all reason and training, and does not permit any logical or reasonable action. It is probably the greatest killer among young and inexperienced divers who are confronted by severe stress – namely a threat to life, whether real or imaginary. The onset of panic is a self-propagating, rapidly accelerating process which takes the diver from anxiety regarding his situation, to uncontrolled, stark terror in which rational reaction to the predicament becomes impossible. There are three dimensions to panic:
- the diver,
- the diving equipment, and
- the environment.

It is the interaction between these three that determines whether a diver has a pleasant and productive dive or dies.

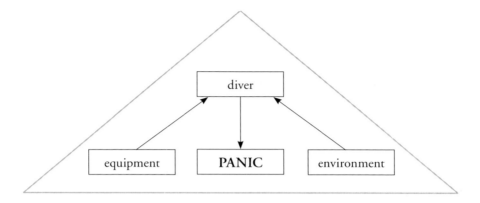

THE DIVER The basic object of diving is the transport of the diver's awareness and individuality into the water. From there, he or she will enjoy exploring a coral reef or cave, working on a rig or salvaging a wreck. Individual personality and inherent apprehension will determine the response to any problem. Different divers will react differently to the same problem. An example will illustrate the point.

> A lone diver has just visited the cave at the bottom of Wondergat, a deep inland sinkhole. The dive was a night dive to 40 metres using a swim line tied to the bottom of a floating shot line. Forgetting to untie his swim line, he ascends up the shot line, not knowing that the swim line, loosely looped in the water, has entangled itself with his scuba cylinder. At 30 metres, he is abruptly brought to a halt as the rope tightens. It is pitch black around him and he does not know why he cannot ascend.

RESPONSES

- Martin Brown, under these conditions, stopped, thought and checked. Using his light, he confirmed that he was on the shot line and that there were no overhangs above him. He then checked his air supply and depth gauge. Looking around and then down by methodically beaming his light, he saw two strands of rope extending down from his backpack. Withdrawing his knife, he cut the strands and ascended safely, mentally kicking himself for forgetting to untie and coil his swim line and for diving without a buddy.
- Cuthbert Quiver, a novice diver who suffered from severe anxiety for which he took tranquillisers, stopped with his eyes bulging into his mask. He had not really wanted to dive but, egged on by his 'friends' over a few beers, he had capitulated. With the sudden halt, he was convinced that some monster was trying to trap him in the dark and, finning furiously, hyperventilating and waving his arms, he let go of his torch which floated to the surface. He then inflated his buoyancy compensator, which pulled him even tighter against the ropes. Screaming through his demand valve and thrashing violently with his limbs, he used up his air supply and drowned, tightly suspended 30 metres from the surface by his BC.

The first dimension of panic, diver awareness and personality, is affected by:

(a) **Physical factors:**
- training and planning,
- fitness and fatigue,
- experience,
- diving problems, e.g. seasickness, vomiting, barotrauma, vertigo, water inhalation,
- alcohol and drug abuse, or
- underlying medical problems, e.g. epilepsy, asthma, diabetes.

(b) **Psychological factors:**
- anxiety and emotional instability,
- phobias,
- visual limitation, e.g. night diving, or
- disorientation due to weightlessness or diffused light.

DIVING EQUIPMENT Diving advertisements and TV films have given female divers an ultra-glamorous and sensuous image, and male divers mega-macho and super-stud appeal. But what divers really are, are people wrapped in tight rubber; their vision limited by masks and with snorkels over their ears; mouths clamped over second-stage demand valves; backs suffering under the weight of heavy cylinders; their breathing made difficult by straps, BCs, wet suits and weight belts; pipes and gauges tangling around them; and liable to stumble over their fins on land. In addition, they have knives on their legs, torches and/or cameras in their hands, plus assorted ropes, tools and other paraphernalia.

On entering the water, divers have much greater mobility and less weight restriction, but any of the above equipment can conspire to place them in peril – and this is the second dimension to panic. A displaced mask, leaky demand valve, empty cylinder, restricting wet suit, very heavy weight belt or lost fin will all cause the diver to react. Reactions range from a rapid assessment and/or handling of the problem, to real distress and anxiety, to panic.

Borrowed or unfamiliar equipment is also a source of danger. The BC control valves may be in an unaccustomed place, the weight belt may be too heavy or have a different clip, making it difficult to ditch, the mask may not fit properly and leak. New or borrowed fins may fall off or cause cramps.

Experience, training and practise in the use of all your equipment are the only solutions to being able to safely handle any equipment difficulties that occur underwater.

THE ENVIRONMENT At this stage, we have a diver, either calm, tense or terrified, fully or inadequately geared up, with greater or lesser expertise, about to jump into the sea, a lake, a sinkhole, a cave, an ice-hole, or plunge through the surf. This is the third dimension to panic.

The sea is vast, bountiful and beautiful. Man is the intruder, yet it is he who calls the sea dangerous. Fish don't complain that the sea is dangerous. The sea has tides, currents, swells, surf, rocks, cold temperatures, poisonous and hungry inhabitants, clear and turbid areas, kelp, caves, boats with propellers and wrecks (which have sharp edges, crannies and traps, unstable plating and sometimes explosives).

If our air-breathing, rubber-wrapped diver knows these things and dives within his limits, the sea is rarely dangerous; it is only merciless to fools. It is invariably the first two dimensions (the diver and his equipment) that cause the problem. The water simply finishes the job. In fact, it is rarely the equipment that fails, but the diver's poor maintenance and/or lack of knowledge and training with his life-support system.

ALCOHOL AND DIVING

The use of alcohol instantly negates any safe dive plan and one does not have to be very drunk to be at risk. Being a socially acceptable custom, and something that is commonly enjoyed by divers at their clubs and on diving holidays, alcohol intake may range from occasional to regular to habitual; but the vast majority of regular alcohol users will deny excess.

The question, 'When last did you take a drink?' if asked on a Tuesday morning at tea-time will often indicate the real situation. 'Yesterday', usually points to a habitual daily intake. 'On Sunday', suggests a weekend drinker; 'I'm not sure', an occasional imbiber; while 'Today', means a serious alcohol problem.

About 80 per cent of adults who drown took alcohol before entering the water. Alcohol, drugs and swimming **never** mix. Look at the reasons.

Alcohol causes:
- overconfidence – risks are taken beyond training, fitness and ability levels,
- inability to react adequately to the situation, resulting in panic,
- hypothermia due to skin flushing and rapid heat loss,
- increased likelihood of vomiting with inhalation of vomit and water, and
- possible suicidal tendencies.

A realistic minimum period of abstinence from any alcohol before diving is 8 hours. If the alcohol intake was enough to cause slight tipsiness, 12 hours must be allowed. With reactions such as vomiting and hangover, 24 hours should elapse before attempting to dive, and copious quantities of water and fruit juice should be taken during that period. Uncontrolled over-indulgence requires medical help and permission to dive must be refused until the problem has been overcome.

PSYCHOLOGICAL INSTABILITY

Assessment of the psychiatric status of a diver is vital, but it is the most intangible aspect of a diving medical, and the most risky side of diving instruction. Emotional stability and mature judgement are fundamental to safe diving. A dive school can teach a student all he or she needs to know in order to dive safely, but when the time comes for open water experience, the undersea environment may expose a sudden intense claustrophobia or anxiety and precipitate panic.

Some student divers may indicate early during their pool training that they are unhappy underwater, and their instructors should pay particular attention to giving these students one-on-one guidance, after-hours if necessary, to promote confidence and improve their underwater skills.

Other students, too shy to mention their problem when the rest of the class seems to be progressing with obvious enthusiasm, may not be forthcoming and the instructor must be on the lookout for them. They often take a long time to tog up, are last in the queue to demonstrate the particular skill being taught, and have great difficulty in achieving neutral buoyancy because they involuntarily keep their lungs half-full at the surface – this increases buoyancy and, instead of exhaling precious air, they require excessively heavy weight belts in order to descend. They empty their air cylinders uncommonly quickly, and tend to perform frequent hasty free ascents from the deep end of the pool. They will appreciate kind, understanding attention from a discerning instructor and, in most cases, will become adequate scuba divers.

NEUROSES AND PSYCHOSES The inherent perils of diving may aggravate existing manic or schizophrenic states, stimulate suicidal ideation in depressive divers with underlying marital, social or financial stress, or cause sudden psychotic or neurotic behaviour in post-traumatic stress disorder (PTSD) victims experiencing sleeplessness and flashbacks of an earlier severe stress, including a possible near-drowning episode. The diving buddy may suddenly be faced with the problem of dangerously abnormal behaviour in his or her diving partner. Diving under these conditions is dangerous and must be strongly discouraged.

Social compatibility can cause problems, too. Many divers, commonly women in the 30–45 age group, take up diving solely to satisfy the demands of their partners. They are secretly very unhappy about diving but decide to give it a try in order to appease mate insistence. There is really a double problem – on the one hand, the male needs to prove mid-life virility with youthful enterprise and, on the other, the heavy apprehension of a partner who is unwillingly training as his dive buddy. In most cases, the disconsolate lady finds, to her unbelieving delight, that scuba diving is stupendous, and becomes an avid protagonist of the sport. In a minority, however, real insecurity and even secret terror persist, but so strong is her willingness to appease that she will continue to dive.

Dive leaders and instructors should be aware of this in new students, and watch out for undue apprehension in qualified diver couples joining a dive trip. If excessive misgivings seem to be present, insist on an up-to-date diving medical with a diving physician. The uncontrollably anxious spouse will usually accept a failed medical with unconcealed relief.

Another socially based cause of potential diver stress and difficulty is loneliness. A significant number of men and women decide to take up diving solely to increase their likelihood of meeting a soulmate. Diving is not the objective – parading in a wet suit and chatting to new acquaintances is the goal. They dive infrequently and have dubious skills, even once some time has passed.

PSYCHOACTIVE MEDICATION Every day, all around the world, millions of anti-depressants, tranquillisers and sleeping pills are used. Stress, even minor, is often greeted with an obliging offer of a 'safe little something for your nerves'. Not one of any of these medications, no matter what anyone personally experienced in their use may say, is ever really acceptable in safe diving. Diving requires emotional stability. These medications are taken precisely because such stability is impaired. They do not cure anything – they merely dull the reaction to the underlying problem. Dulled reaction in an emotionally unstable diver is very dangerous under water.

Throughout the world, many thousands of divers use SSRI (Selective Serotonin Re-uptake Inhibitors) to treat anxiety or depressive disorders. These include fluox-etine, paroxetine, citalopram, escitalopram, fluvoxamine and sertraline. Side-effects, such as epilepsy, drowsiness, sluggishness or increased susceptibility to nitrogen nar-cosis, may suddenly occur. As hyperbaric conditions and SSRIs may both precipitate epilepsy, diving below 18 msw is not recommended. A related group comprises the Serotonin and Noradrenaline Re-uptake Inhibitors and includes duloxetine and ven-lafaxine. The same precautions apply.

Until mid-2008, pseudoephedrine was obtainable as an over-the-counter medica-tion for the management of colds, nasal and sinus congestion and to assist middle ear equalising. It is now a scheduled drug requiring a prescription because drug abusers discovered that it was a precursor in the manufacture of the illicit drug 'tik'.

Illicit drugs, including amphetamines, crystal meth, ecstacy, hallucinogens (such as LSD), opium, cocaine, heroin, so-called 'party drugs' and marijuana are all totally unsafe. Diving and drugs simply don't mix.

ATTENTION DEFICIT DISORDER (ADD)

Also known as attention deficit hyperactivity disorder (ADHD), minimal brain dysfunction and many other names, this condition may present with aberrations in attention, hyperactive behaviour or both. It is more common in boys and, in about half of sufferers, continues into adulthood.

The relevance in diving is plain. The inability to concentrate on the basic laws of physics, physiology, dive planning and safety; the potential for irrational behaviour underwater and the common use of behaviour-controlling medicines by sufferers of ADD all make diving hazardous. In most cases, children with severe ADD who wish to dive should be discouraged from the sport. In mild cases that are being controlled on treatment such as methyl-phenidate, diving may be considered but these children should preferably not use their ADD medication while on a diving holiday.

Adult sufferers who have learned to cope with their disorder require individual assessment before taking up diving.

CONDITIONS IMPAIRING MOTOR AND SENSORY NERVE FUNCTION

The loss, or potential loss, of any modality of the higher faculties is unacceptable for diving purposes, but disability due to loss of motor or sensory function need not necessarily be totally disqualifying, except for conditions such as motor neurone disease and multiple sclerosis.

MOTOR NEURONE DISEASE

This group of disorders of unknown cause results in patchy damage to motor nerve units in the brain and spinal cord which control muscle movement. Nerves supplying sensory information remain intact. A common variant is Amyotrophic Lateral Sclerosis (ALS), also known as Lou Gehrig's disease after the US baseball player who suffered from it. Progressive weakness and then total paralysis occur with loss of reflex activity. There is no known treatment for motor neurone disease and diving must be banned.

MULTIPLE SCLEROSIS

Multiple sclerosis (MS) affects the insulating fatty myelin layer of the white matter of the brain and spinal cord. The cause is unknown, and it presents with initial transient weakness of one or more limbs, sudden loss of vision in one eye, numbness and tingling in a limb, or slowly progressive clumsiness. MS is usually relapsing, with long periods of improvement in remission followed by acute episodes of worsening, alternating over a period of 13–30 years. Eventually, terminal paralysis with uncontrollable spasms and incontinence occur.

Because of the progressive and untreatable nature of the disease, and the unpredictable efficiency of degassing from already damaged areas of brain tissue, diving is not permitted even during the early stages or with remissions. Hyperbaric oxygen therapy (HBO) has not been shown to be of any value in the treatment of MS.

POLIOMYELITIS

Much less common nowadays because of national compulsory immunisation during infancy, poliomyelitis is a viral disease which attacks motor nerve cells in the spinal cord. This results in damage to the motor nerve supply of the limb muscles with resultant wasting and weakness. With certain provisos, diving may be taught to poliomyelitis victims. (See diving with a physical disability, page 86.)

BELL'S PALSY

This condition often presents with sudden paralysis of one side of the face below the level of the eyes. The precise cause is unknown but it is due to paralysis of the facial nerve at the site of its passage through the middle ear on that side. Oral cortisone is usually prescribed and the vast majority of cases recover fully. The difficulty in diving relates to holding a regulator in a half-paralysed mouth, inhalation of water, difficulty in blinking out sea water with mask clearing, and excessively loud bubble sounds on that side with exhalation, as the damping effect of the facial nerve on that eardrum is paralysed too.

PARAPLEGIA

Injury to the spinal cord occurs most commonly after motor vehicle accidents, or trauma from a fall while climbing, parachuting or parasailing. There is usually fracturing of the bony spine resulting in crushing or cutting of the spinal cord. If the damage to the spinal cord is severe, permanent paralysis and total anaesthesia of the body below the level of the spinal cord injury will result. Damage to the cord above the fourth cervical vertebra in the neck is invariably fatal, as all the respiratory muscles, including the diaphragm, are then paralysed, making it impossible for the victim to breathe.

Totally severing the spinal cord lower in the neck will cause quadriplegia with paralysis and anaesthesia of both arms and both legs, and loss of control of bodily functions. Damage to the lumbar spinal cord causes paraplegia with paralysis and anaesthesia of the legs, and variable loss of bowel and bladder control.

Issues relating to the rehabilitation of paraplegics have received massive attention worldwide because the majority of those affected are young people with normal and active brains and, aside from their lower body disability, they have a normal role to play in their society. If the level of transection of the spinal cord is in the low lumbar region, diving after recovery from the acute trauma is often possible and can play an important role in rehabilitation.

Depending on the site of an injury to the spinal cord, different parts of the body are affected.

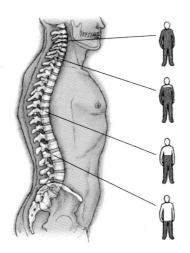

Damage above the level of the 4th cervical vertebrae is invariably fatal.

Damage to the cervical cord usually results in quadraplegia, with loss of all limb functions.

Damage to the thoracic cord may result in quadraplegia or paraplegia, depending on the site and severity of the injury.

Damage to the lumbar cord results in paraplegia (paralysis of the legs).

DIVING WITH A PHYSICAL DISABILITY

For many years, hydrotherapy has been used in the treatment and rehabilitation of physically disabled people. The technique utilises the buoyant effect of water to negate gravity, and facilitates retraining and exercising of weakened muscles and joints. This raises the question: 'Is it safe for physically disabled people to dive?'

There are three primary hazards associated with sport diving. The first two are post-dive tissue bubble formation following an inert gas load at depth, and arterial gas embolism following pulmonary barotrauma. Their prevention, in health terms, requires cardiovascular and pulmonary fitness. Drowning is the third hazard and its prevention requires clarity of higher faculties – the diver must be conscious and fully aware in the subaquatic environment. Any medical condition that predisposes to any of these three hazards must mean a failed diving medical.

But what about people who have had injuries to their limbs or spinal cord – such as amputees, poliomyelitis victims and paraplegics? Aside from their physical or functional loss of limbs, they may technically satisfy all three primary medical requirements for safe diving. All sport divers use fins which, after all, are simply man-made contrivances to assist swimming. Given the possibility that a suitable artifice could similarly be provided to assist a paraplegic who has total paralysis of both legs, should he or she dive?

The answer is – it depends. The first requirement is the absence of any significant medical problem apart from the physical disability. A circulatory disturbance or infection in a paralysed limb will affect tissue degassing after a dive and predispose to bends. Bedsores or areas devitalised by the pressure of sitting or lying will do the same.

Efficient breathing of dense air under hyperbaric conditions requires fully functional muscles of respiration. This sets the limit to the level of spinal cord injury in paraplegic divers. Aside from the diaphragm, which receives its nerve supply from the third and fourth cervical portions of the spinal cord in the neck, there are numerous secondary muscles of respiration in the chest and abdomen essential for effective breathing and coughing. These receive their nerve supply from the dorsal spinal cord (the portion of the cord between the neck and the first lumbar vertebra) and the upper portion of the lumbar spinal cord. Any paraplegic considering diving must therefore not have damage to the spinal cord higher than the second lumbar segment.

In the case of amputees, the reason for their amputation is important. Limb loss following an accident or injury is not as significant as amputation because of arterial disease or the complications of diabetes. Persons with the latter must never dive.

Although suitable prosthetic devices can be constructed to compensate for the accidental loss of both legs, the loss of both arms is almost insurmountable. Should a demand valve become dislodged, it would be impossible to replace it without assistance, and buoyancy compensation requiring manual control of venting and inflation would require buddy support. Under these circumstances two buddies, both dive masters or instructors, are required to assist the disabled diver.

Approval to dive must be tightly qualified in the case of disabled people. There are very few formal diving courses for the disabled so the conditions under which they may be permitted to dive must be individually discussed by the diving physician and the instructor at the particular diving school approached for training.

Before considering whether or not to scuba dive, it is essential that a disabled person can swim competently, and is able to maintain their head above water without any artificial aid whatsoever.

Details of the particular techniques to be used must be carefully considered. In the event of the functional loss of the lower limbs, as in paraplegia, amputation of both legs, or the loss of an arm and a leg, a trio buddy system must be used, allowing two divers to assist the disabled person into and from the water, and also to ensure that either able-bodied buddy can also be assisted in an emergency.

Possible problems and modifications relating to every piece of diving gear must be foreseen and a little ingenuity may need to be applied to compensate for the physical defect. Regular harness straps may slip off weak or wasted shoulders; weight belts may slip off wasted hips. High or low limb amputations, the quality of limb stumps, and their cost, will determine the safety and advisability of using artificial limbs underwater. The loss of one leg may be compensated for by using a fin with a large surface area on the normal leg, but practise is then essential to avoid leg cramps because of the heavier resistance load. A dolphin kick may be needed to avoid swimming in a circle. Finned or webbed gloves may be considered for paraplegic divers.

Buoyancy control must provide not only neutral buoyancy, but vertical and horizontal control. Wasted, artificial or amputated legs significantly alter the body's centre of balance and predispose to swimming in a head-down position or, worse, ascending in that position. Weight must be distributed between weight belts and ankle or fin weights until neutral buoyancy and free axial mobility are achieved. Artificial limbs that are waterproof may help balance and buoyancy.

The question of depth limitation and embarking on decompression-stop dives must be fully discussed between the doctor, the disabled diver and the instructor. The degree of disability will dictate limits. Wet suits must always be worn to avoid skin damage that can occur if trailing paralysed legs come into contact with rocks or coral life. Swimming side-by-side, with the disabled diver between two alert buddies, will help to avert such injury.

DIVING AFTER BRAIN SURGERY

Most diving physicians would bar any diving after major surgery involving the brain. The majority of operations are for head injury, with bleeding inside the skull and brain, or tumours of the brain. The problem is that any surgery to the brain must, in itself, cause damage to nerve fibre tracts simply to reach the objective of the operation. There is a later risk of precipitating a convulsion under water with the higher partial pressure of inspired air oxygen, and any interference with the capillary circulation or venous drainage of the area could predispose to acute cerebral decompression illness. Residual neurological deficits, both physical and psychological, must be carefully considered. Any post-traumatic epilepsy is immediately disqualifying.

CONCUSSION

Very brief loss of consciousness following a relatively minor head injury constitutes concussion. Residual symptoms, such as headache, resolve within a few weeks and diving can probably be resumed after about six weeks. However, unconsciousness lasting more than 30 minutes needs full specialist neurological assessment. If the person is symptom free, has no residual deficits and presents a normal EEG, diving may be considered. The danger of concussion in an apparently normal person is the development of post-traumatic epilepsy within the first few years after a head injury.

HEADACHES IN DIVERS

The three most common causes of headache in non-divers are anxiety, migraine and neck problems that arise following a sporting injury or motor vehicle accident, but managing a headache in divers is often a very difficult medical problem, especially if the doctor isn't diving-orientated. Obviously, any of the above common causes may be involved, but headaches and diving usually follow a pattern. They always occur during or very soon after a dive, and the time of onset and site of the pain nearly always follow a regular format. Sometimes, pain commences during descent or at the bottom depth. More commonly it begins during the ascent or 5-metre stop, and very commonly it begins immediately after surfacing. The pain almost always affects both sides of the head and nearly always involves the back of the head and/or the temples and forehead.

If one excludes a hangover headache, which would be present before the dive and must exclude any diving that day anyway, or a direct blow on the head during an untoward ascent in an underwater cave or tunnel, the following are the usual causes of recurrent headaches in divers.

ANXIETY is a very common cause of headaches in insecure new divers. It causes a typical tension headache with pain over the temples and the back of the head and neck. Anxiety results from the uncertainty felt by the diver coping with unfamiliar and potentially hazardous underwater conditions. This type of headache can commence at any time during, or even before, the dive and usually occurs in divers with a prior history of tension headaches. With ongoing exposure, increasing confidence and improving sub-sea abilities, it nearly always stops.

Novice divers, apprehensive about losing their air supply underwater, frequently grip their teeth very tightly on to the demand valve mouthpiece. This unrelenting grip, if maintained for too long, may cause cramping or spasm of the temporalis muscles and produce severe pain in the temples. This is very similar to the headaches experienced by people who grind their teeth while sleeping. Other dental problems, such as a malaligned bite or a filling that is protruding excessively, may cause uneven distribution of pressure when gripping a regulator too tightly between the teeth – again, a headache is the result.

TIGHT DIVE GEAR, especially masks and wet suit collars, often results in headaches in novice divers. Pulling mask straps tightly to prevent leaking underwater results in a rubber clamp around the head, rather like a very tight helmet. This effect of strap squeezing gets worse with time, but is relieved by taking off the mask after the dive and the headache usually disappears after about an hour.

Wet suit collars that compress the neck are another gear-induced cause of headache. Tight collars compress the jugular veins that drain blood from the skull and cause venous congestion in the brain with reduced removal of cerebral carbon dioxide. A classical carbon dioxide headache can occur. If the collar is extremely close-fitting, not only will the low-pressure jugular veins be compressed, but compression can occur in the high-pressure carotid sinuses that monitor blood pressure in the carotid arteries in the neck. A rise in blood pressure stimulates the pressure sensors in the carotid sinuses and causes a reflex slowing of the heart with a consequent drop in blood pressure. Compressing the carotid sinuses externally achieves the same result – a reflex drop in blood pressure and even sudden unconsciousness, or the so-called carotid sinus reflex.

The third cause of gear-induced headaches involves too-tight wet suits, buoyancy compensators and equipment straps. These limit chest movement and restrict easy breathing, enabling carbon dioxide build-up to occur, followed by headache.

SINUS SQUEEZE occurs when aeration and equalisation of the sinuses is impaired. It results from under-pressurisation of sinuses during descent or sinus overpressurisation during ascent. The site of headache depends on the sinuses affected. There is always a history of nasal and sinus allergy, hayfever, polyps or infection. Any of these can cause obstruction to the ostia, the orifices between the sinuses and the nose, impairing air movement between the sinuses and nose. With increasing or decreasing pressure, sinus barotrauma occurs in accordance with Boyle's Law (see page 21).

Most sinus squeezes affect the forehead and involve the frontal sinuses above the eyes. Pain over one or both cheeks or in the upper teeth is related to the maxillary sinuses. Eyeball pain is caused by ethmoid sinus squeeze, and occipital pain at the back of the head on descent is caused by sphenoidal sinus squeeze. Descent squeeze is relieved by ascent. Ascent squeeze also happens. Pressurised air blocked in a sinus after a normal descent will cause an intense headache on ascent. Treatment is really preventative. Do not dive with a cold or a blocked nose and treat any nasal allergy or infection before diving.

NECK PROBLEMS caused by injuries to the neck, such as a previous whiplash injury to the cervical spine, can result in headache during the dive. This pain occurs at the back of the head and neck and is due to arthritis or damaged discs compressing the spinal nerves of the neck in the hyper-extended position. It occurs because divers swim with their necks extended well back in order to see in front of them while moving horizontally. On land, this would be equivalent to walking around for up to an hour while looking straight up at the sky!

The diver may be completely symptom-free at all other times, the pain only returning when assuming the extended neck position while diving. It usually occurs in relatively older divers who have had ample time to develop arthritic changes in the neck, and it can last for hours or even days after diving. It is often eliminated by wearing ankle weights (and reducing belt weights), enabling the diver to swim at an angle of about 30 degrees to the horizontal and seeing forwards without extending the neck. If you opt for ankle weights, care must be taken not to kick seabed corals and practise is needed to avoid calf cramps due to the increased leg loading.

COLD WATER can cause an intense throbbing headache in cold-sensitive divers and involves the forehead or back of the head. It is akin to the 'brain-freeze' experienced when eating very cold ice cream. The pain is usually delayed until a few minutes into the dive, often worsens with long dives, and continues for a while after ascent. It is usually prevented by wearing a hood and acclimatising the face by cooling it with cold water before diving.

CARBON DIOXIDE BUILD-UP (hypercapnoea) follows inadequate exhalation of the metabolic gas. Total body hypercapnoea occurs with skip breathing, having constricting chest straps and buoyancy compensators, carbon dioxide toxicity on breathing denser gas mixes such as nitrox, and carbon dioxide contamination of the air supply. Local build-up of carbon dioxide in the brain can follow the congestive effect of a tight wet suit collar or hood. The headache either develops gradually during a long dive as blood and tissue carbon dioxide levels slowly increase or, more commonly, commences immediately after surfacing and switching to atmospheric air. A rapid fall in blood carbon dioxide and a pounding headache then occur – one of the so-called 'carbon dioxide-off effects'.

Both an elevated carbon dioxide tissue partial pressure and a sudden reduction of carbon dioxide levels cause headaches. These are severe and throbbing, are not usually relieved by conventional painkillers and last for hours after the dive.

Other gases can cause headaches too: carbon monoxide following contamination of the air supply, and oxygen toxicity following deep diving on oxygen-enriched mixes or using pure oxygen rebreathers.

SALT WATER INHALATION can occur after an episode of coughing under water, or from a flooded mask or demand valve problems during a sea dive. It causes an intense headache, which commences about half-an-hour after surfacing. These headaches are usually accompanied by flu-like aches and joint pains, and are aggravated by exercise and exposure to cold water.

ACUTE NEUROLOGICAL DECOMPRESSION ILLNESS also presents with a headache, usually within minutes of surfacing following a long or deep dive with a heavy nitrogen or other inert gas load. It can also be due to arterial gas embolism following lung barotrauma. **Headache is an extremely serious symptom when it is due to inert gas overload.** It is often accompanied by other manifestations of central nervous system bubble injury, such as blurred vision, weakness or paralysis, confusion and numbness or other abnormalities of sensation. Immediate surface-mask oxygen, urgent communication with a diving doctor and emergency recompression therapy are absolute requirements.

SQUINTING INTO GLARE or sunlight on the water for extended periods during a dive cruise can present with headache due to spasm of the scalp and forehead muscles. The solution is simple. Wear dark polarised glasses when glare occurs.

MIGRAINE can present with very severe and potentially dangerous headaches underwater. All of the above causes of diver headache can precipitate an additional underwater migraine. A blindingly painful headache can be incapacitating, leading to confusion, inability to react to underwater stresses, vertigo, nausea and vomiting through a demand valve.

People prone to severe or frequent migraine should not dive. The likelihood of an attack and the intensity of their pain can be aggravated by diving and can be lethal. Furthermore, the onset of an excruciating headache with vertigo and vomiting after diving poses a huge dilemma in distinguishing migraine from acute cerebral decompression illness, including arterial gas embolism.

Diver headaches continue to be a difficult problem. The causes are frequently multiple, for example, simultaneous anxiety, skip breathing and sensitivity to cold. Sometimes the exact cause or causes in any given diver is very difficult to determine. If you regularly develop a diving headache, consider each of the above causes carefully. If a headache with diving persists despite your best efforts, or the reason for your pain is still unclear, and especially if you suffer from undiagnosed surface headaches too, see a diving doctor or request an opinion from a neurologist – there are many non-diving causes of headache which must be excluded by specialist investigations.

11

UNDERSTANDING THE EARS, NOSE AND SINUSES

After healthy cardiovascular, pulmonary and nervous systems, the next priority for a diver is the ability to actively increase the pressure in the middle ear and passively compensate for pressure changes in the sinuses with depth.

THE EAR

Extending from the cartilaginous external ear to the inner ear deeply buried in the bone of the skull, the ear serves two functions: hearing and orientation. Together, these serve to provide awareness of sound and control the body position.

ANATOMY OF THE EAR

The ear has three compartments:
- external ear,
- middle ear, and
- inner ear.

The compartments are all very different, but they do have common features:
1. They are separated by thin but tough membranes.
2. Each compartment has a passage or tube leading to it.
3. All three compartments are in the bone of the skull and are therefore incompressible (i.e. they cannot change volume without violent objections from the diver).
4. The external and middle ears are normally air-filled. The inner ear, or cochlea, is always **fluid**-filled, and its passage communicates with the cerebrospinal fluid around the brain.
5. Passage obstruction causes squeeze.

The hearing organ is the **cochlea** and the balance organ is the **vestibular apparatus**. They are attached to each other at the **vestibule** and together they comprise the inner ear or **labyrinth**, so-called because of its complex shape.

The vestibular apparatus and cochlea are fluid-filled, the fluid in the cochlea communicating with the cerebrospinal fluid in and around the brain. The cochlea is a spiralled organ containing membranes and hair cells tuned to vibrate in sympathy

Anatomy of the ear

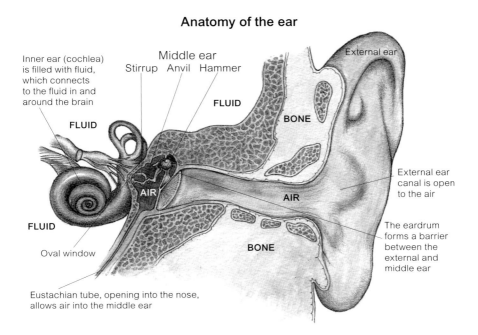

Inner ear (cochlea) is filled with fluid, which connects to the fluid in and around the brain

Middle ear

Stirrup Anvil Hammer

External ear

FLUID

FLUID

BONE

External ear canal is open to the air

AIR

AIR

FLUID

Oval window

BONE

The eardrum forms a barrier between the external and middle ear

Eustachian tube, opening into the nose, allows air into the middle ear

with incoming tones. Different pitched tones cause different hair cells to vibrate. Their vibration is then converted into electrochemical energy and transmitted to the brain as a nerve impulse in the auditory nerve. Being fluid-filled, the cochlea is normally **immune** to Boyle's Law (see page 21) and pressure changes.

Sound reaching the ear from outside passes into the external ear canal, an open pit in the side wall of the skull. This canal is closed off by a taut membrane at its inner end – the **tympanum** or eardrum. The function of the eardrum is to vibrate in air. Behind the eardrum is the middle ear, a small air-filled cavity whose canal, the Eustachian tube, opens to air on the back wall of the nasal cavity.

The middle ear serves to transmit sound from the eardrum to the cochlea, or inner ear. As the cochlea is fluid-filled and the eardrum vibrates in air, a mechanical connecting system exists. It consists of three tiny bones, or **ossicles**, which form a miniature articulated hydraulic press. The **malleus,** or hammer, is attached by its handle to the inside of the eardrum. The head of the hammer has a tiny joint with the anvil-shaped **incus**, which in turn is joined to the **stapes** or stirrup. The stirrup is the smallest bone of the three and weighs just over one milligram, but it is the most important of the three bones because its oval-shaped footplate seals the **oval window**, a hole in the fluid-filled inner ear.

The system is ingenious and works as follows: the tiny vibrations of the eardrum are transmitted to the hammer handle. The head of the hammer thrusts the anvil against the stirrup which rams like a piston against the fluid behind the oval window, setting up pressure waves in the fluid of the inner ear. These pressure waves are then detected by the hair cells of the cochlea. The lever system of the ossicles plus the mechanical advantage of a relatively large-diameter eardrum driving against a tiny footplate magnifies the movement of the eardrum 22 times at the footplate. As fluid is incompressible and the cochlea is embedded in the hardest bone of the body, the system could not work unless there was a weak spot that could give and move a little with the thrusting of the footplate against liquid.

There is the **round window**, a membrane between the cochlea and the middle ear. It bulges as the stirrup shoves. From a diving point of view, the round window is very important. It can rupture with an excessive attempt to equalise on descent, resulting in cochlear fluid and brain fluid leaking into the middle ear and, via the Eustachian tube, out through the nose. This is covered under ear barotrauma (see page 151).

HEARING IN AIR

Nothing designed by man can even nearly compare with the astounding sensitivity and selectivity of the ear. The maximum sensitivity is just short of consciously hearing random movement of air nitrogen and oxygen molecules hitting the eardrum. At the same time, the ear can tolerate the volume of electric guitars loud enough to make the entire body quiver. It can then selectively hear the normal-volume speech of one person in a roomful of people and dismiss the babble of surrounding conversation plus the amplified music of a band in the background. Or it can discriminate and identify the source of a single faulty note from one instrument in an entire orchestra.

Hearing begins with vibration of the eardrum, but vibration is really too coarse a word. What does one call eardrum movement of one millionth of a millimetre – one tenth of the diameter of a hydrogen atom – at high sound frequencies? Even more incredible are the membranes in the inner ear. The movement of these membranes vibrating to convert sound energy into electrochemical nerve impulses is about one ten-billionth of a millimetre!

But the wonder of hearing does not end here. The ear is capable of distinguishing the direction of sound. This may initially seem like a simple task but its complexity is apparent when one considers that, while sound in a room directly reaches the ear, the sound is also being reflected off the walls, floor, ceiling and furniture towards the ear. The point is that the ear is able to disregard all sounds except the first one that reaches it, and unerringly direct its attention to the source.

The range of normal adult hearing is about 100–12 000 cycles per second (cps). In childhood the upper range may be as high as 40 000 cps. The human ear is much less sensitive to very deep bass tones, which is just as well otherwise the body's own vibrations would be heard. Moving the head on the spine would sound like a lumber saw, chewing would be a thunderous experience, and the bedlam of exercise would deter any sporting activity.

The ear also hears by bone conduction, but this is a subjective experience. If one chews potato crisps, the loud crunching noise is due to sound being transmitted to the ears by the bones of the jaw. Someone nearby will not hear the munching because it is not being transmitted through air (unless the chewer really crunches!). When one speaks, the sound the speaker hears is heard by air conduction and bone conduction, but the listener hears by air conduction alone. Many of the low tones produced by the vocal cords are lost during air conduction, and are heard by bone conduction only by the speaker, who firmly believes his or her voice is full and rich and cannot believe the tinny whine when it is heard on a high-tech recording!

HEARING UNDERWATER

Under diving conditions, sound is heard by bone conduction only. The minute vibrations of the eardrum are completely dampened by flooding the ear with water. In air, the relatively slow speed of sound permits its direction to be judged but, under water, its speed is too fast. Both ears receive the sound virtually simultaneously and the ear's ability to distinguish sound direction is completely lost. It is heard quite clearly, but a look-around is needed to find the source.

In air, the speed of sound is about 335 m/sec. In fresh water, it is about 1400 m/sec; and in sea water, 1550 m/sec. This means that sound waves travel faster and better in a denser medium and, in water, the speed of sound is about four times that in air. Water is a better transmitter of sound than air, so sound travels further under water. We have all seen those war movies where the submarine crew sits very quietly, with engines off, while the destroyer above listens for her. Low-pitched sounds carry better than high-pitched ones under water.

Sound transmission in water is further enhanced by reflection off the surface and off the bottom, especially if the sea bed is rocky. Reflection from the surface is very efficient – 99.999 per cent of the sound reaching the surface is reflected back into the water. As a result, transmission of sound from water to air, or from air to water, is very poor. This principle of reflection is also involved in underwater explosions and pressure waves. (See Underwater explosions, page 305.)

HEARING IN A DECOMPRESSION CHAMBER

Pressurised air in a chamber or bell causes speech distortion. The voice becomes more tinny as the pressure increases. The speed of sound increases with the increased gas density and it is thought that more of the voice is transmitted directly through the wall of the throat and less via the mouth. In a helium-oxygen environment, the helium produces a characteristic distortion of speech, the 'Donald Duck' effect, which is attributed to an increased frequency of resonance in heliox mixtures. At great depths, the voice is so distorted as to be unintelligible, and electronic descramblers must be used to adjust the frequency to an understandable form.

ORIENTATION

At the vestibule of the inner ear, the footplate of the stirrup plugs into the oval window. To one side is the cochlea, which is only concerned with hearing. To the other is the vestibular apparatus, which informs the brain about the orientation of the head in space. It continuously provides information about movement – forwards, backwards, up, down or sideways. It maintains equilibrium and, if conditions are confusing, induces disorientation or vertigo. The vestibular apparatus consists of three **semicircular canals**, half-circular fluid-filled tubes all entering a common cistern, the **utricle** and the **saccule**.

These semicircular canals detect movements of the head. They are sensitive to **kinetic** changes, that is, sudden changes in the direction of the head – up, down or sideways, and inform the brain and cerebellum via delicate and specific nerve impulses as to the exact position of the head. The semicircular canals are able to do this because they are orientated in all three dimensional planes. One is sensitive to vertical movement, the second to sideways movement, and the third to forwards and backwards movement.

They operate by inertia, similar to crashing through the windscreen of a car when the brakes are suddenly applied. No movement of the head is possible without causing some ripple disturbance in the fluid within the semicircular canals. As with hearing, hair cells are involved. Each canal has a mound of hair cells projecting into a small cup of gelatinous material. Any movement in a particular plane or combination of planes affects these hair cells. Nerve impulses are immediately generated to inform the brain of the current situation.

The utricle and saccule are **static** sensors. They detect continuous forward or sideways movement. So walking without moving the head will trigger the hair cells of the utricle, informing the brain that forward progression is proceeding. Should one then decide to move sideways without moving the head, the hair cells of the saccule will fire. Diving forwards, downwards and turning to one side will trigger all three semicircular canals, as well as the utricle and the saccule.

The information received by the brain from the vestibular apparatus about the position of the head and its orientation and movement in space elicits a response. It affects the incredibly complex process of balance. The brain receives information from the cochlea regarding the sonic state of the environment. It receives information from the vestibular apparatus about the position and movement of the head. The eyes provide information about the visible conditions, and the skin and joints provide information about the current posture of the body. Within milliseconds, the brain then correlates and processes all this information, adjusts the tone of every muscle in the body, decides on an appropriate response and coordinates hitting a speeding cricket ball for six or a baseball for a home run.

Under diving conditions, many of these sources of information are absent. The effect of gravity on joints and the 'feel' of up and down disappear. With poor visibility, or during night diving, the eyes provide no useful information. The direction of any sound source is indistinguishable. The diver then relies solely for orientation on the vestibular apparatus in the inner ear.

THE SINUSES

The sinuses are a complex maze of air-filled spaces in the bones around the nose. Every sinus has an opening into the nose, allowing movement of air between the nose and sinus. They are named after the bones in which they exist. The **frontal** sinuses are located in the frontal bone of the skull, above the nose and the eyes. The roof of the nose, directly under the brain, is formed by the ethmoid bone and houses the **ethmoid** sinuses. Right at the back of the nose, above the openings of the Eustachian tubes, is the **sphenoid** sinus in the sphenoid bone. To each side of the nose, in the maxillary bones of the cheeks, are the **maxillary** sinuses.

FUNCTION OF THE SINUSES

Together with the nose, the four groups of sinuses form a complicated array of air spaces in the upper face and floor of the brain. Their exact function is obscure. Their openings into the wall of the nose are too small to assist effectively with any nasal humidification of inhaled air. It has been suggested that they serve to lessen the weight of the skull, but as the total weight loss would be much less than the weight of a small hat, this author is sceptical of this explanation. Imparting resonance to the voice has been mooted, but this resonance would be a subjective one, the sound being heard only by the speaker by bone conduction and quite inaudible to the listener who hears by air conduction only.

An interesting theory is that the sinuses are developmental accidents and have no function at all. During facial growth, most of the growth is downwards and sideways as the cheek bones develop to provide support for the teeth. The lining of the nose then simply follows the growth of the enlarging cheek bones to form the maxillary sinuses. As the face develops, the outer layer of the bones of the forehead grow more rapidly to conform to the facial bones and draw up nasal lining to form the frontal sinuses. This explanation would mean that the sinuses are relevant only as sites of possible disease, such as allergy, sinusitis and, for a diver, sinus squeeze (see page 112).

The sinuses

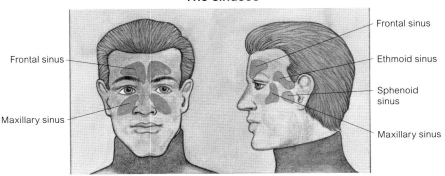

Frontal sinus

Maxillary sinus

Frontal sinus

Ethmoid sinus

Sphenoid sinus

Maxillary sinus

12

DIVING IMPLICATIONS OF EAR, NOSE, THROAT AND SINUS DISEASE

Difficulty in equalising pressure in the air spaces of the skull is the most common complaint of divers. These air spaces comprise the sinuses, the external and middle ears, and cavities in decaying teeth. They are peculiar in that they are all rigidly confined in bone (or tooth) and each has a canal that opens to the atmosphere. Being rigid spaces means that they cannot respond to pressure changes by varying their volume, making them vulnerable to Boyle's Law (see page 21). Any obstruction of their canals while diving will challenge this vulnerability. Being connected to the atmosphere exposes these air cavities to bacteria, dusts and pollens, and the combination of infection, allergy and canal obstruction is the most frequent cause of diving problems.

DISORDERS OF THE EXTERNAL EAR

SWIMMER'S EAR (OTITIS EXTERNA)

The external ear, be it small, large or shell-like, is the Achilles' heel of *Homo scubiens*. The external ear canal is a three-centimetre-long tube which conducts sound waves in the ear to the eardrum. It is an unfortunate fact of diving that, of the numerous orifices possessed by divers, the external ear canal is the only one that cannot be protected or discreetly covered. It **must** be totally exposed to the water. Boyle's Law, unforgiving and ever threatening the delicate middle ear with squeeze, demands that the external ear canal be flooded when a sport diver dives. This means exposure to the polluted, bacteria-rich water of the sea or an unclean dam or lake.

CAUSES OF SWIMMER'S EAR   Only two barriers protect the external ear from bacterial attack by the diving environment – wax and the membrane lining of the external ear canal. But many divers do their best to destroy both by sticking things into their ear canals and having a good scratch around.

WAX REMOVAL   Wax, or cerumen, is produced in the external ear canal. Contrary to popular belief, wax is good stuff. It is not an excretory product of the ear. It is a protective non-wettable substance covering the delicate membrane lining of the canal and preventing it from becoming waterlogged. A soggy membrane is the first step to infection – otitis externa or swimmer's ear.

Wax in the external ear canal should be removed only when build-up threatens to obstruct the canal, preventing free drainage of water from the ear after a dive, and predisposing to external ear squeeze. This is usually heralded by the sudden onset of a deaf feeling in the ear. Ingenious methods of wax mining used by divers include the use of pens, pencils, hairpins, toothpicks, matchsticks, fingernails and the pointed tool of a Swiss knife that is good for removing stones from horses' hoofs. The ubiquitous cotton bud is especially popular. Here is a maxim: **never put anything smaller than your elbow in your ear.** Cotton buds have no place in an ear! They simply plough up the wax and scratch open the membrane, leaving the canal wide open to invasion by aquatic bacteria. Use a cloth to clean away any socially abhorrent wax lurking at the opening of an ear.

If deeper wax must be removed, let a doctor do it and then wait a few days before diving to enable a wax covering to develop again. Divers who dive regularly have very little wax build-up in any event, as frequent immersion rinses most of it away.

DANDRUFF People with dandruff often suffer from maddeningly itchy ears. The need to obtain relief by ear gouging can be almost intolerable, and the incidence of chronic external ear canal inflammation is accordingly high in these individuals. Treatment is available and should be sought. The use of shampoos containing coal and pine tar solutions, or medicated with zinc pyrithione or selenium sulphide will help control the dandruff. Topical antibiotic applications, with or without cortisone, are available for ear canal infections and the treatment of ear canal eczema.

EXOSTOSES Long-term exposure and irritation of the ears by water can lead to the development of bony thickenings, called exostoses, in the bony wall of the external ear canal. These can result in partial or complete obstruction of the external ear canal, leading to occlusion by wax or preventing proper drainage of water from the ear after a dive. The stage is then set for swimmer's ear to develop. Under these circumstances, surgical removal of the exostoses may become necessary.

Management of swimmer's ear

Swimmer's ear differs from the commonly found mixed infections of the ear canal in non-divers in that a particularly virulent bacterium, *Pseudomonas aeruginosa*, is often the causative organism in divers. *Pseudomonas* is a water-loving bacterium and is found in all lakes and dams and even in the drinking water of most cities. A scratched, moist and boggy ear canal is an open invitation to an intensely painful infection. The organism is highly resistant to all oral antibiotics except ciprofloxacin, or daily injections or even hospitalisation for infusions of very expensive and potentially toxic drugs such as gentamycin, and the topical use of ciprofloxacin antibiotic eardrops.

Prevention

1. Keep a plastic bottle of three per cent (3%) saline in your dive bag. After diving, use a clean dropper to rinse the ears with the solution in order to remove debris and organic contaminants.

2. Do not attempt to remove wax by using cotton buds or other foreign bodies. Have wax build-up assessed during a diving medical, or when attending a doctor for an unrelated complaint – it only takes a moment. If there is a significant accumulation of wax, let a doctor remove it.

3. Instil protective drops into both ear canals after diving. These drops either remove water (are astringent) or repel water (are hydrophobic) and include dilute acetates, oil or alcohols as their base. They maintain a dry, slightly acidic ear canal and are readily available at most pharmacies. There are several effective options, depending on sensitivity and availability:
    – olive oil drops – use these prior to diving to maintain a water-repellent surface in the canal,
    – two per cent (2%) acetic acid in aluminium acetate, for use after diving,
    – five per cent (5%) glacial acetic acid in propylene glycol, for use after diving,
    – five per cent (5%) aluminium acetate in water, for use after diving, or
    – Swimseal drops (tea tree oil in a silicone base), instilled before diving are highly protective.

Treatment

Once swimmer's ear has developed, medical help is necessary. Inflammation of the external ear canal presents with severe pain, which is aggravated by gently tugging the external ear. Deafness may also be a feature, due to swelling of the membrane lining. If the diver is in a remote area with **no doctor available** then, depending on the pain and sensitivity, the use of ciprofloxacin drops four times a day into the ear canal is useful. If this is unavailable, any of the following may be tried:
– Neomycin and polymixin in a Vaseline-lanolin base.
– Neomycin, polymixin and hydrocortisone in aqueous solution.
– Gentamycin, betamethasone, tolnaftate and iodochlorhydroquinone in an emulsified base.
– If earache is severe, benzocaine eardrops may be tried. The drops should be warmed by immersing the closed bottle in warm water (taking care not to allow any water into the bottle). Instil 5–10 drops two-hourly and plug the ear with cotton wool.

These medications all require a prescription for their use. If you intend to visit a remote diving destination, consult a doctor before the trip to discuss the management of possible common ailments and to obtain advice and advance permission to use these medications if needed.

If the condition remains unresponsive to treatment or is recurrent, a culture of the causative organism should be taken to identify the bacteria and determine which oral, injectable and topical antibiotics will be effective.

Once swimmer's ear has developed, all diving and swimming must stop to avoid further wetting of the ear canal and flushing out of medication. Only when the canal has healed may diving be continued.

DISORDERS OF THE MIDDLE EAR

The middle ear is the mechanical amplifier of the hearing process. Anything that threatens the integrity of sound conduction in the middle ear must temporarily or permanently prohibit diving.

MIDDLE EAR INFECTION (OTITIS MEDIA)

Bacteria can reach the middle ear in two ways:
— via the Eustachian tube from the nose, or
— via a perforated eardrum.

The first may occur following attempts at equalising during an episode of upper respiratory infection. Equalising drives the infection into the middle ear.

A perforated eardrum usually occurs after a pressure injury (Barotrauma, see page 150). The middle ear becomes filled with blood, mucus and water, and bacterial growth begins. The acute pain and vertigo that result usually subside quickly during the dive, to be replaced by a sensation of deafness after surfacing. Bleeding from the nose or ear is often noticed. Several hours to one day later, the throbbing pain of otitis media begins.

Management of otitis media

Prevention

Do not dive with an upper respiratory tract infection. This commonly causes difficulty with equalisation, making middle ear barotrauma a real possibility. The use of decongestants, either orally or nasally, is not wise either. They may facilitate equalising, but will also assist in driving bacteria into the middle ear. In addition, their effect may diminish during the dive with reverse block on ascent.

Treatment (see also Management of ear barotrauma, page 156)
1. Broad-spectrum antibiotics are indicated, especially after eardrum rupture due to barotrauma. The risk of otitis media is high.
2. WARNING! **Use eardrops only if no history of barotrauma is present and there is no discharge from the ear.** With a perforated eardrum, the use of most antibiotic drops may lead to permanent deafness. Drops containing antibiotics such as polymixin B, neomycin and chloramphenicol, with or without hydrocortisone to relieve inflammation, are available; however, they can cause permanent deafness if the eardrum is perforated.
3. If the eardrum is intact but pus formation occurs in the middle ear, it may be necessary to have a grommet surgically inserted to assist drainage.

Do not dive if you have otitis media, a perforated eardrum or if a grommet is in place. A perforated eardrum takes an average of two to four weeks to heal and this must be confirmed by a doctor before diving resumes. A grommet must first be removed and the eardrum allowed to heal. The only exception could be dry chamber dives where one of the necessary personnel has a perforation. Chronic infections of the middle ear permanently bar diving.

> **Grommets** are tiny tubes that are inserted through the eardrum to drain mucus and pus formed in a middle ear infection or to compensate for chronic Eustachian dysfunction. They usually fall out spontaneously within 3–12 months and the eardrum closes by healing. Diving with grommets is not permitted, as water will enter the middle ear and an infection will invariably follow.

MIDDLE EAR BAROTRAUMA (SQUEEZE)

Mild squeeze that is relieved by ascent and successful equalising should be allowed eight hours before diving again. Even mild squeeze does cause some swelling of tissues in the middle ear and invariably results in difficulty equalising with repetitive dives. Each episode of difficulty compounds the problem. Severe squeeze, with bleeding from the nose and a blocked feeling in the ear, should preclude diving for four weeks; seek medical opinion to exclude a perforation. (See pages 152, 156.)

MIDDLE EAR SURGERY

Surgery to the middle ear includes skin grafting to repair a perforated eardrum, work on the bony chain and replacement of the stirrup. Any procedure that involves the stirrup or the oval window may permanently exclude diving, as there is a high risk that forceful equalising can damage the oval or round windows. Any diving after other surgery to the bones of the middle ear must be discussed by the diver, diving physician and the ear surgeon who did the work.

DISORDERS OF THE INNER EAR

Abnormalities of the inner ear affect hearing or balance. Any abnormality of vestibular function results in a balance disorder and is immediately disqualifying. Vertigo and disorientation under water are perilous.

DEAFNESS

Hearing standards for divers vary in different countries and generally also depend on the type of diving being done. Commercial and military divers have to meet minimum hearing standards and hearing tests should be repeated annually. Among sport divers, however, lower standards are usually acceptable, provided the diver can equalise very easily. The risk of compounding partial inner ear deafness with middle ear damage would make diving unacceptable. A conservative standard would be the ability to hear sounds at 30 dB at frequencies between 500 and 8000 cps. With totally deaf people, sport diving may be approved on condition that very strict provision is made for a meaningful buddy system, for example, a signal line and a normal-hearing buddy trained in signing.

LABYRINTHITIS

This is an acute viral infection of the vestibular apparatus that induces profound vertigo with extreme disorientation, nausea and vomiting. Full recovery must be confirmed by a diving physician before recommencing diving.

TINNITUS

Tinnitus, or ringing in the ears, is common. It is usually caused by acoustic trauma such as gunfire or very loud noise and it may persist permanently. It is thought to be due to damage to the hair cells in the inner ear. Under diving conditions, tinnitus may be caused by inner ear barotrauma or decompression illness and is a significant symptom after diving. Medical assessment is needed.

MÉNIERE'S DISEASE

This condition affects both the cochlea and the vestibular apparatus and is character-ised by recurrent episodes of vertigo, tinnitus (ringing in the ears) and slow, progressive hearing loss. Its cause is unclear but all diving is permanently barred.

SEASICKNESS

There are very few divers who have never suffered from seasickness. The only people who are immune under any sea conditions are those with totally non-functional inner ears – they are stone deaf and have no inner ear balance mechanism. The inner ear is the organ responsible for inducing seasickness. Normal balance depends on harmony between all the sources of positional information received by the brain.

When a diver is sitting on a beach and looking straight out to sea:
- nerve pressure sensors under the skin inform the brain that the ground is beneath the diver,
- the eyes inform the brain of the surrounding view and confirm that the ground is downwards,
- static receptors in the inner ear inform the brain that the diver is sitting still, and
- the semicircular canals inform the brain that the head is being held erect.

If the diver now sits in a boat rolling and yawing from side to side and pitching from fore to aft, the situation is very different. The skin sensors and eyes inform the brain that the diver is assuredly sitting still in a boat, but the inner ear relays that the diver is moving up and down, backwards and forwards, and from side to side at the same time. This conflicting information causes motion sickness. The brain does adapt within two or three days of ongoing exposure, or after short periods of regular exposure, but these can be the most miserable days of a diver's life. Adaptation is often heralded by a gentle rocking feeling when back on land. This memory of movement ('sea legs') is at the same frequency as that of the sea conditions recently experienced.

Development of seasickness

1. **Proceeding out to sea** Maximum pitching of the dive boat occurs when moving out to sea as the boat has to plunge through waves and bob over crests and troughs of incoming swells. The first feelings of being ill at ease appear. Odours such as diesel, petrol and raw fish become noticeable and nauseating. The diver becomes pale and restless and tries to find a place to be alone. Going below deck makes things worse, as does any heat from the engines. Fine beads of perspiration appear on the upper lip and forehead. Saliva production increases, and exaggerated swallowing and yawning occur. Then nausea and vomiting occur, which may be short-lived with full recovery from seasickness, or become ongoing to the point of dehydration and collapse.

2. **Moored on site** The pitching of the bows decreases when moored, but rolling, yawing and moving up and down begin. This may precipitate seasickness and will aggravate an already sick diver's condition.

3. **Underwater** Early symptoms of seasickness usually disappear rapidly once the diver is below the surface. The cold water is refreshing and inner ear confusion stops, but haste to enter the sea can cause trouble underwater if an inadequate or too hurried predive checklist was done. There may be no air in the cylinder, the cylinder valve may still be closed, the regulator may not even be connected to the pillar valve, etc. During the ascent, problems can recur if variable reference points are reintroduced, such as in-water decompression stops on a separate floating shot line or a line attached to the boat. Holding onto this line will ensure a correct and constant decompression-stop depth as the buoy or boat moves up and down on the surface swell, but the bottom, if visible, will approach and recede with the movement. The solution is simple and also applies to heights: don't look down.

4. **Returning to shore** Once back on the boat and returning to shore, the seasick diver invariably recovers. The boat no longer pitches and rolls, and the smooth passage between suddenly gentle swells restores hope that survival is not only possible, but probable.

If a diver has suffered from prolonged vomiting during a day at sea, he or she may become incapacitated as a result of fluid loss and exhaustion and a doctor must be consulted. Dehydration and electrolyte loss can be very substantial, and intravenous fluid replacement and other therapy may be necessary.

Predisposing factors to seasickness

1. **Alcohol** From ruefully remembered personal experience, alcohol the night before is an extremely potent factor in promoting seasickness the next morning.

2. **Food** Divers must eat frugally and intelligently. Overindulgence (which usually includes alcohol abuse) results in a bleary-eyed, flatulent diver braving the morning seas when the best place would be in bed, asleep.
3. **Age** Older divers are less susceptible to seasickness than young divers. This probably relates more to decreased sensitivity of the inner ear to changes in motion than to any innate resistance.
4. **Gender** Seasickness is more common in women. As it is very unlikely that this observation has any truth in real physical terms, it is probable that women simply expose themselves less to exploits that require acclimatisation, such as deep-sea fishing.
5. **Sensory confusion** Sitting in the bow or stern of a dive boat causes maximum disturbance of the inner ear. Pitching and yawing are most marked in these places, which pivot around the central, relatively motionless, middle of the boat.
6. **Psychological factors** It is often said that seasickness is 'all in the mind'. Anatomically, this may be correct, but seasick infants belie such a simple explanation. Fear of becoming sick is definitely relevant and, once one diver begins vomiting, others will follow his or her example. Nervous expectancy and preparedness for seasickness would be closer to the truth.

How to prevent seasickness
1. Eat lightly and do not drink alcohol the night before diving.
2. Ensure that all your equipment is placed in a logical and orderly fashion next to you on the dive boat. Do not leave your mask in one place, fins in another, and your cylinder in a third. Sorting out equipment in a rocking boat will guarantee vomiting if you are predisposed to seasickness.
3. Concentrate on factors that will assist the brain in orientating acceptably. The eyes and body should actively fix on steady bearings:
   – keep the head upright and steady,
   – stare at the horizon ,
   – do not look down at the deck or water, and
   – do not try to read; this removes eye reference and makes things worse.
4. Anti-seasickness drugs generally act by preventing seasickness rather than treating it, so it is logical that they be taken before seasickness starts. It is pointless to tell sport divers not to take anti-seasickness medication because the drugs may cause drowsiness. They will not listen. The fear of uncontrolled vomiting while sitting in a hot wet suit in a rocking boat under a blazing sun makes drowsiness a pleasure, not a side-effect. As the main dangers of drowsiness are sluggish reactions and nitrogen narcosis at shallower than usual depths, a practical compromise is necessary: **do not exceed a maximum depth of 30 msw if any anti-seasickness medication is used.** A seasick diver has no business being at 30 msw in any event. If violent seasickness starts, regardless

of whether or not anti-seasickness drugs have been taken, the diver must forget about any diving that day.

Anti-seasickness drugs

The choice of drug depends on availability and the duration of the diver's exposure to the sea. Unless advised otherwise, take drugs one to two hours before going to sea.

1. **Hyoscine (scopolamine)** This drug blocks the passage of nerve impulses from the balance organs in the inner ear to the vomiting centre in the brain. It is intended for severe sea conditions and is useful for trips to sea lasting less than six hours. It must not be used more than once a day as blurred vision, a very dry mouth and drowsiness then make it dangerous. The dose is 0.3–0.6 mg by mouth. It must not be taken in combination form with other stimulants or antihistamines if diving is intended as severe drowsiness and inability to react adequately to an underwater emergency may result. Hyoscine is also available as a skin patch which slowly releases the drug through the skin over 72 hours.

2. **Dimenhydrinate (dramamine)** Dramamine has been used by divers at depths to 50 msw. The dose is 50 mg six-hourly. It is intended for moderate seasickness and is available without prescription. Sedation has been reported in some divers.

3. **Cyclizine** Available without prescription, cylizine assists with prevention of mild seasickness. The dose is 50 mg four-hourly.

4. **Metoclopramide** Metoclopramide is useful in mild cases of motion illness. The dose is 10 mg three times a day. A prescription is required.

5. **Cinnarizine and domperidone** A combination of two prescription drugs, cinnarizine 25 mg and domperidone 10 mg, is useful in preventing all but severe seasickness. The two tablets are taken together at six-hourly intervals. It is suggested that medication begins 24 hours before diving starts in order to assess individual susceptibility to drowsiness and allow time for acclimatisation to these effects. In this author's experience, divers who actively worked at 30 msw for long periods on the wreck of the *Birkenhead* reported no adverse drowsiness underwater.

6. **Phenytoin** In 1988, Dr William Chelen, a medical doctor and professor of electrical engineering at the US Air Force Institute of Technology, decided to examine the brain wave records of people with motion sickness induced in a rotating chair. It came as a surprise when he found that electroencephalogram (EEG) recordings of these subjects during their motion sickness was strikingly similar to those found with certain forms of epilepsy. Chelen decided to see whether the similarity was more than just electrical and to determine whether the use of phenytoin, an anti-convulsant drug used in the management of epilepsy, would, with short-term use, prevent motion sickness. Phenytoin acts on the brain by stabilising nerve membranes, so preventing a convulsion but allowing normal nerve function to continue naturally.

Would it act similarly with motion sickness? Trials demonstrated that phenytoin was four to ten times more effective in preventing laboratory-induced motion sickness than any other available single agent, but what about side-effects? In the long term treatment of epilepsy, phenytoin does have significant side-effects, but in the motion-sickness trials, lasting only a few days, no side-effects were reported. In particular, no sedation was found, nor was there any effect on a battery of performance tests. The next step was to test phenytoin at sea to determine its efficacy against real seasickness. The idea was to test the efficacy of phenytoin under small-boat conditions, operational sea travel and in hyperbaric chambers. No side-effects such as drowsiness or slowed reflexes occurred, and only one subject reported mild, noticeable but not bothersome seasickness. To determine whether the use of phenytoin would predispose to, or worsen, nitrogen narcosis, chamber dives were undertaken to a depth of 36.6 msw and multiplication tests were performed. No significant difference was found between divers on phenytoin and those on a placebo (sugar tablet), either at the surface or at 36.6 msw.

In August 1994, a trial was undertaken by this author to determine the efficacy of phenytoin (marketed as Epanutin in South Africa) in preventing seasickness in 178 sport divers with a history of severe seasickness, mostly unresponsive to any previous medication. Phenytoin (in lower than normally recommended doses) was administered in daily divided doses, beginning two days before exposure to sea conditions. Ninety-five per cent of the divers reported improvement or no sickness at all. A second trial was undertaken in December 1994 using full recommended dosages, and taking the medication as a single nightly dose in order to simplify the dosage schedule. All the divers in this trial reported dramatic improvement. A few divers reported side-effects of headache, fatigue, constipation and short-lived blurred vision.

The dosage was 5 mg phenytoin per kilogram body weight, beginning the night before diving, taken as a single evening dose or a divided twice-daily dose, and repeated each evening for a maximum of four or five days. After this time the vast majority of people will have acclimatised to sea conditions anyway and do not require any further medication.

WARNING! To date, phenytoin has not been officially registered as an anti-seasickness, anti-airsickness or anti-motion sickness preparation.
Nor does it enable epileptic patients to dive safely. Persons with any form of epilepsy must not dive! Phenytoin must not be taken by people with porphyria, very slow pulse rates, heart problems or low blood pressure. It must also not be taken during pregnancy or while taking any other form of medication whatsoever, as drug interactions may occur.

It is absolutely essential that a doctor be consulted first for advice, and a doctor's prescription is required.

Do not accept this drug from a fellow diver without initial medical opinion.

DISORDERS OF THE NOSE AND THROAT

NASAL ALLERGY AND IRRITATION

The most common ailment among sport divers is nasal allergy and irritation. The combined incidence of all other diving problems becomes almost insignificant when compared with the incidence of grey-blue swelling of the membranes in the human nose. As the nose is the first organ in the breathing process to sample the air, it is exposed to more dust, pollen, fumes and smoke than any other tissue. This is aggravated by the fact that the lining of the nose is designed to humidify air. It is thick, corrugated to provide a large surface area, and covered with mucus-producing cells.

Air streaming through the nose rapidly absorbs moisture from mucus, depositing its burden of pollution onto the sticky film. In some people, this results in allergy or chemically-induced swelling, with severe hayfever or nasal stuffiness. In most cases, the person is unaware of any membrane swelling in his or her nose until the efficient function (patency) of the Eustachian tubes is challenged. This challenge requires a pressure differential and commonly occurs when driving down a mountain pass or descending in an aircraft. The atmospheric pressure (in millibars) outside the ear increases while that in the middle ear remains low. Discomfort or pain occurs, which may be relieved by chewing, swallowing or performing a Valsalva manoeuvre (see page 115). Under diving conditions, the pressure differentials are measured in bars, not millibars, so the problem is vastly worse.

Inability to equalise pressure in the middle ear due to nasal congestion is by far the most common complaint of divers.

Management of nasal congestion

Prevention Without quitting one's job, selling up and moving to a pollution-free island, it is almost impossible to avoid coming into contact with industrial pollution, dusts and pollens. However, one nasal irritant that can be avoided is smoking. Stopping smoking often cures equalising problems.

A deviated nasal septum is often associated with equalising difficulties. When the thin plate dividing the two nostrils is deviated to one side, the interference with air flow through the nose commonly results in more membrane swelling due to turbulent air flow. Surgical straightening of the septum restores normal air flow and often assists chronic sinusitis as well.

Treatment To a large degree, treatment of nasal congestion depends on individual need, diving frequency and the willingness of the diver to comply with long-term treatment. There is no total cure.

In a few cases, an underlying allergy can be pinned down to one or two specific causes, such as cats or pollen. In such cases, desensitisation by injections or via sublingual drops of gradually increasing strengths of solutions prepared from cat fur or pollen mix may help. In most cases, however, the choice lies between decongestants, antihistamines, and nasal cortisone and anti-allergy sprays. Many of these are dangerous under diving conditions.

Decongestants

1. **Oral decongestants** almost invariably contain pseudoephedrine, a drug that mimics adrenaline in action. It shrinks the nasal lining, and improves nasal function and equalising ability. As adrenaline is a powerful natural hormone, mimicking its action can cause side-effects including an increased heart rate, palpitations, high blood pressure, hallucinations, psychotic states, muscular weakness, difficulty in passing urine, sweating, thirst, tremors, dry mouth, breathlessness, disturbances in glucose metabolism, blurred vision and cardiac arrest. Pseudoephedrine should preferably not be taken before a dive to assist equalising.

2. **Nasal decongestant sprays** usually rely for their action on the drugs oxymetazoline or phenylephrine. Their side-effects are not as dramatic as oral decongestants and include local stinging in the nose, headache, a rapid heart rate and high blood pressure. They have one main disadvantage:

    (a) **Rebound congestion occurs** The drugs act by producing intense spasm of the blood vessels in the nasal mucous membrane. This shrinks the lining and stops mucus production, relieving congestion. The nasal membrane, deprived of its normally rich blood supply, dries out and becomes devitalised. As the effects of the drug wear off, the membrane swells again, but this time due to both allergy and drug-induced injury. The swelling is worse than before and results in a totally blocked nose. Repeated sprays cause an ever-worsening cycle of blocking and unblocking, the user becoming virtually addicted to the spray for shorter and shorter periods of temporary relief. This is called *rhinitis medicamentosa*. At this point the spray must be stopped, despite intensely uncomfortable nasal congestion, and a doctor consulted. Decongestant sprays must never be used for more than three to five days.

    (b) Oxymetazoline decongestion nasal sprays are very commonly used by divers. If used about 30 minutes before the dive in a dose of one to two puffs in each nostril, they may facilitate equalising. **However, they will not enable a person who cannot equalise voluntarily to do so!**

Oral antihistamines

Instead of shrinking swollen membranes by squeezing off their blood supply, antihistamines act by preventing the production or effects of histamine. In the allergic process, histamine as well as a number of other compounds are produced by allergic tissues. If histamine production is inhibited, allergic swelling decreases or stops. The problem is that histamine is also used by the brain as one of the normal chemical transmitters in nerve conduction, so the use of antihistamines also affects cerebral function.

Drowsiness, blurred vision, limb heaviness, weakness and ringing in the ears can occur (among other side-effects). These usually make classic antihistamines – such as chlorpheniramine, promethazine and mepyramine – unsuitable for diving.

Newer antihistamines have been manufactured which do not cross the membrane barrier between cerebral capillaries and brain cells, and which exert their effect primarily on nasal mucous membranes. These drugs include loratidine, desloratidine, levocetirizine and astemizole. As they cannot reach the brain they should, in theory, be safe, but drug effects on land cannot be presumed to be the same underwater. If these antihistamines do cross into brain cells with the increased pressure of diving, their effects would be unpredictable.

In this author's experience, many hundreds of sport divers have dived to 18 metres using these products without experiencing any noticeable subjective side-effects.

NASAL ANTIHISTAMINE SPRAYS

Levocabastine and Azelastine sprays are recent newcomers to the nasal range. They are a useful tool in the management of nasal allergy, including seasonal allergic rhinitis. They do need a doctor's prescription and advice on their use.

NASAL CORTISONES

Steroid hormones are normally produced by the adrenal glands in the body. Cortisone is an immensely powerful antihistamine and anti-inflammatory, and these properties are taken advantage of when cortisone therapy is used. But, when used orally for prolonged periods, the side-effects of cortisone are profound; they include decalcification of bone, thinning and weakening of connective tissue and duodenal ulceration. To avoid these side-effects in nasal preparations microgram doses only are sprayed directly where required – onto the nasal membranes. Absorption into the body is limited to minute amounts, but care must nevertheless be taken with prolonged use.

The cortisone sprays include betamethasone, budesonide and beclomethasone, and the more powerful fluorinated cortisones: flunisolide and fluticasone. These products take time to exert their effect so regular use in strictly controlled dosages over several months is needed.

Management of equalising difficulties before a diving trip

Most sport divers dive relatively infrequently and do not suffer any particular nasal or equalising difficulty when on land except, perhaps, for occasional sneezing when the pollen count is high. While they are understandably loath to undertake continuous treatment of their nasal congestion just in case they may want to dive, they do want a regime of treatment to help them when they dive.

The following management regime is useful when planning a dive trip. **However, it must be approved and prescribed by a doctor to ensure that there are no contraindications in a particular diver.** If possible, it should be begun one month before diving. This regime is recommended for adults only.

1. Douche both nostrils with a mixture of ½ teaspoon salt and ½ teaspoon bicarbonate of soda dissolved in 300 ml warm water three times a day and just before bed. Using a medical syringe (without a needle!) is more efficient than sniffing up the liquid from a cupped hand. Douching washes away sticky mucus, clears the nose of particles of pollen, dust, etc. and provides better exposure of the membrane to nasal medication. Douche the nose just before using a nasal spray.

2. Use steroid nasal sprays: either two sprays of fluticasone in each nostril once a day; or two sprays of budesonide in each nostril twice a day; or two sprays of flunisolide in each nostril twice a day.

3. In addition, take one 10 mg tablet of loratidine, desloratidine, levocetirizine or astemizole once a day as a single evening dose for the month before diving.

4. Then, one week before the trip, add pseudoephedrine (available in a tablet in combination with the above or as separate tablets) in two to three divided doses. The total dose per day should be 180–240 mg. Stop pseudoephedrine intake the day before diving begins.

   Note: In 2008, pseudoephedrine became a scheduled drug because it is used by drug abusers in the synthesis of the illicit and highly addictive drug 'tik' (methamphetamine, crystal meth). It is no longer available over the counter and a written doctor's prescription is now essential.

5. Continue regular nasal douching and steroid sprays during the holiday. Loratidine, desloratidine, levocetirizine or astemizole may also be used while diving.

NOSE BLEEDS (EPISTAXIS)

Chronic nasal allergy, abuse of nasal decongestant sprays and drying of nasal membranes by the inert propellant in steroid sprays can cause recurrent nose bleeds. If these become regular, diving must stop until the problem has been attended to. Equalising increases the pressure in one's head and can easily precipitate a severe bleed underwater with accumulation of blood in the mask, forced swallowing of blood, anxiety and panic. High blood pressure must also be excluded as a possible cause. Most cases of recurrent nose bleeds require cauterisation of the bleeding site with a solution of silver nitrate by a doctor.

Management of acute nose bleeds

Most nose bleeds occur from the blood vessels near the front of the nose. The majority are self-limiting and require little assistance, but severe nose bleeds require packing by a doctor. In intermediate cases ,the following usually suffices:

1. Have the person sit erect and with the head tilted **forward** onto the chest. This increases venous back pressure on the bleeding vessel and assists in clot formation. It also stops blood from running into the throat.

2. Compress the nostrils between two fingers for ten minutes.

3. If bleeding persists, plug the nose. Nasal gauze strips or even cotton wool

drawn into a cylinder may be used. Moistening cotton wool with water makes it easier to insert. Feed the plug straight back **parallel** to the roof of the mouth. Do not try to push it upwards into the nose. This is acutely painful and the plug will jam against the internal curled bones on the side wall of the nose. Try to ensure that the nostril is packed as firmly as possible. Continue nasal compression between two fingers.

4. Nasal plugs made of compressed oxidised cellulose are easy to insert and, if available, should be included in a diver emergency medical kit. These plugs swell to many times their compressed dry volume when wetted with blood and are effective. Insert them parallel to the roof of the mouth.

5. Keep the nose plugged for 12 hours. Remove the plug slowly and gently to avoid causing sneezing which may restart the bleeding. Dab away any blood and mucus from the nostrils. Do not blow the nose!

DISORDERS OF THE SINUSES

In diving mechanical terms, the sinuses are no different from the middle ear. They are rigid air spaces connected by an opening into the nose and are subject to the same problems as the middle ear. The only difference is that any pressure differential in sinuses cannot be voluntarily equalised. Their openings into the nose are either clear or blocked. Blockage causes squeeze.

SINUS ALLERGY

Being only extensions of the nasal cavity, sinuses are also affected by allergy and inhaled irritants. These cause diver problems when membrane swelling occurs near or at the openings of the sinuses into the nose. Air flow through the openings may be obstructed, and polyps may be present (these are localised areas of thickened membrane that resemble wet grapes hanging from a stalk). They may act as a ball valve while diving.

Polyps in the nose that obstruct a sinus opening cause squeeze on descent. Polyps in the sinuses that obstruct a sinus opening cause reverse block. Polyps may have to be surgically removed by slipping a looped wire snare over them and snipping off their narrow stalks. Treatment of sinus allergy is the same as nasal allergy and diving restrictions are identical.

SINUSITIS

Infection of the sinuses presents with acute pain over the involved sinuses. In severe cases, an accumulation of pus may occur. This is seen on X-ray as a fluid level of liquid topped by air. The management of sinusitis follows the principles of nasal infection but pus formation requires surgical drainage.

 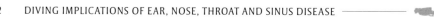

DISORDERS OF THE MOUTH AND THROAT

Infection occurs more commonly in the mouth and throat than anywhere else in the body. Upper respiratory infections include tonsillitis, pharyngitis and laryngitis. These are all relatively easily treated and are important from a diving point of view only because they prevent diving while they are present. The reason for this is mainly related to mouth breathing of very dry air while exercising underwater. The effects are very similar to those experienced by runners who exercise with an upper respiratory infection. Mouth breathing dries and further devitalises those membranes already damaged by infection and inflammation. Deep breathing also draws the infection deeper into the airways and a simple sore throat can progress to bronchitis or pneumonia. Infections of the mouth and gums are similarly aggravated by drying and will get worse.

Divers must care for their teeth. Dental caries is a potential cause of violent pain in divers. If the opening to a dental cavity is obstructed by food or by a swollen gum, the tooth may collapse on descent. If obstruction occurs on ascent, expanding air in the cavity can explode the tooth.

The absence of teeth is important, too. A dental bridge must fit firmly and properly. If it becomes dislodged underwater, it may be inhaled, with disastrous results. People with dentures should dive only if the dentures are well-fitting and they can firmly retain the rubber mouthpiece between their lips. Being accidentally bumped or hit on the face by a fellow diver's fin may dislodge both the mouthpiece and the dentures, and result in sudden respiratory obstruction underwater.

DIVING AFTER A RESPIRATORY INFECTION

'When can I dive after a bout of flu or bronchitis?' is a very common diver query. The answer is that there is no fixed time. Problems that may occur include pulmonary barotrauma due to mucus plugs and membrane swelling, sinus squeeze, and difficulty in equalising the ears. Diving may only continue once any infection is resolved. This means that the productive cough has gone; chest, throat, ear, sinus pain and irritation are all better, and ear equalising is easy once more.

TECHNIQUES FOR EQUALISING THE MIDDLE EAR

Inability to equalise the middle ears on descent accounts for about 95 per cent of diver misery. The saddest thing is that 96 per cent of divers can equalise – they just don't know how to because they have never been taught. A select few divers have the marvellous gift of voluntarily wiggling the Eustachian cushions to equalise. This elite knack warrants an elite name and is called the *beance tubaire voluntaire*, or BTV. For the rest, if a diver can't equalise by blowing or swallowing, he or she usually joins the woefully slow ranks of the AWD (Air-Wasters of Descent).

But don't despair! There are other ways of coaxing the Eustachian cushions to part and allow compressed air to enter the middle ears. With a little practise, virtually all divers can successfully equalise without having to resort to nasal sprays, oral decongestants, antihistamines and a yoyo creep to the coral.

Remember that failure to equalise causes earache, deafness and vertigo, in any combination, due to swelling, as well as haemorrhage in the eardrum and cavity of the middle ear, rupture of the eardrum and, less commonly, rupture of the oval or round windows of the inner ear.

If equalising is your underwater Achilles' heel, try the following techniques. Find the one that works best for you and then perform it ten times a day. Practise it at the surface until it becomes second nature before trying it underwater, and follow this list of equalising dos and don'ts.

DO
- equalise immediately as you submerge,
- equalise at least once per metre of descent,
- descend feet first to bottom depth, and
- halt the descent and ascend two metres immediately if any ear pressure is felt.

DON'T
- forget about you ears while fiddling with buoyancy and gauges,
- wait for ear pressure, let alone pain, to begin before equalising – at a depth of only 2 msw you are already much too deep,
- dive with nasal congestion due to allergy, irritation or infection – have these treated before a diving trip,
- continue to dive if equalising difficulty has caused any deafness, bleeding or vertigo (see a doctor first); further diving will become more and more difficult and will only cause more damage, and
- descend horizontally, or even worse, head-down, until you are sure your new equalising technique works well and reliably for you. It is much more difficult to equalise when inverted.

VALSALVA MANOEUVRE

This is the most commonly used method of equalising pressure during descent. It increases the pressure in the nasopharynx (the nose and throat), opens the valve-like cushions of the Eustachian tube, and drives air up the tube and into the middle ear. The pressure required to open the Eustachian cushions varies from diver to diver, but is in the order of 20–100 cm of water at the surface.

This is equivalent to sitting in a boat and blowing bubbles through a pipe with its far end immersed 0.2–1 metres under water. If you have equalising difficulties and only first attempt to equalise at one msw depth, you have doubled the length of the pipe to two metres, which makes blowing bubbles a heroic feat. At a depth of two msw, a first equalising attempt is equivalent to blowing from the surface through a pipe three metres deep and, unless your surname is Bauer or Draeger, you won't do it because you have to be a human compressor to succeed.

METHOD

1. Clamp off the nostrils with the index finger and thumb of one hand.
2. Press the tongue firmly against the roof of the mouth.
3. Attempt to blow the nose.

Note: Make sure that you can pinch the sides of your nose effectively through your mask.

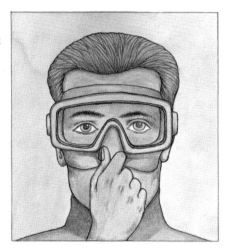

TOYNBEE MANOEUVRE

This is the second most commonly used method. It involves swallowing to separate the Eustachian cushions. The great advantage of mastering this technique is that it also relieves imminent middle ear barotrauma of ascent. If a diver develops sharp ear pain due to expanding middle ear air being unable to vent through the Eustachian tube during the ascent, performing the Toynbee manoeuvre will open the Eustachian tube. **A diver developing air pain during ascent must swallow, not blow, to equalise middle ear pressures. Do not perform a Valsalva manoeuvre during ascent! It increases the pressure in the nose and opposes middle ear venting!**

METHOD

1. Clamp off the nostrils with the index finger and thumb of one hand.
2. Swallow.

FRENZEL MANOEUVRE

With this technique, pressure in the nasopharynx is increased by blocking off the nose, the mouth and the throat, and then using the back of the tongue to compress and force air into the Eustachian tubes. It requires simultaneous contraction of the muscles of the floor of the mouth and throat. This author has found this almost impossible to explain and, as a consequence, devised the following simple method of instruction. It needs practise.

METHOD
1. Clamp off the nostrils with the index finger and thumb of one hand.
2. Press the tip of the tongue hard against the lower front teeth.
3. Say 'kick' from the back of the throat and simultaneously try to blow the nose.
A continuous string of 'kicks' during each exhalation will provide very rapid and repetitive equalising during the descent.

LOWRY TECHNIQUE

This often works where all other techniques fail and is especially useful for divers who are plagued by constant equalising difficulty and who always have to spend a great deal of time getting to bottom depth. It is a combination of the Valsalva and Toynbee manoeuvres and is a very powerful equalising mode, but requires much surface practise to perfect.

METHOD
1. Clamp off the nostrils with the index finger and thumb of one hand.
2. Press the tongue firmly against the roof of the mouth.
3. Blow very gently, maintain the blow and then swallow **simultaneously**.

EDMONDS TECHNIQUE

With this method, the lower jaw is thrust forward so that the lower teeth protrude well in front of the upper teeth. A Valsalva, Toynbee or Frenzel manoeuvre is then done.

Try all these techniques and then choose the one for you. With a little practise and perseverance you, too, can find joy in descent.

13

VISION UNDER WATER

Divers are observant souls and when they enter the sea, they use their eyes. They notice three things – things are darker, colours are different and things look bigger.

THINGS ARE DARKER

Even in the clearest ocean water, such as around the British Virgin Islands or the Maldives, only 20 per cent of the surface light reaches 10 metres below the surface, and a mere one per cent reaches 85 metres depth. This means that the bright illumination of the sunny day above is very reduced and the harsh shadows of the surface recede, making the contrast between objects much less.

COLOURS ARE DIFFERENT

Sunlight or white light includes a spectrum of visible light from red to violet. Clean water has a maximum transparency to blue wavelengths of light and absorbs the other colours. Coastal waters allow the yellow-greens through. The other colours are absorbed by suspended material such as plankton and pollution. Reds and oranges are absorbed first. To see **true colours**, even at 10 metres, underwater lights are needed. This absorption and scattering of light by suspended particles limits vision and diffuses illumination and, with poor visibility, the light intensity appears the same in all directions.

On descent or ascent, the surface and seabed disappear and a diver may feel suspended in a featureless green, blue or grey watery sphere. This may cause loss of orientation with up, down and sideways all having the same light intensity. Only a dangling pressure gauge or the direction of ascending bubbles show down and up.

THINGS LOOK BIGGER

When a beam of light passes through transparent substances of different optical densities, it is bent at the interface between them. Light reaching the surface of the eye (the cornea) is bent or refracted into the eye. It is an air-tissue interface, the cornea being optically denser than air. Having passed through the cornea, light is then fine-focused by the lens onto the retina at the back of the eye. The air/cornea interface is the main site of focusing. Most of the necessary bending of light waves occurs here.

Within the eye, the lens is surrounded by liquid with only minute differences in optical density and very limited refracting ability. A normal cornea is essential to clear vision. If a diver decides to snorkel down to check an anchor without using a

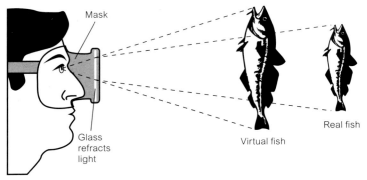

Mask

Glass
refracts
light

Virtual fish

Real fish

Wearing a mask can make objects in the water seem closer and larger than they are.

mask, his or her eye would not be able to focus as a water–cornea interface would be present. Their optical densities are too similar and no effective refraction can occur; instead, everything would be blurred. This is the reason for using a mask while diving, as well as to protect the eye.

A mask enables a diver to focus, but why should things appear larger? The reason is the introduction of a water-glass interface. Light passes from water into glass and then from glass into the air inside the mask. The light is bent at each interface so that the mask acts like a pair of low-power binoculars. An apparent image is formed, which is closer and larger than the real image – about 25 per cent closer and 30 per cent larger. But wearing a mask or helmet does cause problems:

LIMITED FIELD OF VISION The field of vision is limited by the size of the mask and its distance from the face. The further from the face (the eye) the glass is, the narrower will be the field of vision. It is rather like looking through a tunnel. The longer the tunnel, the smaller the field.

If a diver wears a mask above the surface of the water, there would be air just outside the mask and air within. This cancels any refraction by glass, just as things are not magnified when looking through a window. The field of vision is limited only by the size of the mask as no effective refraction occurs.

Underwater however, refraction between the water outside the mask and the air inside it reduces the field of vision. There is a limit to the degree that light can be bent: beyond a certain point, any light reaching the surface of the mask from one side will be reflected off the surface of the glass and none will reach the eye. This limit is an angle of 48.6 degrees on each side, making a total visual field of 97.2 degrees. Beyond this, all the light is reflected back into the water. A magnified image is paid for with a narrower field of vision.

MASK SQUEEZE A mask contains an air space, which must obey Boyle's Law (see page 21). As pressure increases with depth, mask volume decreases. This has the novel effect of attempting to suck out the diver's eyes and is called mask squeeze. For this reason, all diving masks include the nose so that air can be vented through the nostrils to compensate the pressure increase without a decrease in mask volume.

SHORT-SIGHTED DIVERS

It is fine to use a mask and depend on the water-glass-air interface to enable one to see under water, provided one has normally curved corneas. But what about those thousands of frustrated divers who have very curved corneas and are short-sighted? Their visual images are focused in front of their retinas, making a beautiful red fern coral look like a gaudy blob or a stone fish a brown blob until a poisonous spine is virtually up a nostril. What options are open to them?

Management of short-sightedness (myopia)

Five thousand years ago, the Chinese tried to cure myopia by sleeping with sand bags on their eyes. They understood that their corneas were too curved and were trying to flatten them. Nowadays there are three possibilities open to divers:

1. the use of prescription lenses in a mask,
2. the use of soft contact lenses, or
3. undergoing corneal surgery.

1. PRESCRIPTION LENSES These are the simplest means of correcting submarine myopia. Lenses are specifically ground and polished to the user's needs and then fixed to the glass of the mask. These adjust the angle of light waves reaching the over-curved cornea of a myopic eye, making it possible for a great white shark to be focused very nicely onto the retina. The mask should be a good one, fitting the user's face comfortably and easily as it will become a 'designer model', suited to one person only.

2. CONTACT LENSES These are probably the most convenient means of visual correction for divers. They may be soft or rigid gas permeable (RGP) lenses. Errors of refraction are corrected at the surface of the eye, making a specially modified mask unnecessary. Aside from avoiding the owl-like appearance of prescription lenses, they do have some real disadvantages, however. They have to be sterilised and cleaned, sensitive eyes will not tolerate them, and eye irritation and potentially serious and even blinding infection are potential complications. A downside is the risk of having one's mask inadvertently dislodged or kicked off during a dive. This will eliminate the surface tension that is needed to retain contact lenses in place and they may float off, to be lost forever in the sea. Disposable, cheap, soft contact lenses are ideal and divers who use contacts should ensure that they carry spare lenses.

    The cornea has no blood supply. It receives its oxygen by direct absorption from the air to which it is exposed. During decompression after hyperbaric conditions, the excess nitrogen absorbed diffuses directly from the cornea into the atmosphere. Being permeable to nitrogen and oxygen, contact lenses allow these interchanges of gases to occur. The older PMMA contact lenses do not permit speedy nitrogen diffusion with decompression, and corneal swelling or even bubbling is a potential hazard. Because of this, hard impermeable lenses are not safe for diving.

3. CORNEAL SURGERY There are three main options: radial keratotomy, LASIK (Laser in-situ keratomileusis) and Photorefractive Keratectomy (PRK). Whatever the option chosen, the subject must not be too short-sighted. Refractive errors are measured in dioptres (a unit of measurement of the refractive power of a lens equal to the reciprocal of the focal length in metres). A normal cornea requires a zero dioptre correction. A myopic cornea requires positive correction, but a maximum of six dioptres is generally acceptable for surgical intervention. Only adults should be operated on – myopia is usually maximal at about 20+ years. The candidate must be realistic in his or her hopes. The operation may provide only partial correction, not eliminating the need for lower prescription glasses.

    Complications include sensitivity to excessive light or glare, risk of infection, inability to drive at night due to oncoming headlights refracting in the scars and causing starbursts, and fluctuations in focus that can require the use of glasses on one day and not on another. The cornea may be overcorrected, causing the image to be focused behind the retina, the exact opposite of myopia, resulting in the patient still requiring glasses, this time for long-sightedness. Blindness or serious loss of vision are very uncommon.

    (a) **Radial keratotomy** This was the first surgical procedure developed and involves reducing the sharp curvature of the cornea by making tiny, radial, spoke-like cuts on the outer edge of the cornea. These weaken the periphery of the cornea which bulges outward because of the internal pressure of the eye, pulling on and flattening the central corneal area. The result is a cornea with a central shallow curvature and a peripheral sharp curvature. As the central area of the cornea over the iris is used for vision, the refracted image then falls closer to or on the retina.

    For those divers who undergo the procedure, awkward questions arise concerning nitrogen uptake and degassing in corneal scars. Increased pressure at depth should not be a problem, provided mask equalising is meticulously done. But beware of mask squeeze! The effect of relative vacuum on the distorted and weakened curvature of a keratotomised cornea could be much more severe than that on the even curvature of a normal (albeit myopic) cornea. Pressure distortion could have unpredictable consequences after radial keratotomy. At least three months should elapse before diving after this surgery.

(b) **LASIK** In the 1990s LASIK (Laser in-situ keratomileusis) was introduced to correct myopia. It is a surgical procedure in which a flap is cut in the cornea and pulled back to expose the corneal bed. This exposed surface is then ablated to the desired shape with a carbon dioxide or ultraviolet excimiter laser, following which the flap is replaced. Infection and corneal bubble injury may theoretically occur but the procedure appears to be safe in divers as no hyperbaric complications have been reported. After uncomplicated LASIK surgery, at least one month should elapse, with the ophthalmologist's approval, before diving again.

(c) **PRK** Next came Photorefractive Keratectomy (PRK), a procedure free of corneal incisions and also utilising ultraviolet excimer laser, with much fewer complications than radial keratotomy, and enabling divers to return to the water only a fortnight after uncomplicated surgery.

Recovery from other eye surgery options

1. Full-thickness corneal surgery requires six months off diving to allow the cornea to heal fully.
2. Pterygium removal, squint (strabismus) correction and eyelid plastic surgery – allow two weeks after all sutures have gone.
3. Surgery that involves the introduction of gas or air into the eyeball requires two months after all the gas has been completely absorbed.
4. In the case of cataract removal, the time varies:
   - scleral tunnel incision: one month,
   - corneal valve incision: two months, and
   - non-corneal valve incision: three months.

VISUAL STANDARDS FOR DIVERS

The minimum visual requirements for diving are surprisingly lax. Only enough is required to ensure an accurate buddy system, the ability to react to danger, safety around boats, and the capacity to read clearly pressure gauges and a timing device on the arm. So both far and near vision are required.

Far vision is commonly measured by the diver's ability to read letters on a distant chart. The Snellen chart has varying-sized rows of letters. A normal eye can read the line designated 6/6 or 20/20 from a distance of 6 metres (20 feet). The largest letter is designated 6/60 (20/200), meaning a normal (or far-sighted) eye can see it from a distance of 60 metres (200 ft).

Short-sighted people are unable to read the 6/6 line, but can make out one of the larger lines (6/9, 6/12, 6/18, 6/24, 6/36, 6/60). Using their glasses or contact lenses provides the correction. If fully corrected, they can then read the 6/6 line.

Being unable to visualise the 6/60 letter, even with corrective lenses, represents legal blindness as it means a loss of visual acuity of more than 80 per cent. Military and commercial standards vary but, for sport divers, at least one eye should be correctable to 6/9 (20/30).

Near vision is measured by the ability to read simple print, such as a newspaper. Here normal and short-sighted people cope, but far-sighted people need corrective lenses. Far-sightedness (hypermetropia) is just the reverse of short-sightedness. The curve of the corneal surface is too shallow and the visual image is focused behind the retina. Far-sighted divers generally don't use contact lenses because they would then only be able to read their gauges – everything else, including their buddy or a coral reef, would be blurred. Unless it is severe, far-sightedness is not generally corrected under water as bifocal mask lenses would be needed. These divers must ensure that the dials on their gauges and timing devices are large and luminous enough to be read under gloomy subsurface conditions. Some divers have solved the problem by using a corrective lens in one eye to read their gauges and using the other uncorrected eye for distance vision!

As one ages, the lens of the eye stiffens and its ability to fine-focus the image from the cornea on to the retina decreases. This usually becomes apparent after 40. Things close by become blurred and written material has to be held further and further away until the print becomes too small to read anyway. This is called presbyopia (Greek for 'old man's eyes'). Although the cornea is curved normally, the effect of the lens stiffening is similar to far-sightedness. Magnifying corrective lenses have to be used for reading on land, and underwater readouts must be large and bright.

Colour vision is the ability of the eye to distinguish between red and green when tones of these colours are presented in complex patterns. The Ishihara test uses coloured dots. Dotted numbers are seen against differently coloured dotted backgrounds. Inability to see these numbers is called colour blindness and is an inherited trait. Colour vision is completely irrelevant as far as sport scuba diving is concerned. The reason is simple – starting with red, colours are absorbed by water and disappear anyway as soon as one is more than a few metres deep. Below about 10 msw the sea is brown, green and blue.

Above water, colour vision is necessary if selecting colour-coded gas cylinders and communication wiring, or if navigation is required, particularly at night.

14

DIVING IMPLICATIONS OF MUSCULOSKELETAL DISEASE

The musculoskeletal system comprises the bony skeleton and the muscles that move articulating bones. Diving requires coordinated muscle action, plus strength and ease of joint movement. Conditions that would absolutely preclude diving are those that predispose to lumbar spine disorders, bone death (osteonecrosis), and ailments that may mimic, mask or provoke acute limb or joint decompression illness.

CRAMPS

Divers unused to swimming with fins often experience sudden spasm of leg muscles, usually the calves and soles, but sometimes the thighs and abdomen. The pain is extreme, makes swimming almost impossible and raises the spectre of drowning.

Prevention This involves physical fitness, regular swimming practise with fins, ensuring that fins do not have drag in excess of the strength of the diver, ensuring that wet suits are not too tight, and maintaining good nourishment and hydration.

Treatment The spasms are usually short-lived and often relieved by passive extension of the muscle in spasm.

LUMBAR SPINE DISORDERS

Man is the only creature on earth who always stands erect on two feet, maintaining a vertical spine against the unrelenting drag of gravity. Man is also the only creature who suffers from chronic backache. No one is immune and over 80 per cent of people will suffer from lower backache at one time or another in their lives. Of all the possible causes for permanent disability claims in the insurance industry, the commonest by far is back pain. It affects people of all sizes and shapes and in every occupational group – labourers and academics, fat and thin, muscular and scrawny, short and tall, male and female.

The spine is a stack of 26 bony vertebrae, each separated from the next by a fibrocartilaginous pad or disc. The discs act as elastic spacers, keeping the vertebrae apart and providing the spinal nerve roots, which arise directly from the spinal cord, room to pass between vertebrae and out of the spine. The discs also allow the tilting of one vertebra on another. Each individual tilt is small but the sum is the forwards, backwards or sideways movement of the spine.

In the vertical position, each disc supports the mass of the body above it, so the lowest discs, in the lumbar spine, bear the brunt in terms of compression force. Should compression on a lumbar disc become excessive, the disc tears and ruptures, with extrusion of the soft centre of the disc. The space between the two vertebrae decreases and the spinal nerves between them become pinched. Once a disc tears it stays torn; cartilage does not heal and repair itself like bone, muscle or skin, and any damage to a disc is permanent. But things can get worse: the spinal cord lies directly behind each disc and if extrusion of the disc pulp is backwards, the spinal cord itself becomes compressed – and a bed in an orthopaedic ward is guaranteed.

The problem is that, aside from crawling to keep the lumbar spine horizontal or living under zero-gravity conditions, there is little one can do about an inherent situation. Furthermore, if one is tall, there is more leverage and strain on the lower back. If one is brawny with big shoulders, it's even worse. If one is fat or has a comfortable belly, the same applies. The ideal vertical person is a petite pygmy.

From the point of view of your back, diving is both good and bad. It is good because neutral buoyancy is as close as anyone can get to zero-gravity conditions and absolute freedom from spinal strain. It is bad because divers have to lift, lug, haul and shove before they can achieve the luxury of weightlessness.

A little understanding of the mechanics of the lumbar spine will help to prevent undue stresses and avoid unnecessary damage. The lumbar spine is most stable in extension (leaning back) and least stable in flexion (leaning forwards), so the way to prevent damage is obvious – **don't bend forward and lift simultaneously.** Unfolding the normal inward curve of the lumbar spine by bending forward to pick up a bar of soap in the shower, or to tie a straggling shoelace, is a very common cause of acute lumbar disc damage and recurring backache for life. If just supporting the weight of the upper body by an unstable flexed lumbar spine is enough to rupture a disc, then attempting to lift a heavy cylinder, compressor or dive bag while bending over is lumbomechanical Russian roulette.

The solution is to use your head and then your legs. Face the object squarely. Get close to it, spread your feet and bend your knees. Keep your back straight and your upper body vertical to the ground. Hold the object firmly with both hands and straighten your knees, using the power of your thigh muscles and being careful not to lean forward. Use the same technique when putting an object down.

If you can't easily lift an object by squatting and using your legs, it's too heavy for you and you are also going to get a hernia, because squatting opens the hernial canals, while straining to lift completes the job.

Another way to nuture your back is to be aware of your posture. Don't slouch when sitting, rather walk tall and exercise your back. Strong back muscles provide muscular support and help to stabilise the lumbar spine. Brisk walking and extension exercises are the best. Deadlifts are worst and are well-named because bending over with straight legs and jerking up a heavy weight will inevitably crush your discs. Ensure an adequate intake of calcium in the diet. One gram a day will help to reduce the risk of osteoporosis, the condition characterised by progressive vertebral decalcification and softening of bone. If your diet is restricted by choice or design, speak to your doctor about your calcium and vitamin intake and, if you are female and fiftyish, about the advisability of female hormone replacement.

LUMBAR SPINAL SURGERY

Lumbar pain in a known back-sufferer after a dive may be difficult to distinguish from DCI (see page 128). Once disc protrusion has occurred, especially protrusion into the nerve root canals or spinal cord, surgery is usually inevitable. Once the operation is over, and providing it was successful and no complications such as sepsis occurred, you should allow three to six months before returning to diving. The presence of inserted stainless steel or titanium plates or clips does not affect diving but further severe pain, nerve involvement or weakness would bar any diving.

DYSBARIC OSTEONECROSIS

Dysbaric osteonecrosis (DON), also known as asceptic bone necrosis or bone rot, is an area of bone death and was first described in compressed air workers in caissons in the early 1900s. The connection between a history of joint bends and subsequent X-ray signs of death (necrosis) in bone was first made by a Chicago neurologist, Peter Bassoe, in 1913. Exposure to hyperbaric conditions does not have to be deep. The disease has occurred following caisson work at only 11 metres. Exposure does not even have to be repetitive. It occurred in three of five men who escaped from the submarine *Poseidon* in 1931, after being trapped at 38 msw for nearly three hours. The condition occurs very rarely in sport divers who dive up to 50 msw and who follow recommended sport diving tables and ascent rates.

PREDISPOSING FACTORS

DON occurs most frequently among older male commercial divers with a long diving history. The incidence increases with depth and dive time, being least common with short, shallow air dives, and most common with deep helium saturation dives, especially if the diver has a history of joint bends. Other predisposing factors are high blood fats, obesity, diabetes, peripheral vascular disease, haemoglobin disorders, alcoholism and the use of cortisone.

CAUSES OF DYSBARIC OSTEONECROSIS

DON is a disease of the long bones, that is, the arms and legs. Anyone who has eaten a marrow bone knows that there is a lot of fat in bone marrow. A lot of fat means a lot of possible nitrogen uptake with diving. Marrow bones are limb bones. The bones of the ribs, skull, pelvis and spine have very little fat and therefore less nitrogen storage capacity. Marrow could explain the reason for the condition ocurring in arms and legs. Food for thought? If one looks for common factors to try to explain DON in divers, three factors emerge:

1. fat metabolism is involved,
2. adequate blood supply and oxygen carriage by blood is important, and
3. conditions causing bone decalcification are relevant.

Interference with the blood supply causes the death of bone, fat and marrow cells supplied by the blood vessels involved. Breakdown of fat results in the liberation of free fatty acids. These acids attack calcium in bone and form dense soaps in the dead area. After some weeks, new blood vessels grow into the area from nearby normal bone and healing begins.

There is a definite relationship between DON and one's exposure to inadequate decompression, missed decompression, acute decompression illness and experimental diving. As a diver's breathing mixture consists of an inert gas and oxygen, both inert gas bubbles and oxygen toxicity have been blamed for DON.

INERT GAS BUBBLES   Bubbles may appear in arteries, capillaries or veins inside a bone, impairing the available blood (oxygen) supply to the bone after a dive. Bubbles may also occur in the bone marrow, outside blood vessels. On ascent, pressure drops and volume increases. The enlarging bubbles then compress the blood vessels from without but within a rigid bone and produce the same effect – interference with oxygen supply and hypoxia of bone. Even without a very heavy gas load, inadequate release of inert gas inside bone may occur after a dive. If lung degassing is impaired due to disorders of ventilation, perfusion and diffusion, then bubbling can result. Decompressing after a dive with the limbs in a very flexed position, such as sitting on folded or crossed legs, is not wise as it kinks the knee and hip veins, and prevents easy venous transport of inert gas to the lungs for exhalation.

OXYGEN TOXICITY   A high partial pressure of oxygen to the brain causes reflex constriction of blood vessels. People who breathe hyperbaric oxygen become pale. Reflex constriction of blood vessels in bone, if intense, could have the same effect as obstruction with bubbles – the tissues beyond the spastic vessels can become hypoxic. In addition, a too-high oxygen partial pressure may interfere with local metabolism in bone, disrupting glucose utilisation and the essential supply of energy to bone and marrow cells. High oxygen concentrations and pressures can cause the formation of free oxygen radicals. In its normal form, oxygen exists as two oxygen atoms linked together with no residual electrical charge. At a high partial pressure, this link may break, resulting in positively and negatively charged oxygen ions. These are intensely chemically active and may damage bony fibrous tissue (collagen) and fat and marrow cells in bone. Tissue damage then causes swelling within the tight confines of a bone and interferes with circulation, nitrogen release and bone nutrition.

VASOACTIVE SUBSTANCES Damage to fat cells may result in the release of vaso-active substances – chemical triggers that can result in clotting or sludging of blood inside the blood vessels in the area and further bone damage.

CLASSIFICATION OF DON

DON only affects long bones and, as the diagnosis is made after viewing an X-ray of a bone, the disease is classified according to its X-ray appearance. It can affect the extreme end of a bone (the metaphysis) just below the joint surface. As a result, the joint surface may gradually collapse with pressure of use. Loss of the smooth curved articular surface and subsequent arthritis occur. These are called Type A lesions and occur more commonly at the large joints of the shoulder, hip and knee. DON can also occur in the head, neck or shaft of a bone behind the metaphysis. These are called medullary or Type B lesions, and rarely cause too much trouble, as healing usually occurs as with a fracture of a limb.

The difference between DON and a bone fracture is that in DON the diver may be totally unaware of any activity in his bones, as it is usually a painless procedure until joint distortion occurs. X-ray changes are late signs of DON. They may take three or more months or longer to develop. To detect DON before gross joint collapse occurs, computerised scanning techniques are used. A tracer dose of radioactive technetium 99 (Tc 99) is injected, and scanning detects 'hot spots' in damaged bone; but practical considerations and cost limit the usefulness of isotope studies to symptomatic cases.

Whether divers should routinely have their long bones X-rayed has been a hotly debated point. In the UK, it is recommended that commercial divers working below 12 msw have X-rays of their long bones before any hyperbaric exposure, and then again every two years, as well as immediately after and again four months after any joint bend. Divers are understandably loath to undergo repeated irradiation and they argue that debilitating DON is rare. The incidence varies greatly from country to country: in a survey of more than 4 000 British divers, the Decompression Sickness Central Registry of the UK's Medical Research Council reported a six per cent incid-ence of bone necrosis. Of these, the vast majority had shaft or only suspected joint involvement. Only one per cent of commercial divers had definite joint involvement and, of the one per cent, very few had actual gross damage to the joint surface.

So in the UK series, DON with serious joint damage or disability was rare. How-ever, Chinese commercial divers have reported an 80 per cent incidence – which only goes to show how fiendish Oriental nitrogen can be!

DIVING AFTER DON

Once Type A DON with joint involvement has occurred, diving must be stopped. Type B involvement of the head or shaft of a bone will heal and diving may continue after healing. Unexplained DON is a problem because it may indicate susceptibil-ity to DON. If it occurs in a diver who always dived within the rules, future diving should be limited to diving to a maximum depth of 18 msw.

CONDITIONS THAT MIMIC OR MASK
ACUTE LIMB DECOMPRESSION SICKNESS

A number of disorders can present with joint pain and can be confused with acute limb decompression illness after diving. The problem is compounded because any pre-existing inflammation or swelling of a joint will interfere with capillary circulation, diffusion and the transport of inert gas after a dive, and predispose to a bend in that joint. The diver will then assure everybody that the pain is due to an old sports injury and is old-hat and of no particular diving significance. While he or she swallows an anti-inflammatory tablet or a painkiller, joint DON begins, never to be recognised as such because the subsequent destruction will be attributed to ongoing or repeated inflammation and only-to-be-expected arthritis.

GOUT

Acute gout is caused by an elevated uric acid level in the body and presents with exquisitely painful swelling and redness over a joint. The smaller joints of the hands and feet are usually involved but major limb joints can be affected. It is barely conceivable that anyone experiencing an acute gout attack would want to dive, but it is very important that the diver waits for all swelling to subside once the acute pain has been treated and ensures that the blood uric acid level is properly controlled.

RHEUMATOID ARTHRITIS

This illness belongs to the auto-immune group of diseases, such as systemic lupus erythematosis, where the body produces antibodies against its own tissues and then responds with inflammation to the resulting damage. It is a process of auto-destruction and may result in severe deformity and crippling of joints. It usually first involves the small joints of the fingers but can affect any joint or connective tissue. Like gout, the inflammatory process in rheumatoid arthritis can mimic or predispose to acute decompression illness.

Unlike gout, rheumatoid arthritis is usually progressive and the treatment often involves ongoing use of drugs such as anti-inflammatories, methotrexate, gold salts, Immuran and cortisone. These alone usually bar diving, and ongoing pain and joint deformity make diving risky.

VENEREAL DISEASES

Syphilis, gonorrhoea and non-specific urethritis (NSU) are not simply diseases of the reproductive system. Their effects can be generalised and arthritis is not uncommon. Once again, bends and DON are hazards, and diving must wait until treatment is complete and any joint swelling has subsided. Chronic or tertiary syphilis may produce gross joint destruction and diving is then disallowed. Late syphilis often presents with severe neurological involvement.

BONE INJURIES

Diving is not permitted during the healing of any bony fracture. Difficulty with togging up, wetting a plaster cast, infection by aquatic bacteria and worsening the fracture by diving activity make this necessary. Healing of the bone and its associated blood vessels must be complete, and the length of time required will depend on the severity of the injury and the presence of any complications, such as infection. A conservative approach is usually taken with fractures of limb bones, especially the weight-bearing bones of the legs, because of the possibility of developing acute limb decompression illness and DON at an incompletely healed fracture site. Metal implants and plates are acceptable.

If no complications occur, allow the following period of time to elapse before resuming diving:
– femur (thigh bone) and hip or knee transplants: 6 months,
– fractures of the tibia (shin bone): 6 months,
– fractures of the fibula (lower leg bone): 6–10 weeks,
– fractures of the humerus (upper arm bone) or a humeral head (shoulder) transplant: 6–10 weeks, and
– fractures of the radius or ulna (forearm bones) or wrist implants: 6 weeks.

If a sprain, not a fracture, has occurred and the diver is wearing a plastic cast with water-repellent liner to allow bathing, diving may be considered if mobility is good and the requirements of diving can be met.

Before diving can be resumed after limb bone fractures, all swelling must have subsided and X-rays must be done to confirm that healing is complete.

Fractures of the sinuses bear mention in that the thin bones of the maxillary, ethmoid and frontal sinuses are also the walls of the eye socket. It depends on how you look at the injury: is a fracture of a paper-thin bone that separates an eye from a sinus cavity a fracture of the eye socket or a fracture of a sinus? In any event, a Valsalva manoeuvre (see page 115) or reverse block on ascent can drive air in a sinus into the tissue around the eyeball (orbital surgical emphysema).

SCOLIOSIS

A side-to-side curvature of the spine is called scoliosis. From a diving point of view, it is only significant if it impairs breathing, predisposes the diver to CO_2 retention or pulmonary barotrauma (see page 160), or causes pain or equipment problems. Surgery may then be needed.

BONE INFECTIONS

Infection in bone usually follows an injury, with or without a fracture, that breaks the skin and exposes underlying bone. Disrupting the integrity of the skin provides a route for bacterial invasion and, if a bone is injured too, the likelihood of bone and bone marrow infection (osteomyelitis) is high and may become chronic. Any bone infection must be completely cured before diving resumes.

SOFT TISSUE INJURIES

Any significant bruise, sprain or strain that causes swelling or pain on movement should be allowed to heal before diving is recommended, as reduced mobility and interference with degassing may occur. This may require only a few days, or several months in the case of severe tearing of the ligaments of an ankle or knee. Painless full function must first be restored.

MUSCULAR DISORDERS

There are a number of relatively uncommon muscle disorders, most of which are familial, which present with insidious and progressive muscle weakness with or without obvious wasting. Some present during childhood and others during adult life. They are collectively known as the **muscular dystrophies.** In some cases, the degree of wasting and weakness is very slight. In others, the patient may be wasted, deformed and bedridden. The different types are characterised by the muscle groups first affected; for example, the calves or the shoulder girdle muscles. As a general rule, people with muscular dystrophy must not dive, but if the degree of disability and weakness is slight, a decision to dive may be made by the diving physician and the muscle specialist.

Another rare disorder which causes weakness and easy fatigability of muscle is **myasthenia gravis.** It usually effects the muscles of the face and throat, as well as the muscles of respiration. The primary defect is a chemical abnormality at the precise site where nerve impulses are transmitted to muscle fibres. Nerve signals from the brain ordering a particular group of muscles to contract are blocked and the muscles do not respond. As the disease may affect muscles of the respiratory system – one of the vital systems needed in diving – people with myasthenia gravis may not dive.

15

DIVING IMPLICATIONS OF GASTROINTESTINAL DISEASE

Aside from being the site of alcohol absorption, the gastrointestinal system is important from a diver's point of view because it is subject to common ailments such as
diarrhoea and vomiting, and pain in the abdomen may mimic acute decompression
illness. Being open to the air via the mouth, it is also subject to barotrauma. Diving
should be stopped if any abdominal symptom is present. Abdominal pain under water
can be incapacitating; vomiting can result in water inhalation and, together with
diarrhoea, predispose the diver to dehydration and acute decompression illness.

Some conditions temporarily exclude diving until treated. All ongoing or intermittent chronic diseases of the gastrointestinal system causing pain, vomiting, diarrhoea
and fluid or blood loss permanently bar scuba diving.

PEPTIC ULCERS

Gastric ulcers affect the stomach, and duodenal ulcers involve the duodenum, which
drains the stomach via the pyloric valve. Collectively they are called peptic ulcers. They
are erosions in the inner membrane lining of the stomach or duodenum and can deeply
penetrate or even perforate the underlying smooth muscle wall of the gut. Their cause
has been attributed to a number of factors including stress, excessive hydrochloric acid
production by the stomach, inadequate acid production, abnormalities of the immune
system, and the side-effects of medicines such as aspirin, cortisone and non-steroidal
anti-inflammatory drugs (NSAIDs). An interesting finding has been the presence of
the bacterium *Helicobacter pylori* in the floor of many duodenal ulcers, adding an infective agent to the list of causes.

Scuba diving is contraindicated with active acute or chronic gastric or duodenal
ulceration. Pain may mask acute abdominal decompression illness, and spasm of the
muscles of the stomach may predispose to gas trapping and stomach barotrauma
of ascent (see page 167). Healing should be complete and proven by direct optical
examination of the stomach and duodenum by gastroscopy.

GALLSTONES

Bile is produced in the liver and stored in the gall bladder. It contains bile salts which
emulsify fats during digestion, and bile pigments which are the breakdown products
of haemoglobin released during normal red blood cell replacement in the body. Bile

also serves as a route for excreting many end-products of normal metabolism and ridding the body of drugs, toxins and medications. During a meal, the gall bladder contracts, sending a flow of bile into the duodenum to assist digestion.

Gallstones occur when bile pigments in the gall bladder come out of solution in bile. This is often preceded by an episode of gall bladder inflammation (cholecystitis). The initial deposit of inflammatory cells and pigment slowly grows by accumulating further layers of pigment. There may be only a few or up to hundreds of gallstones present but the individual is usually unaware of the growing stone crop until one of them jams in the duct leading from the gall bladder to the duodenum. The chances of this happening are about two per cent each year. Violently painful biliary colic results and the invariable outcome is the surgical removal of the gall bladder.

Diving may be permitted with silent gallstones, as most cases are only diagnosed incidentally while X-raying or scanning the abdomen for an unrelated complaint. In any event, many divers with gallstones will not even know they have them. Once an attack of acute inflammation of the gall bladder occurs, or a stone makes its presence felt, diving should stop until the gall bladder has been removed and all symptoms have disappeared. In commercial diving, six months off diving work after surgery is recommended. Among sport divers, any earlier clearance to dive must be obtained from a diving physician.

SPASTIC COLON

Also called irritable bowel syndrome (IBS), the main feature of this condition is colicky abdominal pain. Although diarrhoea or constipation may also be present, all investigations are essentially normal. Pain is attributed to incoordinate contractions and spasm of the muscle in the bowel wall. There is usually a strong history of emotional, financial or work stress.

Divers with a history of spastic colon must exert great caution during an acute attack or if they are on medication. Although most antispasmodics are considered safe by many diving physicians, disturbances in vision and blood pressure control, as well as drowsiness, can occur. Because of a strong emotional overlay, many people with spastic colons are also using tranquillisers or antidepressants, and great care and consideration are then needed in the decision about diving safety.

GASTROENTERITIS

Viral infection of the gastrointestinal tract is extremely common. Occurring most often during spring and early summer, it almost vies in frequency with winter colds and coughs. Nausea, vomiting, abdominal cramps and diarrhoea, in any combination, occur. A common bacterial variety is a 24-hour episode of diarrhoea and vomiting due to coliform bacteria following stool contamination of food. It is invariably self-limiting. The importance of these symptoms from a diver's point of view is threefold:
1.   Cramps can cause underwater incapacity.
2.   Fluid loss predisposes to acute decompression illness.

3. The condition can occur while on holiday in a remote area and the diver must be able to cope with the situation. Divers must be aware of the potential for developing gastroenteritis and should obtain a prescription and discuss the safe use of any of the following medications (see below) with his or her doctor before embarking on a diving trip to a remote destination.

Management of gastroenteritis

1. Stop all diving.
2. Stop any dairy product intake and the consumption of fatty foods. All food should be bland, and boiled, baked or lightly grilled. Boiled chicken, fish, rice, pumpkin, potatoes and thin, clear soup are examples of suitable foods.
3. Encourage fluid intake. Replacing lost body fluids is the cornerstone of treatment. Water, weak black tea, soda water, and fruit juice diluted 1:1 with water are examples.
4. If nausea or vomiting persist, antiemetics are required. Many are available and include dimenhydrinate, metoclopramide, domperidone, cyclizine and prochlorperazine. If vomiting is the major feature, oral use of these drugs may be ineffective as they will be rejected almost as soon as they are swallowed. Rectal suppositories of cyclizine or prochlorperazine may then help. If frequent diarrhoea makes this impractical, an intramuscular injection by a doctor of an antiemetic such as cyclizine or prochlorperazine may be required.
5. Abdominal cramps are commonly handled by the use of antispasmodics such as hyoscine and atropine sulphate.
6. Diarrhoea can usually be controlled by dietary restriction and adequate fluid intake. If persistent, loperamide or diphenoxylate with atropine sulphate are usually effective. Binding agents containing the clay kaolin, apple pectin and milk of bismuth may also help. If ineffective, you can try the combination of kanamycin sulphate, aminopentamide, pectin, bismuth subcarbonate and activated attapulgite (marketed as Kantrexil in South Africa).
7. In severe cases, hospitalisation is required for intravenous replacement of fluid and electrolytes (such as Ringer's lactate plus added potassium chloride) to combat dehydration and electrolyte loss.

BACTERIAL DIARRHOEA

Bacterial diarrhoeas (salmonella and shigella enteritis) are most commonly spread by the stool-oral route – eating food contaminated by flies or prepared by infected food handlers with poor personal hygiene. In divers, contamination can also occur after entering sewage-contaminated water. Enteric fever is caused by the salmonella species. The shigella species causes bacterial dysentery and, if water-spread, shigella can survive up to three days in sea water. Diarrhoea may be profuse and mucus and blood may be present, with severe cramping, pain and fever. Nausea and vomiting are common.

Management of bacterial diarrhoeas

Prevention

1. Try to determine whether any particular bacterial dysentery is currently prevalent in an area before embarking on a dive trip.
2. Ask your doctor about the advisability of taking suitable antibiotic therapy, such as norfloxacin, with you on the trip.
3. Avoid eating dubious foods, including potentially contaminated fruits and vegetables, and drinking local water in areas with primitive sanitation.
4. Take an adequate supply of bottled water, or boil or chlorinate water before drinking. Remember that the ice-cubes in your drink may be contaminated!
5. Avoid diving in areas contaminated by sewage.

Treatment

1. General management is on the same lines as gastroenteritis (see page 133).
2. If fever becomes a persistent feature, or mucus and blood appear in the stool, medical assistance is necessary as the various bacteria have different sensitivities to antibiotics.
3. If medical help is unavailable, oral norfloxacin (400 mg twice a day for three days) generally provides cover against all salmonella and shigella dysenteries. Previous discussion with and permission from a doctor is necessary, and norfloxacin must not be used before puberty.

PARASITIC DIARRHOEAS

These occur commonly in primitive or outlying areas. Two parasites are primarily involved: amoebic dysentery is caused by the single-celled organism *Entamoeba histolytica* and can present with severe, bloody and profuse diarrhoea, followed by rapid collapse. Emergency medical help is necessary. Giardia infections are caused by the parasite *Giardia lamblia* and diarrhoea, bloating and severe cramps occur. The basic treatment of both amoebiasis and giardiasis is metronidazole, but additional fluid and electrolyte support and intravenous therapy may be needed.

HEARTBURN

Heartburn is caused by the reflux of acidic stomach contents into the food pipe (oesophagus). This is called gastro-oesophageal reflux disease or GORD (spelled GERD in the USA). It presents with burning in the upper abdomen and behind the breastbone, bloatedness, biliousness, an acidic taste in the mouth and sometimes frank regurgitation of food.

It is often precipitated by overindulgence in food, coffee or alcohol or consumption of chillies or curries. Obesity, anti-inflammatories and smoking worsen it. Foods that cause reflux should be avoided before diving, as should the other aggravating factors.

Should acid spill-over from the oesophagus into the airways occur, bronchospasm presenting as asthma may result. A tight wet suit, weight belt and body straps can also cause reflux, as can ascent after swallowing to equalise on descent. If food regurgitation occurs under water, inhalation or choking may happen.

HIATUS HERNIA

The term 'hernia' refers to the protrusion of any portion of the gut through a defect in any part of the wall of the abdomen. A hiatus hernia occurs when a segment of the stomach, near the entry of the foodpipe into the stomach, slides or rolls through a weakness in the diaphragm and into the chest cavity. This weakness exists where the foodpipe penetrates through the diaphragm to reach the stomach. It presents with a feeling of fullness in the upper abdomen, or frank heartburn, and commonly occurs at night in bed. Sitting up helps, as gravity then causes the herniated part of the stomach to fall back.

The importance of a hiatus hernia in divers relates to gear. Tight suits, straps, weight belts and buoyancy jackets may press on the abdomen and encourage herniation. Divers who equalise by air swallowing (aerophagia) may also develop difficulty if air trapping occurs at depth in a roll of herniated stomach. Acute pain due to expanding air on ascent may occur. Divers with hiatus hernias should ensure their gear fits comfortably, and those who develop upper abdominal or low chest pain during or after diving should speak to their doctors about the possibility of a hiatus hernia.

In most cases, dietary care, losing excess weight and the occasional use of antispasmodics and antacids controls the hernia. Only rarely is it so severe that surgery is required – a procedure called a Nissan fundoplasty is then generally curative.

OTHER HERNIAS

There are several other potentially weak sites in the front of the abdominal wall through which the bowel can herniate. The most common places are the groins, the navel and the mid-abdomen after childbirth, when the exertions of labour strain the vertical rectus muscles straddling the middle of the abdomen, leaving a gap between them (divaricated recti).

Commercial divers may not dive with a hernia as their work inevitably demands heavy lifting. Sport divers need to be able to lift their compressors and cylinders and should therefore have their hernias repaired. The wound must be fully healed before diving resumes (three to six months, depending on the amount of boat handling, lugging and lifting done). The same would apply to any abdominal surgery.

COLOSTOMIES

Some diseases of the bowel, such as cancer and Crohn's disease, may be of such a severe nature that the bowel or rectum has to be removed. The lower end of the remaining bowel is then brought through the front wall of the abdomen and joined to the surface of the skin. Emptying of the colon is done into a special bag placed over the opening. Diving is not a problem, but care must be taken not to injure the delicate site of anastomosis by straps or a weight belt.

ULCERATIVE COLITIS

This disease of unknown cause manifests as ulceration of the inner lining of the bowel and presents with diarrhoea, blood in the stool, abdominal pain, weakness and weight loss. It is treated symptomatically with drugs such as sulphasalazine, olsalazine, mesalazine and cortisone. In some cases, the colon has to be removed.

Ulcerative colitis is a relapsing condition with periods of relative normalcy followed by episodes of acute recurrent bloody diarrhoea. Diving is generally prohibited, especially during acute attacks.

CROHN'S DISEASE

Also a disease of unknown cause, Crohn's disease results in patchy inflammation of the gut with thickening and scarring. It interferes with normal bowel motility and presents with pain. It may proceed to malignancy. Removal of the affected bowel sections is commonly required. Diving is generally prohibited in sufferers unless remission is excellent.

PANCREATITIS

The most common cause of an inflammation of the pancreas is long-term alcohol abuse, although a single episode of excessive alcohol abuse can also lead to irreparable damage to the pancreas. The pancreas produces digestive enzymes and damage results in abnormalities of digestion and food absorption. Liver damage due to alcohol is usually present too. Diving is prohibited.

Pancreatitis may follow penetration of a peptic ulcer through the back wall of the stomach or duodenum into the pancreas behind. It can also occur if a gallstone blocks a common bile and pancreatic duct. Further diving would then depend on treatment and healing of the ulcer or gall bladder problem and the return of normal pancreatic function.

HEPATITIS

Acute viral infections of the liver are not unusual and usually proceed to complete healing and recovery and subsequent life-long immunity. The most common viruses causing the condition are Type A and Type B hepatitis viruses, although Types C, D and E also occur. The disease presents with jaundice – the staining of body tissues, including the skin and whites of the eyes, with bile pigment as a result of obstruction of the normal bile flow from the liver and spillover of bile pigment into the blood.

Hepatitis A is spread by direct contact with infected persons, and hepatitis B by blood contact, contaminated needles and syringes, and sexual contact. Vaccines immunising against hepatitis A and B are readily available. Three injections, given over a few months, are required to ensure permanent immunity.

It is highly recommended that every diver be immunised against hepatitis B, as the chances of contamination by infected blood during an emergency diver rescue or resuscitation attempt are very real.

A vaccine for Hepatitis C does not yet exist and the possibility of infection via sharing of regulators has been raised. Cleaning them with disinfectant after diving is recommended.

Hepatitis is a considerable insult to the liver and diving should only be renewed six months after liver function tests have completely returned to normal. Hepatitis B may progress to chronic hepatitis, the person being apparently well but being an active carrier and capable of spreading the disease. Diving is then permanently prohibited.

In severe cases of acute hepatitis of either type, permanent damage to the architecture of the liver may result, leading to scarring and cirrhosis of the liver. With chronic liver disease, obstruction to normal venous flow occurs with opening of venous shunts. Multiple arterio-venous shunts predispose to venous bubble spillover into the arterial system and arterial gas embolism. Diving is permanently prohibited.

GENITOURINARY DISEASES

Aside from chronic renal failure and kidney transplants, disorders of the genitourinary system usually do not permanently bar sport diving. Common urinary tract infections, such as cystitis, can be treated with antibiotic medication, but urinary tract obstructions or kidney stones may need medical intervention and treatment. Surgery usually means a six-week layoff from diving.

Sexually transmitted infections require conventional treatment. These include syphilis, gonorrhoea, chlamydia and genital herpes and, unless the complications of advanced disease, such as arthritis are present, do not bar diving.

16

DIVING IMPLICATIONS OF HIV/AIDS

During the mid-1970s a killer virus spread silently and unnoticed to all continents. Between 1981 and 1985 the virus was identified and information about a new, lethal and incurable sexually transmitted disease reached an unbelieving world. AIDS, or Acquired Immune Deficiency Syndrome, now threatens to be the greatest and most frightening epidemic the world has ever known. The disease is caused by the Human Immunodeficiency Virus (HIV) and two distinct types of HIV diseases have been found, HIV-1 and HIV-2.

The HIV-2 epidemic originated and is still concentrated in West Africa, but has spread beyond its borders following the emigration of HIV-2-afflicted locals or by tourists who had sexual contact with infected West Africans. Initially, the HIV-1 epidemic was most prevalent among the homosexual population and intravenous drug abusers of North America, Brazil, Western Europe, Australia and New Zealand. A second pattern of spread – from bisexuals to the heterosexual population – occurred in sub-Saharan Africa, South America (particularly in Brazil), and in the Caribbean. A third, more recent spread, occurred through North Africa, the Middle East, Eastern Europe, Asia and the Pacific.

By mid-1992, the World Health Organisation (WHO) estimated that 10–12 million people throughout the world were HIV-positive. Most will die prematurely. In 2006 the figure was 39.5 million, and the incidence is still increasing.

The overwhelming majority of cases (about 60 per cent of the world total) are in sub-Saharan Africa, where much of the spread has been attributed to infected prostitutes passing the disease to transport drivers working the central to southern Africa routes. The highest incidence of HIV occurs in Kenya, Zaire, Uganda, Tanzania, Zambia, Malawi, Mozambique and Zimbabwe where the disease is spreading at a horrific rate, with some estimated figures approaching well over half of the sexually active population in some areas of these countries.

In South Africa, the incidence of HIV is highest in KwaZulu-Natal and lowest in the Western Cape.

METHODS OF SPREAD
1. Vaginal, anal or oral sexual contact with an infected partner.
2. Sharing contaminated needles among drug abusers.
3. Blood transfusions with HIV-infected blood.
4. Infection of the newborn by an HIV-positive mother.

5. Tattoos, acupuncture etc. with contaminated needles.
6. Needle-stick or scalpel injury in medical staff working with HIV-positive patients.
7. Giving CPR to an HIV-positive victim with blood in their airways.

The disease is only spread by infected blood or sexual contact. Mosquitoes have not been shown to carry the HIV virus. Kissing or saliva contact does not cause infection, unless there is blood in the saliva, nor do sweat or urine contact. Touching, sneezing, coughing, working together, or sharing food utensils, towels, combs etc. cannot cause the spread of AIDS. Dry blood is not infective – the virus is dead.

THE DISEASE PROCESS

There are several types of white blood cells in the body. Some act as scavengers, actively ingesting and destroying foreign bacteria and viruses. Others, such as the lymphocytes, are involved in the immune system. There are two main groups of lymphocytes – the T lymphocytes and the B lymphocytes. Once the HIV virus is in a new host, it invades a particular type of T lymphocyte: the T4 helper lymphocyte. These normally function by inducing B lymphocytes to produce antibodies, and other specialised cells to release substances toxic to invading organisms. Inside the T4 cell, the HIV virus invades the cell genes and incorporates itself right into the DNA genetic material of the T4 cell. The cell loses its helper function and is repro-grammed into an HIV factory. During the initial few months following infection with the disease, proliferation of the HIV virus is explosive, with the takeover of tril-lions and trillions of T4 cells. The diagnosis depends on the detection of antibodies produced by the body in response to HIV invasion, and the virus attacks the very heart of antibody production – the T4 helper lymphocyte. So the victim first remains HIV-negative on testing. This initial period of HIV-negativity is called the **window period**. The person will test HIV-negative because antibodies are below detectable levels, but he or she will be enormously infective to others because of the prodigious duplication of HIV virus that occurs during the window period.

Only after about six weeks will the person convert to HIV-positivity on testing a sample of blood, urine or saliva. It must be clearly understood that this test only measures **antibodies** produced by the victim. It does not test for the virus itself, and only blood is infective. At this point, the profound replication of the virus dimin-ishes and may appear dormant for many years, but incidental infections demanding antibody production may reactivate HIV proliferation for a while.

Finally, the immune system fails and full-blown AIDS appears. It does not present as a disease in itself, but it allows other infections to manifest. Diseases such as tuberculosis may be acquired for the first time or become reactivated if long dormant. Other opportunistic diseases, which virtually never gain a lethal foothold in a healthy individual, appear. These include certain parasitic, bacterial, viral and fungal infections, as well as some cancerous tumours.

Management of HIV/AIDS

This comprises prevention of initial infection and appropriate drug control of HIV-positive persons. There is no cure, but with an effective and properly maintained treatment regime, an HIV-positive person can continue to live a productive life. However, once HIV-positivity becomes full-blown AIDS, the death rate is 100 per cent. HIV infection is escalating at a phenomenal pace now that it is well entrenched around the world, and sexual promiscuity has become a lethal game. Condoms, previously used to prevent pregnancy, must now be used to prevent death.

DIVING AND AIDS

HIV-positive persons should probably not dive, at least not without informing their buddies of the situation. There is a moral obligation, because a rescuer may have to resuscitate a bleeding HIV victim. Ideally, this should also mean wearing a Medic-alert necklace informing an unknown rescuer that the victim is HIV-positive and that precautions are necessary, but the ethical, personal and social ramifications of acknowledging that one is HIV-positive are still raging in most countries.

Non-contact non-return mouth-to-mouth airways are available for emergency use, but the problem with CPR is its urgency. A suitable airway would have to be immediately on hand at all times – on the dive boat, at the shore base, and perhaps even in the buddy's BC pocket. Suitable gloves, plastic aprons and goggles are also necessary to avoid inadvertent blood contact through existing skin injuries or via the eyes, should the victim be coughing or spluttering blood.

The dilemma is a truly dreadful one for rescue personnel and any first-responder, because an emergency can occur at any time on land or sea. There are instances where unwitting rescuers have paid with their lives for saving an HIV-positive victim.

Once full-blown AIDS is present, diving must be totally barred.

17

DIVING IMPLICATIONS
OF ENDOCRINE DISEASE

Endocrine disease involves the hormone-producing glands of the body – the pituitary, adrenal, thyroid, parathyroid, pancreas, testes and ovaries. Uncontrolled endocrine disease presents with serious symptoms and signs and results in immediate unfitness to dive. Diabetes mellitus is a common condition that, like asthma, has been a bone of contention between divers and doctors for years.

DIABETES MELLITUS

For many years, it was considered unsafe for diabetes sufferers to dive, but this is no longer necessarily the case. Diabetes mellitus is a disorder associated with an abnormally high level of glucose in the blood. In young people, it usually presents with a history of excessive thirst, dry mouth, weight loss despite a voracious appetite, the need to urinate excessively frequently, or unheralded coma. In older people, the symptoms are often not so dramatic and the diagnosis is either made during a routine check-up by finding sugar in the urine, or after the doctor becomes suspicious and investigates because of recurring infections, such as boils or conjunctivitis.

The disease is caused by failure of specialised cells in the pancreas (called the islets of Langerhans) to produce enough insulin, the primary glucose-reducing hormone.

DIABETES OCCURS IN TWO DISTINCT FORMS:

1. **Insulin-dependent diabetes mellitus** (IDDM) occurs mostly in children and young adults and requires regular injections of insulin for control. The difficulty with insulin-dependent diabetes is that the sufferer is poised on a balance with coma on either side. Inadequate insulin can lead to coma due to an excessively high blood sugar level (hyperglycaemia). This typically takes several hours to develop. Excess insulin or forgetting or failing to eat after an insulin injection results in a very low glucose level (hypoglycaemia) which also causes coma. Hypoglycaemic coma occurs rapidly and brain cells, which are totally dependent on an adequate glucose supply, start to die.

2. **Non-insulin-dependent diabetes mellitus** (NIDDM) begins later in life and usually can be controlled by dietary restriction alone, or added oral therapy to

stimulate the pancreas to produce insulin. Coma generally only occurs after inadvertently taking too many oral tablets.

SHOULD DIABETIC PERSONS SCUBA DIVE? Controlling diabetes has become very sophisticated, with many diabetics using portable electronic glucometers to monitor their blood glucose levels, and achieving excellent control by strict attention to diet, insulin injections or oral medication, and exercise.

In June 1994, a meeting was held in New Orleans between members of the Council on Exercise of the American Diabetes Association and the diving committee of the Undersea and Hyperbaric Medical Society (UHMS) to examine the question of diabetes being a disqualifying condition for divers. It was only in 2005, at a workshop on diabetes and recreational diving sponsored by UHMS and Divers Alert Network (DAN), that a guideline for diabetic sport divers was produced by Dr Neal Pollock of Duke University Medical Centre (Durham, North Carolina, USA). It was emphasised that this is a list of guidelines only and not rules. Each interest group must use them as they best serve their community's needs. This author has drawn up a protocol based on these guidelines (see below).

PROTOCOL GUIDELINES FOR SPORT DIVING BY DIABETICS

This protocol must be regarded as the minimum requirements to adhere to before recreational diving is even contemplated by a diabetic. It does not condone diving by brittle, unstable or uncontrolled diabetics or permit anyone with any diabetic complications to dive.

THE FOLLOWING DIABETICS MUST NOT SCUBA DIVE:
- Diabetics under the age of 18 years.
- Qualified divers who have commenced insulin treatment within the last six months.
- New divers who have commenced insulin treatment within the last 12 months.
- Diabetics with a history of loss of consciousness or who have required the assistance of others within the last 12 months.
- Those with diabetic complications, i.e. involvement of the eyes, kidneys, peripheral nerves or arteries, or the coronary arteries.
- Individuals who cannot 'feel' that their blood sugar is low (hypoglycaemic unawareness). Most diabetics develop recognisable symptoms when their blood sugar falls, such as excessive sweatiness, extreme paleness, intense hunger, a rapid pulse or heart palpitations, sudden anxiety or uneasiness, exaggerated yawning and headache. They learn to recognise these symptoms for what they

mean and are able to take urgent corrective steps in the form of oral glucose. With hypoglycaemic unawareness, coma may be the first presenting feature.

- Those who have poor or inadequate control of their diabetes, i.e. an average blood glucose of more than 8 mmol/litre or less than 4 mmol/litre or an HbA1c above 8 per cent.

GUIDELINES FOR THE DIABETIC DIVER

1. The diabetic diver must be fit, well educated about diabetes, and be well controlled on diet, insulin or oral treatment.
2. There must excellent appreciation of the roles of exercise, stress and body temperature in blood glucose control.
3. This control must be regularly monitored (at least six-monthly) by a diabetes specialist.
4. An annual medical must be had with a diving doctor, including a resting and effort electrocardiogram.
5. The diabetic diver must be proficient at using and interpreting a blood glucometer and must carry it with him or her at all times.
6. Two diabetics must not form a buddy pair.

GUIDELINES FOR THE BUDDY, INSTRUCTOR, DIVE MARSHAL AND BOATSPERSON

1. These persons must be taught, by the diver, about diabetes and notified immediately should any problems occur after diving. They should be given a basic pamphlet or booklet about diabetes. This invariably means that a diabetic diver develops a network of knowledgeable buddies with whom he or she always dives.
2. They must be shown how to use and read a blood glucometer.
3. They must be taught what to do in the event of hypoglycaemia.
4. They must be informed of the dive plan and that the plan must be strictly adhered to. As the saying goes, 'plan the dive and dive the plan'.

ACTION BEFORE DIVING

1. Both the diabetic and the buddy must be well hydrated by drinking 500 ml water before the dive.
2. Ensure some carbohydrate intake about one hour before diving.
3. Monitor the blood glucose level 60 minutes, 30 minutes and immediately before the dive on the boat. It must be slightly elevated at about 8 mmol/litre for all three measurements.
4. The diver must ensure that mask oxygen (or better, demand valve oxygen) is available on the boat.
5. The diver must ensure that a supply of oral glucose and two injectable glucagon kits are available on the boat.

6. The diver should carry glucose tablets (or some form of oral glucose e.g. squeeze tube) in a sealed collapsible container in a pocket of the BC in case he or she gets 'lost' or experiences an impending hypoglycaemia situation.
7. The diver should carry a flare, flag or other method of attracting attention.
8. Making an 'L' using the thumb and index finger of either hand has been recommended as a signal for possible hypoglycaemia.
9. Seasick diabetics **must not dive**, or must abort their dive. Vomiting ejects food reserves and predisposes to hypoglycaemia after insulin.

ACTION DURING THE DIVE

1. The buddy and the diabetic diver must be alert for any signs or symptoms of impending hypoglycaemia. This will usually present as peculiar or uncharacteristic behaviour. The dive must then be aborted. At the surface, inflate the BC for positive buoyancy and the diver must take the oral glucose that has been stashed in the BC.
2. Diabetic divers should not dive deeper than 30 msw. Nitrogen narcosis will make any evaluation of impending hypoglycaemia impossible.
3. The dive should last less than an hour, never require mandatory in-water decompression stops, and heavy underwater work should be avoided.
4. Do not ignore any unusual symptoms or signs that occur after diving! This is essential in order to differentiate between hypoglycaemia, arterial gas embolism and acute decompression illness!

ACTION AFTER THE DIVE

Measure the blood glucose on the boat immediately after diving. If it is low, the following steps should be taken:
1. If the diver is fully conscious, he or she should take oral glucose and inhale 100 per cent oxygen by mask or demand valve (preferred). Full recovery is usually rapid.
2. DO NOT give oral glucose to a confused or comatose individual – the chances of inhalation and choking are enormous. Be alert for sudden vomiting and possible inhalation of vomit. This will requiring clearing the airway and possible CPR.
3. Place the affected diver in the left lateral recovery position (see page 232).
4. Administer continuous 100 per cent oxygen. Be ready for CPR (see page 235).
5. Monitor the blood glucose. If it drops below 3,6 mmol/litre:
   - If a trained person is at hand, inject 1 mg glucagon or give 50 ml of 50 per cent glucose solution intravenously.
   - If no trained person is available, inject 1mg glucagon – this can be given subcutaneously, intramuscularly or intravenously. Any will do.

- Monitor the blood glucose after 10 minutes. If there is no improvement in consciousness and the **blood glucose is still low**, inject another 1 mg of glucagon.
6. If the blood glucose is normal, then diabetes is probably not the cause of confusion, weakness or coma. Regard and manage the case as arterial gas embolism (see page 164). Maintain oxygen administration and urgently notify an emergency rescue service and hyperbaric centre.

OTHER ENDOCRINE DISORDERS

Pituitary and adrenal gland diseases are immediately disqualifying for diving. These glands are involved in every vital function and diving becomes very dangerous.

Thyroid disease has to be considered carefully. An underactive thyroid predisposes to very rapid hypothermia and all its complications, and drastically reduces a diver's ability to cope with exercise stress. An overactive thyroid predisposes to uncontrollable abnormalities of heart rate and rhythm under water. If the thyroid derangement is mild and well controlled, diving may be considered.

18

FLUID BALANCE

The total amount of water in an average male diver's body is approximately 70 per cent of his body weight. In women, the figure is about 10 per cent less due to a relatively higher body fat content. In the average obese person, the body water figure is lower still. About two thirds of body water exists within cells (intracellular), which make up the vast bulk of body tissues and organs. The remaining third is outside cells (extracellular) and occurs in body fluids – blood plasma, tissue or interstitial fluid, lymph, the cerebrospinal fluid bathing the brain and spinal cord, the lubricating fluid in joints, and the fluid in hollow organs, glands and the eyes.

Whole blood contains only about one-tenth of the total body water but this circulating volume is critical to life, supplying oxygen and nutrients to the tissues and removing carbon dioxide and waste products for elimination by the lungs and kidneys. Not surprisingly then, the blood volume is maintained at remarkably constant levels. It is really a balance between the fluid in blood and fluid in the tissues.

When circulating fluid is lost, for example by haemorrhage, the blood volume rapidly replenishes itself from fluid in the tissue spaces outside the giant network of capillary blood vessels. This obviously dilutes the blood but, unless excessive, it does maintain circulating volume, blood pressure and ongoing vital functions. The reverse happens if there is any tendency for the blood volume to rise, such as at a beer festival or post-dive party. Excess circulating fluid first passes into tissues and later from the body as large volumes of urine.

Under normal conditions, the body maintains a perfect balance: water intake balances water output. A complex biofeedback system exists, involving the pituitary and adrenal glands, the hypothalamus in the brain, and the regulation of sodium, potassium and acid/base electrolytes by the kidneys.

WATER INTAKE

Body water is replaced in two main ways:
1.) by ingesting liquids, semi-solids (such as fruit) and solid food (even lean, cooked meat comprises about 65–70 per cent water), and
2.) by the water formed during the metabolism of food:
   - 100 grams of fat yields 107 grams of water,
   - 100 grams of starch yields 55 grams of water,
   - 100 grams of protein yields 41 grams of water,
   - 100 grams of alcohol yields 117 grams of water.

In an average adult, the total amount of water needed from all sources is about 2500 ml a day, which usually means drinking about one litre of water or beverages. The rest is supplied by solid and semi-solid food and metabolism. If water intake is inadequate, the sensation of thirst occurs.

WATER OUTPUT

About 1500 ml of water are lost in urine per day, 500 ml in insensible perspiration (at average temperatures and humidity), 350 ml in expired air from the lungs and a further 150 ml in faeces. Insensible perspiration is not sweat and the skin remains dry to the touch. It is the evaporation of water from moist tissues under the skin, occurs constantly, and is an important method of heat loss by the body. Under hot conditions or during exercise, however, the rate of production of water from tissues under the skin increases markedly and the sweat glands begin secreting.

If humidity is high and air movement low, sweating becomes even more obvious, not necessarily because more sweat is produced, but because evaporation of sweat is reduced. In hot climates, sweat production can reach three litres daily, and in very torrid climates, as much as 10 litres.

DEHYDRATION

If water output exceeds intake, total body water is reduced and a negative water balance is said to occur. This is called dehydration. There are several causes, all of which are important to divers – and not only because dehydration reduces stamina and ability. It also increases the likelihood of acute decompression illness following a normal dive profile.

CAUSES OF DEHYDRATION:

- Inadequate water intake, especially under hot conditions, and when combined with muscular exercise or with fever, can rapidly result in dehydration.
- Excessive water loss occurs with persistent vomiting (e.g. seasickness, food poisoning and bulimia), prolonged diarrhoea and excessive sweating or urine production (including the use of diuretics in a misguided attempt to achieve a slim summer figure), especially if a restricted water and electrolyte intake is also present.
- A diver dressed in a full wet suit who remains under a blazing tropical sun for any length of time is especially prone to heavy sweating, but the presence of insulating rubber makes evaporation off the skin and consequent cooling impossible. Aside from dehydration, the stage is then set for a rapid rise in body temperature and heat stroke.
- The kidneys filter blood and produce about 120 ml of filtered fluid per minute. If all the filtered fluid were passed as urine, over seven litres of urine, rich in electrolytes and glucose, would be passed per hour and death would soon occur. This obviously doesn't happen. A water-conserving hormone called antidiuretic hormone (ADH) is produced by the pituitary gland and it causes

reabsorption of all but one millilitre of water per minute in kidney filtrate. Alcohol stimulates an increased urine output by impairing the release of ADH. Although the quantities of fluid imbibed as beer may be great, the volume of urine produced will be even greater, causing negative water balance.

- Inadequate replacement of electrolytes following vigorous exercise, excessive vomiting or diarrhoea worsens dehydration. Depending on the cause and nature of the electrolyte loss, the body is then subjected to a relative excess of other remaining acidic or basic electrolytes. The end result is the same: the kidneys attempt to excrete the relative excess of acidic or basic electrolytes and this means an increased urine production that in turn further aggravates dehydration. Athletes have been aware of this for years and drink isotonic fluids rather than water for fluid replacement during exercise.

EFFECTS OF DEHYDRATION

Each and every effect of dehydration reduces a diver's capacity to handle a dissolved nitrogen gas load safely.

- Loss of weight occurs. This is due to a reduction in body water as well as a breakdown of fat tissues and carbohydrate stores in an attempt to provide metabolic water for continued physiological function. While weight loss may be considered aesthetically desirable, the problem, from a diver's point of view, is that it results in a reduced volume of total body water for dissolving absorbed nitrogen gas during a dive. Even a moderate loss of body water can convert a safe tabled or computerised dive profile into one favouring DCI.
- Disturbances in acid-base balance occur, usually toward the acidic side. Acid metabolites, such as lactic acid, accumulate. Kidney circulation slows, resulting in a decreased urine output and retention of additional acids such as phosphoric acid. Body water can only hold a limited amount of dissolved substances in solution. As acidic products increase in tissues, so the capacity decreases to retain nitrogen gas in solution during decompression.
- A rise occurs in the concentration of normally excreted products such as urea and creatinine. The water loss also causes an increased concentration of normal components of blood such as plasma proteins and even glucose. Once again, the effect is a reduced carrying-capacity of a dissolved nitrogen load in divers.
- Body temperature rises. A reduction in the volume of circulating fluid means less heat transfer to the skin. Under hot conditions, nitrogen gas is less soluble in water.
- The pulse rate increases but blood output by the heart decreases. This delays tissue degassing and elimination of an inert gas load.
- In severe cases, dryness, wrinkling and looseness of skin occurs. The face has a haunted and pinched expression due to recession of the eyeballs and loss of subcutaneous fat and water from the deeper layers of the skin.

Finally, exhaustion and collapse occur.

MANAGEMENT OF DEHYDRATION

The primary message is prevention. Alcohol must only be taken in very moderate amounts and at least eight to twelve hours should elapse between drinking and diving. All divers should ensure an adequate intake of fluids and electrolytes prior to diving. Drinking 300–500 ml of plain water or any other non-carbonated liquid before diving is easy, sociable and very beneficial.

Very seasick divers must not dive. Aside from the dehydrating effect of prolonged vomiting and the increased liability to DCI, disorientation, a reduced swimming ability and a very doubtful response to underwater stress are present. Exposure to the sun while in a wet suit should also be minimised

Flying after diving is a common source of concern to divers. The reduced pressure predisposes to DCI, while the cabin humidity on a commercial flight is only eight per cent, as opposed to an average comfortable humidity of about 70 per cent. Breathing this dry air for any length of time also depletes body fluids. Drinking alcohol on a flight simply increases urine output and aggravates any dehydration and likelihood of DCI. (See page 179.)

If any symptoms of dehydration occur before a dive – and this is not a difficult diagnosis to make as severe thirst is usually present – do not dive, and ensure the liberal replacement of fluids, preferably with an isotonic drink. (In cases where there is simultaneous severe fluid and electrolyte loss, thirst may not be present, but the diver will be in a state of collapse and any thought of diving would be ridiculous. In such cases, intravenous fluid replacement with a solution such as Ringer's lactate is needed, as well as advanced in-hospital treatment to correct the acid/base imbalance.)

Dehydration is an insidious condition during its early stages because, aside from being thirsty, nothing else is obvious. Few divers would abort a dive just because they felt thirsty beforehand, but remember that your safe dive profile is about to evaporate. Dry suits are the closest a diver should ever get to the word 'dry'. Dive wet!

19

BAROTRAUMA

Barotrauma is a pressure injury. It results from forced volume changes in closed air spaces (such as the lungs or sinuses) and occurs when these air spaces cannot otherwise comply with pressure changes in accordance with Boyle's Law (see page 21). There are two possibilities:
- increased pressure causes descent barotrauma, and
- decreased pressure causes ascent barotrauma.

DESCENT BAROTRAUMA

As a diver descends, the pressure around him or her increases. If this increase cannot be equalised in an air space, its volume must decrease. If the air volume cannot decrease (for example, an air space within bone or a face mask), then tissues will swell and blood vessels may burst in order to accommodate the required decrease in air volume and to equalise the pressure. This is called **squeeze**.

ASCENT BAROTRAUMA

This is the reverse problem to barotrauma of descent. On ascent, an **increase** in volume occurs, along with a drop in pressure. If expanding gas cannot escape, explosive destruction of tissue can result. An air space must be present for pressure/volume effects to occur. Such spaces occur in:
- the ear,
- the sinuses,
- the lungs,
- decayed teeth,
- the gut, and
- diving equipment.

EAR BAROTRAUMA

A real understanding of ear barotrauma requires some knowledge of the anatomy and working of the ear. This has been presented in chapter 12 (see pages 92–94).

EXTERNAL EAR BAROTRAUMA OF DESCENT (EXTERNAL EAR SQUEEZE)

While diving, the external ear floods with water up to the eardrum. If water cannot enter the external ear due to wax lumps, ear plugs, or a tight hood or mask straps, a relative vacuum forms between the obstruction and the eardrum, and external ear squeeze occurs on descent.

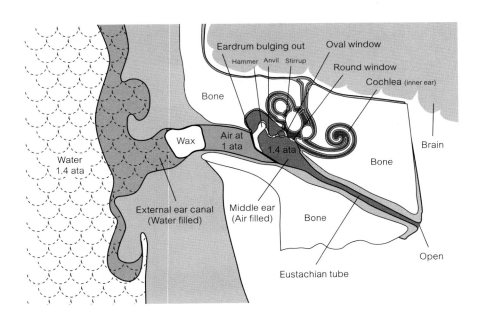

Example

> Flora only took up diving because her boyfriend, Jimmy, told her she'd like it. Setting off on a dive excursion, she has one ear completely blocked by a hard lump of wax. As she descends to 4 msw she develops sharp pain in the ear which is not relieved by equalising. She becomes very agitated and ascends noisily.

At 4 msw the pressure is 1.4 ATA. The pressure in Flora's external ear is still 1 ATA. Her eardrum bulges outward to accommodate the decrease in volume, causing pain. A similar experience occurs with ear plugs, which must never be used in diving. Wet suit hoods should fit easily and be able to admit water.

MIDDLE EAR BAROTRAUMA OF DESCENT
(MIDDLE EAR SQUEEZE)

The middle ear, which contains the three tiny bones involved in hearing (the anvil, hammer and stirrup), is always air-filled and communicates with the air in the back of the nose via the Eustachian tube. The Eustachian tube allows air to move into and out of the middle ear. At the surface it functions continuously, because oxygen in the air of the middle ear is constantly being absorbed by the membranes of the middle ear, creating a vacuum that the Eustachian tube corrects.

On descent, the Eustachian tube tends to block, and the increased pressure in the water-filled external ear pushes the eardrum inwards.

Air must be introduced into the middle ear to equalise the pressure. This can be done by swallowing, moving the jaws around, or performing a Valsalva or Toynbee manoeuvre (see page 115). These have the effect of opening the valve-like mouth of the Eustachian tube and letting air into the middle ear. This must be done continuously during descent, and especially frequently (at least once per metre) during the first 10 msw where volume changes are greatest.

If equalisation is omitted or delayed, the pressure in the nose presses the lips of the Eustachian tube together, blocking and then locking them. Equalisation is then impossible and the diver must ascend until equalisation is possible.

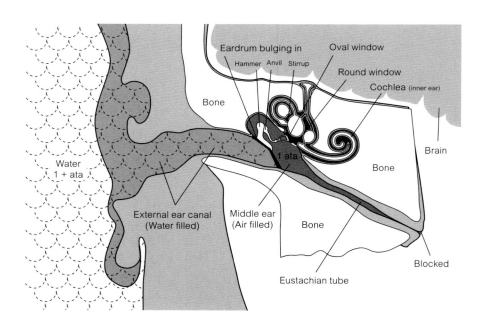

Omitted equalisation

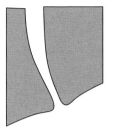

Open Eustachian tube

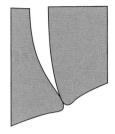

Blocked Eustachian tube

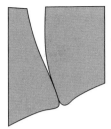

Blocked and locked
Eustachian tube

IF EQUALISATION IS NOT DONE: At 2 msw (1.2 ATA), the volume in the middle ear decreases by one-sixth; at 5 msw (1.5 ATA), by one-third, etc. This causes pain, due to inward bulging of the eardrum, swelling of the membranes lining the middle ear and, if continued, bleeding into the cavity. This is middle ear squeeze (barotrauma of descent). Any bleeding in the middle ear commonly drains out of the Eustachian tube and presents as a trickle of blood from the nose after the dive.

Ear pain on descent, followed by a nose bleed on ascent, means that significant middle ear descent barotrauma has occurred. Repetitive dives will aggravate any damage and bleeding can easily recur. The diver may find that equalising becomes easier with repetitive dives but this is because there is blood, tissue swelling, or both, in the middle ear. This reduces the air volume in the middle ear and causes apparent improvement and ease of equalising ability.

But, after each dive, the ear will feel blocked or even deaf because of liquid interference with the middle ear's 22-times amplification system. This deafness may seem to disappear during the next dive, but this is only because hearing operates under water by bone conduction. The middle ear is damped when the external ear canal is full of water. However, on surfacing and returning to hearing by air conduction, deafness will recur.

If the diver persists in his or her descent without equalising, the eardrum may rupture. Pain and a loud noise herald the event then, as cold water enters the middle ear, pressure is equalised and pain disappears. Sudden vertigo and nausea may occur from the abrupt temperature drop in the middle ear, but this is usually temporary, as the water in the ear quickly warms.

CAUSES OF A BLOCKED EUSTACHIAN TUBE
1. Failure to attempt equalising.
2. Upper respiratory infection e.g. a cold.
3. Nasal allergies e.g. hayfever.
4. Smoking.
5. Nasal polyps.
6. Use of oral isotretinoin in acne treatment.

Example

Flora has her ears syringed and decides to try diving again. Unfortunately, she is allergic to her dive buddy Jimmy's aftershave, *Sweaty Passion*, and begins to sneeze as her nose congests and blocks. Back at 4 msw, she just cannot equalise, gets ear pain once again and surfaces very loudly. She has exchanged external ear squeeze for middle ear squeeze.

Squeeze may also be experienced in aircraft, especially unpressurised ones. On descent, the air pressure increases and air must enter the middle ear to equalise the pressure. This can be assisted by chewing during descent, swallowing, or holding one's nose and blowing. Only very rarely is pain experienced during ascent in an aircraft. In this case, the air pressure is decreasing, and the middle ear vents through the Eustachian tube. Any obstruction causes barotrauma of ascent as described below.

NOTE: Mammals that dive, such as whales and seals, cannot and do not need voluntarily to equalise their middle ears on diving. They are protected against squeeze because they have large veins in their middle ears which simply distend with blood on descent to compensate air volume drop. Their round windows are buttressed with fibrous bands which give great strength.

MIDDLE EAR BAROTRAUMA OF ASCENT

On ascent, the gas in the middle ear expands and the excess gas vents through the Eustachian tube. If the tube blocks, this escape cannot occur. Obstruction is usually caused by a plug of mucus or blood from a previous squeeze.

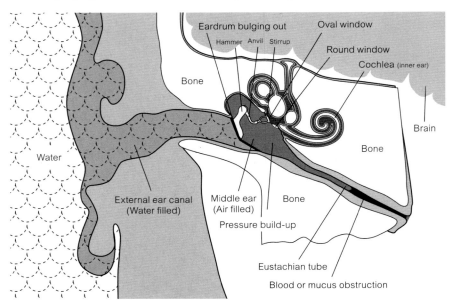

INNER EAR BAROTRAUMA OF DESCENT

The inner ear is the organ of hearing and balance. It is a fluid-filled space with its passage communicating with the fluid bathing the brain. As such, it is normally immune to pressure and volume changes, because no air spaces are involved.

Inner ear barotrauma occurs only with descent when the diver attempts to equalise with excessive force. Any increase in the pressure within the skull is transmitted to the fluid in the inner ear. The round window is the flexible membrane between the inner and middle ear that permits effective cochlear fluid movement with stirrup vibration in the oval window (see Hearing in air, page 94). If the pressure of an equalising attempt becomes too high, the round window bulges and bursts into the middle ear; this is called a round window fistula.

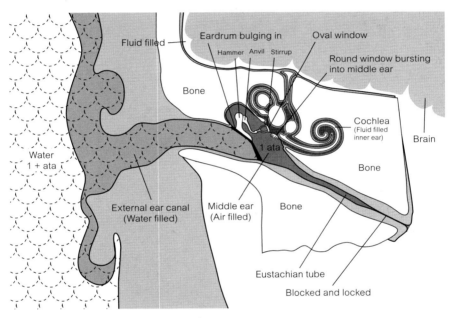

Example

Ever-willing Flora has been persuaded to try diving one more time. At her favourite 4-metre depth, she still can't equalise because Jimmy persists in using *Sweaty Passion*, his offensive aftershave, and her nasal lining is now grossly swollen. Bravely, she endeavours to blow her head off with an enormous equalising attempt. The pressure in her head builds up with the force of her blowing. This is transmitted through the fluid around her brain to the inner ear. The round window bulges, then bursts into the middle ear. Flora experiences immediate severe pain, vertigo and ringing in her ear (tinnitus). Clawing her way to the surface, she finds she is totally deaf in the ear and, screaming curses at Jimmy, she gives up diving for good in order to relieve her allergy.

Round window rupture is a medical emergency. Cerebrospinal fluid in and around the brain will leak through the hole in the inner ear into the middle ear and then drain into the Eustachian tube. From there it reaches the nose and presents as a drip of clear brain fluid from a nostril. The nose is not sterile and the possibility of infection spreading from the nose via the inner ear to the brain is very high. At this point, meningitis beccomes an extreme hazard.

The sudden development of a clear nasal drip accompanied by deafness and vertigo after a maximal equalising attempt must be regarded as inner ear barotrauma. Seek immediate medical help. Do not blow the nose! Do not attempt any equalisation! Do not fly in an aircraft!

In the event of inner ear barotrauma occurring, surgery may be required to repair the ruptured round window.

Management of ear barotrauma
Prevention
1. Ear barotrauma, especially middle ear squeeze, is very common among novice divers, who are often too concerned about monitoring depth, cylinder pressure and buoyancy to think about their ears. Pain is the signal to equalise, but their Eustachian tubes are already blocked or locked. They ascend a few metres to relieve the pressure, equalise, then descend to their next pain level in a yo-yo descent to the bottom. Equalisation must be a constant process from the surface. If it is properly done with every exhalation, the diver will have no sensation of pain with increasing depth – only a reassuring clicking of the eardrums.
2. Don't dive if you are unable to equalise at the surface because of a nasal allergy, cold or smoking. Have these treated first, and stop smoking! (See Management of nasal congestion, page 108; Management of equalising difficulties, page 110.)
3. Wax lumps should be removed by a doctor before a diving trip. Do not use earbuds for cleaning ears. They damage the delicate membranes of the canals and open the way for infection.

Treatment
Any combination of deafness, a persistently blocked ear, tinnitus, vertigo or earache following difficulty with equalising under water indicates ear barotrauma. Inner ear barotrauma must be suspected if partial or complete deafness, vertigo, nausea or vomiting, and loss of balance occur. Medical help is essential to establish the exact problem and treat the damage.
1. **Stop further diving.**
2. **Do not** use anaesthetic or antibiotic eardrops. It is essential first to exclude eardrum rupture. If the drum has been perforated, the antibiotics used in most eardrops can cause permanent deafness. Consult a doctor.
3. Oral painkillers may be used to alleviate earache.
4. Local heat, such as a warm hot-water-bottle, may be soothing.

5. Take one 60 mg tablet of pseudoephedrine three times a day for five days.
6. Spray one puff of oxymetazoline nasal spray into each nostril three times a day, or instil three drops of oxymetazoline nasal drops into each nostril three times a day, for five days.
7. Oral antibiotics are indicated after eardrum or round window rupture.

SINUS BAROTRAUMA

Like the middle ear, the sinuses are air spaces in the bone of the skull with openings to the nose. Blockage of any of these openings occurs for the same reasons (see also Disorders of the sinuses, page 112):
1. Upper respiratory infection e.g. a cold.
2. Nasal allergies (e.g. hayfever).
3. Smoking.
4. Nasal polyps.

The sinuses do not have the valve system of the Eustachian tube, so active equalising is not possible. Exactly as with the middle ear, there can be sinus barotrauma of descent and ascent.

Example

Jimmy is trying to impress his new love, Phillipa. *Sweaty Passion* has finally given him nasal congestion too, so at 6 msw he develops a tearing pain in the forehead above his nose. Equalising his mask gives him a little relief, and he takes Philippa down to 12 msw to watch the sea cucumbers play. On ascent, the pain improves, and on surfacing, he smiles at Phillipa, not knowing that his mask has a fluid level of green mucus and blood. Jimmy has had a frontal sinus squeeze, or **sinus barotrauma of descent**. As with middle ear reverse block, sinus barotrauma of ascent can also occur.

Sinus barotrauma of descent

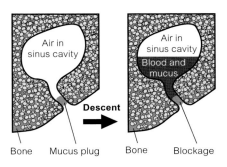

Air in sinus cavity

Air in sinus cavity

Blood and mucus

Descent

Bone   Mucus plug   Bone   Blockage

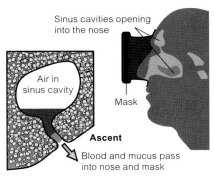

Sinus cavities opening into the nose

Air in sinus cavity

Mask

Ascent

Blood and mucus pass into nose and mask

DENTAL BAROTRAUMA

Teeth are incompressible, so the presence of gas pockets within them will cause problems with diving. This air can only arise from dental decay or from fillings that have trapped air in the tooth.

DENTAL SQUEEZE

On descent, the pressure on the tooth increases. If the enamel over the cavity is thin, the tooth can implode.

DENTAL BAROTRAUMA OF ASCENT

Gas that has entered a tooth cavity at depth may become trapped by a fold of gum tissue. On ascent, pressure decreases, volume increases and the tooth can explode.

Management of dental barotrauma
Prevention
1. Divers must take care of their teeth. All fillings must be firm and healthy.
2. Inform your dentist that you scuba dive. He or she should then pay particular attention to potential trouble.

Treatment
This is directed at pain relief before seeing a dentist.
1. Use oral painkillers.
2. If the pain is very severe, try pressing a small wad of cotton wool soaked with alcohol on the tooth. This could be whisky or other spirits.
3. Oil of cloves is also useful. Grip a small wad of cotton wool soaked in the oil between the jaws at the site of the affected tooth.
4. If available, lignocaine spray will provide some relief (two sprays every three hours onto the tooth).

EQUIPMENT BAROTRAUMA

Any piece of diving equipment containing an air space is a potential cause of diver barotrauma. Most are minor injuries only, but some can kill.

MASK SQUEEZE

Mask squeeze occurs for two main reasons:
- the diver fails to equalise his or her mask, or
- the mask is too large.

It is interesting that divers who struggle to equalise their middle ears very rarely get mask squeeze; while divers who do develop mask squeeze generally do so because they can equalise their middle ears *too* easily – for example, by a small movement of the jaw from side to side. This is enough to open their Eustachian tubes and allow air under pressure to enter the middle ears. But it allows no air to pass through the nose into the mask because the rubber nosepiece is firmly pressed by water pressure against the openings of the nostrils. Voluntary snorting or blowing is required to push air past the nose seal and into the mask.

Divers with middle ear equalising problems snort vast amounts of air into their masks as they hold their noses and strenuously blow. A puff of nasal air always occurs on releasing the nose while blowing to equalise.

Large masks are unnecessary and ill-advised. They are unnecessary because the refraction of light at a water-glass-air interface limits the angle of view to 97.2 degrees anyway (see Vision under water, page 117). A large mask protruding further from the face will only reduce this angle of view by providing a small tunnel to peer through. The ill-advisedness lies in the large volume of air that is required to equalise pressure changes on descent. This becomes even more apparent on a breathhold dive when the amount of air available for mask equalisation is both limited and shrinking with every metre of increasing depth.

Treatment of mask squeeze is non-specific. Aescin and heparinoid gel help relieve swelling, but take care to avoid the eyes. Stop diving until all bruising clears.

SKIN BAROTRAUMA

This occurs most commonly when dry suits or baggy wet suits are worn. Pockets of air are trapped between folds in the suit, and descent causes these spaces to contract. The skin is sucked into the folds and welts or bruising can occur. No treatment is required and the diver is invariably pain-free.

HEAD AND BODY BAROTRAUMA OF DESCENT (DIVER'S SQUEEZE)

This is the greatest potential fault of freeflow systems using a copper or hard hat. With freeflow systems, air or a breathing mix is supplied through a hose from the surface to the diver. A constant excess of gas is delivered to flush out exhaled carbon dioxide and prevent accumulation of the gas.

If a freeflow, or Standard, diver's hoses break, or he descends too fast, the surrounding water pressure increases more rapidly than can be maintained by his air supply. In the worst case, his whole body and suit will be squeezed up into his copper helmet. A non-return valve on the helmet prevents this in the event of hose rupture, and careful control of descent is mandatory.

SUIT BAROTRAUMA OF ASCENT ('BLOW UP')

This occurs classically with a Standard Diving Suit (see page 15), but it can result from accidental underwater inflation of any buoyancy accessory – dry suits, buoyancy compensators and counterlungs in closed-circuit rebreathing units.

'Blow up' in scuba divers most commonly occurs as a result of neglecting to dump air used for buoyancy control at depth once the ascent has begun. Failure to vent expanding air causes the dry suit or BC bladder to inflate like a balloon (Boyle's Law, see page 21), and the diver then rockets to the surface (Archimedes' Principle, see page 26). This can cause pulmonary barotrauma of ascent, arterial gas embolism, acute decompression illness, diver entrapment in a tightly inflated suit, and diver injury, for example, a forceful collision with the bottom of the dive boat.

PULMONARY BAROTRAUMA

Pressure-volume damage inside the fixed space of the chest is the **most dangerous** of all pressure injuries in scuba divers. The two most vital life-support organs in the body – the lungs and the heart – are directly affected, and significant derangement then effects brain function. As with all barotraumas, a fixed gas space (air in the lungs) is involved, with obstruction of the passage (the bronchial tree) to atmosphere. The problem may be with descent or ascent.

PULMONARY BAROTRAUMA OF DESCENT
(CHEST SQUEEZE OR LUNG SQUEEZE)

Chest squeeze cannot occur while breathing normally on scuba. Regulated air pressure maintains lung pressure at ambient. Among sport divers, the condition is limited to breathhold divers who descend beyond their depth limit, and depends on two things:
–   the diver's residual volume, and
–   the distensibility of blood vessels.

As residual volume is the fixed volume of the bronchi and bronchioles in both lungs, it follows that at residual volume depth all the air in all the alveoli is now in the bronchial tree. All the alveoli are completely flattened, the rib cage is tremendously compressed, the diaphragm is sucked up high into the chest, and the lungs are a solid mass of tissue penetrated by more rigid tubules pressurised to the particular depth.

Further descent cannot be compensated for by a decrease in alveolar volume. The large veins in the chest begin to dilate with blood to accommodate for continued air volume decrease as maximum breathhold depth is reached. Then rupture of veins, haemorrhage and death occur. Further descent results in crushing and collapse of the ribs and chest.

CAUSES OF CHEST SQUEEZE

1.   Breathhold diving, especially attempts at depth records.
2.   Excessive speed of descent with freeflow Standard Diving equipment, also leading to diver's squeeze into the helmet.
3.   Losing surface pressure with Standard Diving equipment and the absence of a non-return valve on the helmet.

Treatment
1. Treat for shock (see page 283),
2. Give 100 per cent oxygen, and
3. Summon emergency medical help.

PULMONARY BAROTRAUMA OF ASCENT
(BURST LUNG)

Pulmonary barotrauma of ascent is precisely the reverse of lung squeeze. The diver begins with normal lung volumes that are safely balanced at depth pressure and then develops overpressurisation and bursting of lung tissue on returning to the surface. It is usually the alveoli that distend and burst because they are the thinnest-walled (one cell thick). Inadequate exhalation of expanding gas distorts their normal grape-like configuration and they distend like blown-up rubber gloves, with their capillary network tautly stretched around them.

With total lung involvement, the ribs are forced out tightly and the diaphragm is driven down into the abdomen. The ultimate release of pressurised gas is not a gentle process. When the elastic limit of the lungs is reached, shredding of the lung tissue occurs with rapid liberation of pressurised gas.

CAUSES OF BURST LUNG

The following are the usual causes; except for the lung disorders, all are related to inadequate underwater techniques. (See also page 182.)
1. PANIC, with an attempt at an emergency ascent.
2. Free ascents, especially uncontrolled free ascents, and submarine escape training.
3. Skip breathing, with a diver attempting to conserve air by breathholding and being unaware that he or she is ascending.
4. Buddy breathing at depth becoming uncoordinated and leading to panic.
5. Inability to gain comfortable and relaxed control of the regulator during ditch and recovery training, resulting in the exercise being abandoned in favour of a hurried return to the surface.
6. Apparatus difficulties, such as a high regulator resistance to inhalation because of an almost empty cylinder.
7. Water inhalation, causing choking, panic and laryngospasm, with frantic attempts to reach the surface.
8. Lung disorders, such as asthma and chest infections with a high resistance to outflow, or mucous plugs blocking bronchioles.

All of the above cause internal air to be trapped, resulting in inadequate exhalation. The degree of damage and the effects on the diver depend on the speed of the ascent, the size of the pressure differential, whether the injury is localised to a small area of the lungs or generalised, and the presence of any underlying lung disorder, such as asthma or a respiratory infection.

Pulmonary barotrauma of ascent

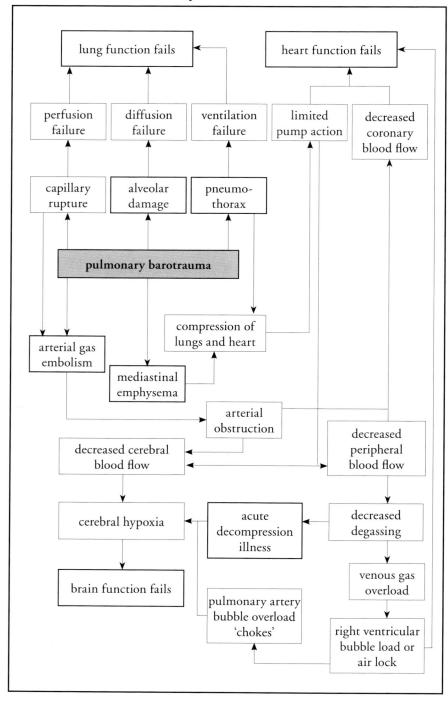

Pressurised gas, bubbling or gushing out of torn alveolar units, can cause any combination of the following four presentations:

1. LUNG TISSUE DAMAGE Alveolar and surrounding connective tissue damage results in a reduction in the number of functional alveolar units. If extensive, this decreases ventilation ability. Rampant membrane disruption causes diffusion failure, and the inevitable accompanying damage to the capillary supply causes perfusion insufficiency, failure of gas exchange and respiratory failure. **Presentation** At the surface, pressurised gas gushes through the trachea and larynx and whistles out of the mouth as a high-pitched cry. The diver is breathless, has chest tightness or pain, and coughing produces blood-stained sputum. If damage is extensive, death will occur.

2. MEDIASTINAL EMPHYSEMA Alveolar rupture may be followed by gas tracking along the slack tissue layer around bronchi and blood vessels to reach the root of the lung, the major bronchi and blood vessels, and the heart – all located in the mediastinum – the very centre of the chest. The trapping of gas here is called **mediastinal emphysema**. Further tracking can occur – under the pericardium, the fibrous sac lining the heart – to cause a pneumopericardium with free gas around the heart; down through the diaphragm and into the peritoneal cavity, to cause a pneumoperitoneum with free gas around the intestines and swelling of the abdomen; or up into the neck as far as the jaw. Here it can be felt as a 'crackling' under the skin. This is called **subcutaneous or surgical emphysema**.

   In scuba diving, the most common cause of mediastinal emphysema is ascent with a near-empty air cylinder. The high resistance to inhalation results in long, slow inspirations with air expanding in the lungs all the while as the diver ascends to enable the regulator to deliver the last vestiges of air. It is imperative that divers do not delay ascent until the cylinders are virtually empty. Begin ascending when the cylinder pressure gets to 50 ATA.
   Presentation As free gas may be present in connective tissue planes anywhere from inside the abdomen to the jaw, the effects on the individual diver may vary. With extensive gas tracking, the onset of mediastinal emphysema is instantaneous but, in milder instances, the presentation may be delayed for hours. In most cases, the effects of air in the neck and mediastinum are felt, and the onset is delayed. The neck feels 'full', the voice is hoarse or brassy, and chest discomfort and breathlessness are present. Coughing may worsen matters by driving more gas into the mediastinum. The effects of compression become felt. Shortness of breath increases and the diver becomes blue (cyanosis). Pressure on the oesophagus causes difficulty in swallowing; compression of the great veins and heart results in a fast, thready pulse with a drop in blood pressure, going on to a decreased blood supply to the brain, unconsciousness and shock.

Bear in mind that the free gas in the tissues is not stable air. It is post-dive gas and the surrounding tissues may have a substantial dissolved nitrogen load. At the surface, the free gas obeys Boyle's Law and expands until its pressure is ambient. Degassing of tissues is also occurring and nitrogen will be delivered to adjacent free gas which will increase in volume. Delayed worsening must therefore be anticipated.

3. ARTERIAL GAS EMBOLISM Simultaneous alveolar and capillary rupture can result in a direct hook-up between the respiratory and cardiovascular systems. Gas in the lungs can be vented directly into the blood to reach the general body circulation. This is an **Arterial Gas Embolism (AGE)**.

AGE does not occur while the lungs are tightly inflated during the ascent from depth because the low-pressure capillaries surrounding the alveoli are stretched and compressed flat by the tightly distended alveoli. It follows the first exhalation after lung-tearing. Blood-flow through capillaries then resumes and alveolar air is sucked into them with each inspiration. Once inside the blood, gas bubbles form and pass via the pulmonary vein to the left atrium and ventricle. Within the heart, the powerful pumping of the left ventricle may churn larger bubbles into many tiny bubbles which, in turn, are sprayed into the aorta and reach the coronary or cerebral arteries, or the arteries of any organ or tissue in the body. Bubbles do not have to be large to be lethal, nor is a large volume of gas required. Bubbles as small as 0.03 mm in the coronary or cerebral arteries can cause grave trouble and, when AGE is accompanied by mediastinal emphysema or lung tissue damage, the diver is in very dire straits.

But, if the diver has significant coexisting decompression commitments, AGE combined with obstruction of the blood supply to an organ or tissue will prevent effective degassing and the removal of nitrogen from the area affected. Under these conditions, even a minor tissue gas load, that would not normally require any in-water decompression stops, can cause acute decompression illness. Carbon dioxide build-up in oxygen-starved tissues will also drive excess dissolved nitrogen out of solution in those tissues. Computer and dive table predictions regarding safe decompression no longer apply, as they are based on a normal blood supply to tissues. Never assume that a diver who develops AGE after a short non-repetitive shallow dive cannot develop acute decompression illness – he or she can, and precisely in the area already damaged by AGE. **Presentation: A diver who develops any untoward neurological symptoms immediately after a dive must be presumed to have AGE. This is a diving medical emergency. Do not wait to see what develops! Begin first-aid treatment and summon trained medical help urgently!**

Cerebral Arterial Gas Embolism (CAGE) is the most common manifestation of AGE, probably because arterial bubbles resulting from lung-bursting will rise to the head in a vertically-ascending diver. This then causes brain injury.

(a) Brain damage presents in three ways:
- impairment of the higher faculties, resulting in confusion, disorientation, unconsciousness and convulsions,
- impairment of motor function, leading to weakness, abnormal gait, incoordination and paralysis, or
- impairment of sensory function, resulting in blurred vision, blindness, loss of balance, vertigo and numbness.

(b) Heart damage presents with tightness in the chest or constricting chest pain, sweating, extreme paleness, faintness, a rapid, weak pulse with an irregular rhythm and breathlessness.

Both types of damage may progress to death.

4. PNEUMOTHORAX In this event, compressed gas ruptures through the pleural lining of the lung, enters the pleural space and the lung collapses. The effects are identical to those of a tension pneumothorax (see page 66). **Presentation:** A pneumothorax is usually a sudden event that presents during the ascent or soon after the dive. The usual features are sudden pain on the involved side – worse on breathing in; the need for rapid shallow breaths with inability to breathe deeply; a feeling of tightness in the chest; and the development of shock.

Examples of pulmonary barotrauma of ascent:

Konrad, aged 32, was a scuba diving instructor. He had a cold but had no-one else to take his Openwater 1 class on their first sea dive. After diving for 40 minutes at 12 msw, he surfaced, feeling well. About two hours later, he felt weak, had difficulty in getting enough air and had mild chest discomfort. He went to see his doctor when his voice became tinny. The examination revealed subcutaneous emphysema and a chest X-ray showed air in his mediastinum and neck.
Diagnosis: Pulmonary barotrauma of ascent with mediastinal emphysema.
Treatment: He recovered speedily on 100 per cent oxygen alone.

Harry was on holiday on a tropical island. The water was warm so he dived without his wet suit. At 20 msw he accidentally brushed against a reef of fire coral. Startled by sudden intense pain in his leg, he made for the surface. While swimming toward the moored dive boat, he realised that his chest was painful and his breathing was becoming difficult. His dive leader immediately took him to the local doctor who, worried about possible AGE, decided to recompress Harry in a chamber. Breathing pure oxygen at 18 msw, Harry's discomfort disappeared. However, during decompression, the breathlessness recurred at 10 msw and Harry was recompressed to 18 msw, this time with only little relief. Any attempt to reduce the pressure caused severe breathlessness and pain. Really worried now, the doctor called his partner who examined Harry in the chamber and diagnosed a pneumothorax. A one-way needle valve was used to drain the free air in Harry's pleural cavity and decompression was safely accomplished while Harry breathed pure oxygen.

Stan was an inexperienced diver doing his first night dive. On ascent, he became panicky at 12 msw and inflated his BC. He rocketed to the surface, gave a high-pitched cry, coughed up blood and lost consciousness. He was quickly rescued from the water, but he had stopped breathing. Cardiopulmonary resuscitation (CPR) was commenced and an emergency rescue service was summoned. All attempts at resuscitation were futile, however, and Stan was pronounced dead by the emergency doctor.

Diagnosis: Pulmonary barotrauma of ascent with cerebral arterial gas embolism.

Management of pulmonary barotrauma of ascent
Action
1. Have someone notify the nearest recompression facility to prepare the chamber and summon a diving physician.
2. Administer continuous 100 per cent oxygen via a demand valve. This is to ensure that any further bubbles will be oxygen, not nitrogen, and to increase the available oxygen to the brain and tissues.
3. Some authorities recommend the 'knee-elbow' position immediately and up to 10 minutes after surfacing. Beyond this time, it **should not** be used. The diver is placed on his or her knees and elbows with the left shoulder lower than the right. The objective is to gravitate bubbles away from the brain. The position should be maintained for 10 minutes, then the diver should be laid flat.
4. Keep the diver quiet and as relaxed as possible. Further movement or coughing may increase lung damage or cause more air to be vented into the blood.
5. Keep the diver flat. Do not use the Trendelenburg position (head down with the body and legs elevated about 30 degrees), as this will encourage bubbles to enter the coronary arteries with resulting additional heart damage.
   If the diver is unconscious, he or she should be placed in a 15 degrees left lateral position (the Recovery position, see page 232), with the head turned to the side to avoid inhalation should vomiting occur.
6. Cardiopulmonary resuscitation may be needed. (AIDS awareness! See page 234).
7. Set up a Ringer's lactate intravenous lifeline if a trained person is at hand. The casualty needs to be urgently transported to the nearest hyperbaric centre by the fastest means – road, helicopter or low-flying aeroplane.

8. Recompression therapy is needed. However, **do not recompress a pure pneumothorax** – it will convert to a life-threatening tension pneumothorax. If there is no neurological AGE, then chest drainage and **oxygen at surface pressure** are required. If both neurological AGE and a pneumothorax are present, then chest drainage followed by recompression are both needed.

GASTROINTESTINAL BAROTRAUMA

Gas in the stomach and intestines expands on ascent and, if air is swallowed during the dive, painful and occasionally dangerous distension may occur.

CAUSES OF GASTROINTESTINAL BAROTRAUMA

1. Swallowing air to equalise, especially in the head-down position, when air will enter the stomach.
2. Drinking carbonated beverages under hyperbaric conditions. This occurs occasionally during chamber pressurisations but more commonly among sport divers trying to prove their diving expertise by drinking champagne under water while coordinating a thumb over the opening of the bottle!

Management of gastrointestinal barotrauma

The condition is usually self-limiting, being relieved by belching or passing flatus. The discomfort may also be eased by removing any constricting belts or straps, or unfastening tight wet suits or BDs.

20

EMERGENCY ASCENTS

The incidence of sport divers becoming low on air or depleting their air supply remains unacceptably high. Emergency Ascent Training (EAT) has long been a controversial issue in the training of sport divers, as it has resulted in deaths. In April 1977, five major US training centres made a policy statement under the aegis of the National Scuba Training Committee (NSTC) in the USA. These centres were NAUI, PADI, SSI, YMCA and NASDC, and there was general recognition that, despite the potential risks of lung or ear injury, EAT is necessary during basic diving training.

EAT is a life-saving diving skill that allows a diver to safely reach the surface when out of air or to escape drowning. In most cases, emergency ascents are performed not because of a true out-of-air situation or equipment failure, but because of human error. Diving schools spend a great deal of time and effort training divers to avoid an emergency situation in the first place but, for moral, psychological and practical reasons, it is important that a student knows and has actually practised what to do in an emergency, should the need arise. (It is worth noting that virtually all training accidents occur during the **first** exposure to open water.)

Carrying a spare cylinder of air is recommended for deep diving (below 30 msw), cave diving, penetration wreck diving, staged decompression diving and any diving where entanglements are likely. However, the availability of an alternative air supply from a spare cylinder, a pony bottle or a buddy does not obviate the need for avoiding out-of-air situations. Nevertheless, just knowing that one can reach the surface and has already safely practised surfacing from depth without an air supply eliminates an enormous amount of the fear and insecurity that novice divers have to deal with. Obviously, avoidance is the best policy though, and divers should always carry a cylinder pressure gauge and monitor it closely during the dive.

EAT should be confined to a maximum depth of 9 msw and should be conducted vertically with a safety-line. The number of students per instructor should be limited in order to minimise the number of free ascents that instructors also have to perform. It goes without saying that oxygen resuscitation equipment, and personnel trained to use it, must be on-hand during all emergency ascent training exercises at scuba diving courses.

The NSTC agreement covered two primary aspects:
1. The underwater situation must be evaluated, and
2. A choice of possible actions must be taken.

EVALUATING THE SITUATION

In an out-of-air situation, choosing an appropriate course of action depends on many variables, including:

- depth and visibility,
- distance from, and focus of attention of, others,
- nature of activity (swimming, stationary, photography, spearfishing, etc),
- available breathhold time,
- training level and extent of experience of all diver/s involved,
- stress level of each diver,
- obstructions to the surface,
- water movement (current or tide),
- buoyancy of the diver,
- equipment,
- familiarisation of skills and equipment between divers,
- apparent reason for air loss, and
- decompression requirements.

These variables must be covered during a scuba diving course, as must their relationship to selecting an appropriate emergency ascent procedure. Risk stems mainly from loss of self-control, panic and too rapid an ascent. It is crucial to teach confidence as well as to provide adequate training. The problem is that this training requires between 7 and 14 exercises to reach the overteach curve.

Due to the scare tactics often used in lectures, many dive students are excessively apprehensive about developing arterial gas embolism (see page 164).

Dive schools must coordinate their teaching so that students trained under the auspices of different centres or dive schools would make the same decision under a particular set of circumstances. Training must provide divers with safe, effective emergency procedures to follow when their diving instructors and supervisors are no longer available. Divers must be taught that, before they enter the water for any dive, they should coordinate with their dive group the emergency procedures to be used in the case of a sudden loss of air at depth.

POSSIBLE COURSES OF ACTION

Confirm the existence and nature of the apparent air loss.

- Stop, and think consciously.
- Attempt to breathe. If successful, proceed with a normal ascent.

Many out-of-air situations lie with the diver and/or the situation rather than an equipment malfunction or actual depletion of air supply. For example, a flooded mask may be interpreted as being out of air; hyperventilating due to stress may fill the lungs but, because of verging panic, the diver does not realise this and still tries to inhale. When he or she cannot do so, loss of air supply is inferred.

If a true out-of-air situation exists, there are **five possible courses of safe action**; three requiring dependent action and two independent action (see page 170).

Dependent action

1. Using an **octopus rig** is the optimum choice, allowing the diver and buddy to ascend, each with their own second stage. They must stay fairly close together and maintain eye contact. Divers should be encouraged to include an additional second stage regulator on their rigs. Remember, though, that if one diver is out of air, his or her buddy has probably got a very limited supply too. So don't hyperventilate and waste remaining air. A double emergency may result! Stay calm and breathe as normally as possible during the ascent.

2. **Buddy breathing** under emergency conditions is a less desirable choice. Effective buddy breathing needs regular practice and is too difficult for most divers to remember and then use under extreme stress while ascending.

> In March 2007, the South Pacific Underwater Medicine Society (SPUMS) published this policy statement on EAT developed at a 1993 workshop:
> **Buddy breathing as a form of emergency ascent appears to cause an unacceptable level of risk to participants, both in training and in an actual emergency. Consequently, the Society advises divers to discontinue buddy breathing and instead practise less risky out-of-air procedures such as the use of alternative air sources. The Society believes that buddy breathing should be neither taught nor practised.**

Despite this, buddy breathing remains a source of emergency air supply training. If utilised, the recommendations are:
- First establish a satisfactory breathing cycle at depth.
- Continue buddy breathing while ascending at a reasonable rate to the surface. **Both** divers must remember **not to breathhold** while the other uses the regulator.

3. **Buddy breathing followed by a controlled emergency swimming ascent (CESA).** This is a semi-dependent choice that allows the out-of-air diver time to compose himself and prepare for a safe CESA. If this method is chosen, buddy breathing must commence at the bottom and continue until the dependent diver signals that he is ready to perform a CESA. Do not use this method while ascending. Once air-sharing on ascent commences, it must be continued to the surface.

Independent action

Independent action should only be performed if dependent action is impractical or impossible. Accidents have happened under circumstances that could have been avoided if the diver had stopped to think before he acted. For example, an out-of-air diver who swam 27 metres horizontally underwater to reach his buddies in 17 metres of water; or the diver who swam 8 metres **deeper** from the 16-metre mark, only to discover, when he reached his buddy, that he could not get air from him.

1. The recommended independent emergency option is a **controlled emergency swimming ascent (CESA)**, in which the out-of-air diver swims to the surface, looking upwards, with the second stage regulator **in the mouth**. There are two ways of developing arterial gas embolism during a CESA:

   (a) **Breathholding** embolises the panicky diver, as expanding air stresses the lung as a whole.

   (b) **Forced exhalation** embolises the careful student who obeys his or her instructor too implicitly and exhales fully and completely during ascent. **Forced exhalation markedly reduces the calibre of small airways near alveoli and even collapses some small airways.** This traps expanding alveolar air and causes alveolar tearing and AGE at the surface. Even gentle exhalation can close an airway that is partially blocked or in spasm due to asthma, a scar, cyst or tumour or a mucous plug due to inflammation or cigarette smoking. Relax and breathe normally through the regulator during the ascent – it will always deliver air as the ambient depth and pressure decrease.

   The message is: WATCH YOUR BUBBLES!
   - Do not breathhold!
   - Do not actively forcibly exhale. Gentle humming or rapid shallow panting are enough to ensure an open airway.
   - Do not remove the regulator from the mouth. An involuntary inhalation will result in water inhalation and either initiate the drowning process, or cause laryngospasm and AGE with further ascent. With the regulator in place, an inhalation will nearly always provide additional residual cylinder air as surrounding depth and pressure decrease.
   - If bubbles are streaming from your regulator, your lungs are safely depressurising. If no bubbles are present, you are breathholding. Total exhalation also reduces the diver's buoyancy and makes active ascent more difficult.

2. A **buoyant ascent** is the last option. Either the weight belt is dropped or the BC is inflated. A buoyant ascent must only be attempted when the diver seriously doubts that he can reach the surface by swimming. Note that the rapid ascent rate will cause an even more demanding and rapid flow of air from the lungs than a CESA. So watch your bubbles!

To summarise, in a low-on-air situation, the first choice of action is a normal ascent. If possible, take independent or dependent action. Independent action is usually quicker and simpler and does not put another diver at risk, but it may not be feasible. Dependent action can provide for slower ascents and a safety stop, but it requires another diver, an octopus rig, or an additional air supply, such as a pony bottle.

21

DECOMPRESSION

In simple terms, decompression is a time-dependent process whereby excess nitrogen or any other inert gas that is absorbed by the body during a dive is exhaled during ascent and after surfacing.

TISSUE UPTAKE OF INERT GAS DURING COMPRESSION

When a diver breathing air is exposed to increased pressure under water, each contraction of the right ventricle of the heart sends a surge of venous blood to the lungs for oxygen renewal and carbon dioxide extraction, a process that also results in the diver's blood becoming loaded with nitrogen. The prodigious size of the alveolar-capillary area in the lungs ensures virtually instant saturation of lung capillary blood with nitrogen at the now higher partial pressure (see Henry's Law, page 26, and Dalton's Law, page 24).

This nitrogen load is carried within the arterial system to the body tissues where capillary-tissue gas transfer occurs. With time and repeated recirculation of the blood volume to the lungs, the tissues will eventually have the same nitrogen partial pressure as the alveoli. The tissues are then in equilibrium with the alveoli and are said to be **saturated** at that partial pressure of nitrogen. At this point, no further uptake of nitrogen will occur.

This occurs on land, too. For example, a person living at Lake Titicaca, in the Peruvian Andes, at an altitude of 3 600 metres above sea level will have a nitrogen partial pressure of about 0.51 ATA in his or her tissues. On arrival at the coast for a diving holiday, tissue nitrogen will equilibrate over 24 hours to the higher coastal air nitrogen partial pressure of 0.79 ATA.

Tissue uptake of a gas depends on five things:
1. solubility of the gas in a tissue,
2. blood supply to the tissue,
3. time,
4. depth, and
5. gas gradient.

1. Solubility

Different tissues have different solubilities for the same gas. For example, nitrogen is about five times more soluble in fat than in water. This means that fatty tissues can dissolve about five times more nitrogen than blood can. It also means that fatty tissues take a long time to saturate, and blood, with its lower solubility for nitrogen, rapidly saturates.

2. Blood supply

Although the total capillary-tissue exchange area in the human body is colossal – around $10\,000\,m^2$ in an average individual – our blood volume is about six litres, so only a limited amount of inert gas can be carried in the blood at any one time. It is also only the arterial portion of the blood that transports the higher partial pressure of inert gas from lungs to tissue during descent and while at bottom depths.

In addition, some tissues, such as muscle, the brain and the spinal cord, have a rich blood supply and saturate quickly. Others, such as fat, have a much poorer blood supply. Fat has a high solubility for nitrogen and a poor blood supply and therefore saturates more slowly than any other tissue but, once saturated, a large nitrogen load is present, which then desaturates very slowly.

3. Time

As tissue saturation depends on blood circulation, time becomes an important factor because blood circulation requires time. Each minute, an average heart circulates about four to six litres of blood through the systemic circulation, and an identical amount through the lungs. Long exposures to pressure therefore cause greater nitrogen uptake than shorter periods.

4. Depth

At depth, partial pressures of inhaled gases increase (Dalton's Law) and the amount of inert gas diffusing from alveoli into blood increases proportionally (Henry's Law). The deeper the dive, the greater the gradient from alveoli to blood to tissues.

5. Gas gradient

At the seaside, a diver is exposed to nitrogen at 0.79 ATA. Body tissues saturate with nitrogen at 0.75 ATA because, in the alveoli, inspired air is mixed with outgoing carbon dioxide and water vapour which dilute air nitrogen a little. Should a diver dive to 50 msw, the nitrogen partial pressure in his air supply increases six times to 4.74 ATA. So, at the beginning of his 6 ATA exposure, the gradient between alveoli and tissues increases by 4.74 minus 0.75 ATA or 3.99 ATA.

It is important to appreciate what this really means. A pressure of nearly 4 ATA is not just a number; it is a **huge** pressure differential – enough to burst a motor car tyre! The diver can only survive because the total gas pressure inside his lungs and the water pressure around the body are exactly balanced and equal. But the absolute amounts of nitrogen – in the air supply and in solution in the tissues – are now very different. A pressure head of nearly four atmospheres of nitrogen gas in the alveoli is separated from the blood in lung capillaries by only two membranes of extreme delicacy – each one cell thick. Nitrogen gas speedily diffuses through this insignificant and almost ridiculous barrier, passes into solution in blood, and is carried to the tissues and loaded there.

With time, the concentration of nitrogen in muscle, say, increases to 2.74 ATA. The gradient is then 4.74 minus 2.74 ATA or 2 ATA, so nitrogen absorption into muscle slows. The uptake is **exponential** and a progressive slowing of uptake occurs as the gradient falls. Initial uptake is very vigorous and speedy; later uptake progressively slows, then stops when the gradient disappears at saturation.

INERT GAS LOSS BY THE TISSUES – DECOMPRESSION

The biggest difference between the loading and unloading of tissues with inert gas is that tissue gas loading is **passively receptive** whereas decompression is **actively driven** by tissue gas pressures and can be explosive. While a tissue may be remarkably tolerant to a horrific gas gradient during uptake, Henry's Law can either gently drive a gas from a tissue and along a small gradient to the lungs for exhalation, or send the gas bubbling and boiling out of solution inside a tissue if the gradient is too high. As soon as free gas is present, Boyle's Law operates and expands the free gas volume to ambient pressure. This is the picture of acute decompression illness. The complete process is equivalent to preparing soda water – the water passively absorbs carbon dioxide from the gas cartridge during pressurisation, but sudden release of pressure by rapidly opening the bottle causes instant bubbling. The purpose of using decompression tables is to establish gentle gas gradients which avoid bubbling.

DECOMPRESSION THEORY

In the early 1900s, John Scott Haldane, a Scottish doctor, physiologist and president of the British Institute of Mining Engineers, did much of the basic work on decompression. He proposed two hypotheses:

FIRST HYPOTHESIS Both nitrogen uptake and release from the tissues follow an exponential gas gradient, and all the tissues in the body can be represented by five theoretical model tissues having half times of 5, 10, 20, 40 and 75 minutes.

Blood is the fastest tissue, with a half time of five minutes. This means that during a dive, saturation of blood with nitrogen can be considered in blocks of five minutes. In the first five minutes, blood will absorb half of the maximum volume of gas it can dissolve at that depth. It is half-saturated in five minutes. During the next five minutes, blood will absorb half as much again, i.e. one quarter. It will be three-quarters saturated. After another five minutes, half of a quarter, or one-eighth, will be absorbed and blood will be seven-eighths saturated, then fifteen-sixteenths, and so on. The same applies to the slower tissues, except that they half-saturate in blocks of 10 minutes to 75 minutes. After six half-times, a tissue is saturated.

Release of gas during decompression follows a reverse exponential gradient. Blood would lose half of its excess dissolved nitrogen in the first five minutes; half of the remainder in the next five minutes; etc. After six half-times, a tissue will be desaturated. Blood desaturates in 30 minutes.

SECOND HYPOTHESIS Divers can tolerate a doubling of the nitrogen partial pressure in their tissues on returning to the surface after a dive and still not suffer from acute decompression illness. Haldane called this **supersaturation**.

He believed that ambient pressure could be halved, causing the tissue tensions to be twice that of environmental pressure without bubble formation. That is, decompression could be done in safety from, for example:

2 ATA to 1 ATA (10 msw to the surface),
4 ATA to 2 ATA (30 msw to 10 msw), and
5 ATA to 2.5 ATA (40 msw to 15 msw).

This 2:1 ratio, or **critical ratio** hypothesis, forms the basis of many current stage decompression tables. Haldane recommended its use to 50 msw; it is not adequate for deeper dives.

In practical terms, combining Haldane's two hypotheses means that different tissues control safe ascent at different times. Ascent rates, and the depth and time of decompression stops, must ensure that at no time is any tissue loaded with inert gas by more than 2:1.

At the beginning of ascent, the five-minute tissue will dictate safe ascent. When it is desaturated to below 2:1, the 10-minute tissue will begin to set the safe ascent limits, and so on. A decompression stop with any tissue saturated to more than double the water pressure will cause bubbling in that tissue.

Haldane was actively opposed by a British physiologist, Sir Leonard Hill, who believed that decompression should be continuous and uniform. Hill's technique, called a **linear** decompression, is now used in decompression from saturation, rather than Haldane's **staged** decompression.

However, for very long deep dives, the five-model tissue half times are insufficient and others have been added by different scientists, some even using half times of up to 12 hours! The 2:1 ratio was also found to be too simple, because some model tissues have different critical ratios at different depths.

The concept of '**M values**' was introduced in the 1960s by Robert Workman, a doctor with the US Navy Experimental Diving Unit (NEDU). This stipulates the maximum ratio of supersaturation for each model tissue at varying depths.

BEHNKE'S OXYGEN WINDOW The big question with Haldane's work was 'Why can tissues retain gas at double the ambient pressure without bubbling in the first place?' Work by US physician Albert R. Behnke showed that one reason is oxygen use by tissues. As oxygen is used by a tissue, its partial pressure falls in the tissue. This means that the total gas pressure in the tissue drops. A 'space' is formed which nitrogen can fill – the so-called **oxygen window**.

HILL'S UNSUPERSATURATION Okinawan pearl divers, diving off Australia, used to perform dives to 90 msw on air for 60 minutes, twice a day, six days a week, without any theoretical tables. Using only experience, they developed their own tables which are about 30 per cent shorter than the US Navy tables, use deeper in-water stops and no stops shallower than about 9 msw. Hill studied these and, in 1966, proposed the concept of **unsupersaturation**. Venous blood and tissues have a total gas pressure which is less than ambient air at the surface – nearly 0.1 ATA less, due mainly to low oxygen. They are technically gas vacuums. So if a diver ascends one metre, nitrogen can take up the 0.1 ATA to saturate the tissue. A nitrogen gradient to the alveoli is then established, and more nitrogen is vented. This restores another 0.1 ATA of unsaturation for nitrogen occupation.

These two concepts – the oxygen window and unsaturation – permit the tables that enable a diver to ascend safely with nitrogen supersaturation but little or no bubble formation. The **oxygen window** can be increased enormously by breathing pure oxygen (0 per cent nitrogen) during decompression. If no nitrogen is inhaled, a very high gradient for elimination of nitrogen is set up. The gradient becomes the difference between the tissue nitrogen content and zero in the inhaled gas – that is, the maximum possible gradient at the surface. If the diver enters a recompression chamber at this point and breathes pure oxygen at pressure, the gradient will increase further, actively driving oxygen into, and nitrogen out of, the tissue cells. In addition, the extra chamber pressure effectively keeps all potential bubbles in solution.

This is the basis of all oxygen decompression tables and oxygen therapeutic tables for arterial gas embolism and acute decompression illness.

BUBBLE BEHAVIOUR

Consider a bubble inside a tissue. Inside the bubble is gas under pressure. Let's call the pressure in the bubble Pb. If the pressure around the bubble is less than Pb, the bubble will grow. But if the surrounding pressure is greater than Pb, the bubble will shrink.

The pressure around the bubble consists of:
– ambient environmental pressure (Pressure ambient) – Pa,
– tissue pressure on the bubble (Pressure of tissues) – Pt, and
– surface tension of the bubble (Pressure of tension) – Pτ.
The total pressure on the bubble is Pa + Pt + Pτ.

- if Pb is greater than Pa + Pt + Pτ, the bubble will enlarge,
- if Pb is smaller than Pa + Pt + Pτ, the bubble will shrink,
- if Pb equals Pa + Pt + Pτ, the bubble is stable, and
- if Pb is much smaller than Pa + Pt + Pτ, the bubble will redissolve.

It is apparent, therefore, that to treat or eliminate a bubble (i.e. a bend), one must increase Pa or Pt or Pτ or all three. To date, there is no way of increasing the surface tension (Pτ). Increasing Pa (ambient pressure) can be done by recompression in a chamber. Substances having high molecular weights, such as dextran, are also available for increasing the osmotic pressure in the blood in an attempt to increase tissue pressure in blood (Pt).

WHERE DO BUBBLES APPEAR? Bubbles can originate anywhere, but are mostly found in the venous system, which drains and transports inert gas from all tissues to the lungs during the degassing process. In addition, veins are very low pressure systems, so venous Pt is low. In contrast, the arterial system has the highest Pt because of left ventricular pump pressurisation and the lowest inert gas load because arterial blood has been subjected to lung degassing of nitrogen.

Venous bubbles pass through the right side of the heart and into the pulmonary arteries, arterioles and capillaries. Direct transfer of gas from bubbles to alveoli can then occur. Although there is always some venous bubble transport after any dive, under normal conditions most of the inert gas load is transferred in solution to the lungs for exhalation.

If the number of venous bubbles reaching the right ventricle is excessive, or if they coalesce to form big bubbles, an air-lock may occur in the right ventricle, leading to death. Similarly, the pulmonary arteries could become overloaded with bubbles, causing right heart failure and shock; in diving terms, this is known as the 'chokes'. Shunts between the right and left sides of the heart can shift bubbles en route to the lungs back into the arterial circulation as nitrogen emboli (see pages 44–45).

Bubbles do not have to reach the chest to cause trouble. They can be problematic anywhere. Obstruction in spinal veins can cause paralysis. Bubbles can form directly in brain tissue, causing acute cerebral decompression illness; in joints, causing limb bends; in the fluid-filled labyrinth of the inner ear, giving rise to deafness or vertigo. If bubbles form in arteries, they can embolise, for example to the brain, exactly like arterial gas embolism after pulmonary barotrauma (see page 164).

22

ACUTE DECOMPRESSION ILLNESS

Acute decompression illness is associated with the development of free gas or bubbles in the blood or tissues as a result of a decrease in ambient pressure. It is also called decompression sickness (DCS), which is classified into Type I and Type II DCS. This author prefers the more descriptive definition of acute decompression illness (DCI), which incorporates arterial gas embolism.

Acute decompression illness (DCI) is caused by:

– the formation of inert gas bubbles after a dive
– pulmonary barotrauma of ascent (see page 161).

Both result in tissue damage or obstruction to blood flow which then interferes with the oxygen supply to the area involved.

FACTORS PREDISPOSING TO INCREASED BUBBLE FORMATION

1. **Missed or incomplete decompression** These result in an excessive tissue inert gas load on return to the surface.
2. **Repetitive dives** If the required surface interval time is reduced or residual nitrogen time is not included in the next total dive time, nitrogen overload may occur.
3. **Exposure to heat** Heat promotes tissue degassing, so a hot shower after diving can cause bubbles to form, even if a correct ascent schedule was used. Gases are more soluble in cold solutions than in warm ones.
4. **Exposure to cold** Cold promotes tissue upgassing. If a diver is inadequately protected by a wet or dry suit and develops some degree of hypothermia, he or she will absorb more inert gas during the dive. Circulation also slows down, causing a later, slower return of nitrogen to the lungs for degassing.
5. **Excessive movement** Exercise after diving may dislodge bubbles which are harmlessly lodged and are degassing, causing them to embolise. Exercise also increases tissue temperature, causing an increase in bubble size (Charles's Law, see page 22), or actual bubble development.
6. **Dehydration** A drop in total volume of body fluids results in less available fluid for inert gas dilution and more rapid saturation of the remaining fluid. This can arise from excessive sweating, restricted fluid intake, vomiting, etc.

7. **Rapid ascents** Even if decompression stops are not required, rapid ascents may cause too steep a nitrogen gradient for nitrogen solubility in venous blood. That is, more nitrogen is released from the tissues than venous blood can hold in solution to the lungs.
8. **Obesity** A greater mass of tissue is available to absorb inert gas.
9. **Increased age** The efficiency of tissue blood supply in degassing may decrease with age.
10. **Increased carbon dioxide** Inadequate ventilation due to skip breathing, deep air dives, dense breathing mixes, a contaminated air supply, a faulty regulator or excessive underwater exercise can lead to a high level of carbon dioxide in tissues. This 'closes' the oxygen window and reduces nitrogen tolerance. Smoking, which raises carbon monoxide levels in blood and tissue, does the same thing.
11. **Alcohol excess** Alcohol is a diuretic, and overindulgence causes increased urine output, with consequent loss of body water and dehydration. It also predisposes to vomiting, with similar results. Flushing of the skin predisposes to heat loss and hypothermia, with increased nitrogen absorption at depth.
12. **Physical injury** Injury to an arm or leg, for example, causes tissues to swell and distorts capillary-tissue function. Degassing of the tissue is slowed and bubble formation can occur.
13. **Altitude** Flying after diving, with the further drop in atmospheric pressure, will increase the size of existing bubbles (Boyle's Law, see page 21) or trigger new ones. If a medical emergency makes it essential to transport a diver by air, the aircraft should be pressurised, or should fly as low as possible.
14. **Females** Initial reports suggested a higher incidence of acute decompression illness in women than in men. The usual explanation is that women naturally have a greater amount of subcutaneous fat, but more recent studies have not shown any significant difference in divers using conservative modern tables.
15. **Limb flexion** Sitting with the legs crossed or flexed after diving may cause problems by kinking the veins in the knees and groin. This may occur, for example, when one drives home at the end of an active diving weekend.
16. **Previous decompression illness** If a diver experiences recurring bubbles, they frequently appear at a site of a previous injury or bubble formation, such as a shoulder, elbow or knee. This may be due to the previous distortion or damage to tissue-capillary function, resulting in inadequate inert gas elimination.
17. **Increased viscosity of blood** This occurs in conditions such as sickle cell anaemia or the carrier trait.

In most cases, a combination of factors is responsible for increased bubble formation. Common examples of relatively innocent behaviour that can result in bubble development after a technically correct dive include things like standing in the sun in a wet suit after a repetitive dive, going for a jog on the beach or on a hike a few hours after a dive, or diving with a sports injury to a knee or shoulder.

FACTORS PREDISPOSING TO
DECREASED BUBBLE FORMATION

A great deal of extremely interesting work is currently being done to determine which factors might actually reduce bubble formation in sport divers.

1. **Slower ascents and deep stops** In sport divers, it is the fast tissue gas tensions that are critical for bubble generation during and after the ascent. The most serious signs and symptoms of DCI in scuba divers involve the spinal cord, with a tissue half time of only 12.5 minutes. John Haldane (see page 174) suggested 18 m/min (60 ft/min) as a safe ascent rate. Recent work measuring bubble formation using sonic Doppler methods suggests that 10 m/min (33 ft/min) is not only safer but that current sport diving tables **below 25 msw** might not allow adequate degassing from these fast tissues, resulting in heavier gas loads and bubble formation.

    It has been proposed that the use of a deep stop will significantly reduce fast tissue bubble formation and the risk of neurological DCI. In 2008, a series of experiments led by Peter Bennett and Alessandro Marroni of DAN involved two dives to 25 msw for 25 and 20 minutes respectively, with a 3½ hour surface interval. Fewest bubbles and the lowest nitrogen gas loads were detected when an ascent rate of 10 msw/min was used with a 2½ minute stop at 15 msw (50 fsw) plus the customary stop for 3–5 minutes at 6 msw (20 fsw).

2. **Strenuous pre-dive exercise** In 2004, after a series of experiments, Croatian researcher Zeljko Dujic and his co-workers reported that taking a single bout of aerobic exercise 24 hours before a dive significantly reduced the formation of circulating venous gas emboli (VGE) on decompression after diving. Circulating bubbles were detected with a precordial Doppler, which measures the number of bubbles passing through the heart, at 30, 60 and 90 minutes after surfacing.

    Then, in 2007, Jean-Eric Blatteau and co-workers showed that 45 minutes of running two hours before a **non-repetitive dive** also significantly decreases bubble formation after diving to 30 msw, suggesting that aerobic exercise has a protective effect against DCI. The number of bubbles in the right hearts of the test divers was reduced, protecting them from decompression illness. However, the exact amount of exercise necessary to reduce venous circulating bubbles remains unknown, and how exercise exerts its protective effect also remains unclear. It has been suggested that, rather than altering the nitrogen elimination rate, exercise may reduce the number of existing gaseous nuclei that are required for initiating bubble formation in tissues and blood vessels. Pre-dive exercise, in the form of outdoor running for 45 minutes two hours before diving, may form the basis for a new way of preventing serious decompression sickness. However, this would only be feasible in physically fit divers having the time to exercise before a dive; the optimal type (if any) of aerobic exercise performed has not yet been demonstrated.

3. **Nitric oxide** Experiments using laboratory rats in a simulated chamber dive showed that undertaking exercise 20–24 hours before a dive reduced bubble formation, thereby increasing survival rates. Aside from the postulated reduction in the number of existing gaseous nuclei, nitric oxide (NO) may be involved in this protection. Blocking the production of NO in tissues **increases** bubble formation, but providing a long-lasting NO donor both 20 hours prior to and immediately before a dive **reduces** bubble formation. In the human experiments conducted by Zeljko Dujic in 2004, the use of a short-acting NO donor, in the form of a nitroglycerine spray (used by angina sufferers to relieve chest pain), reduced bubble formation after standard dives and shortened decompression time in scuba divers. Whether the use of nitroglycerine will have any practical use in the prevention of DCI in sport divers is still very speculative.

DIVER DISBELIEF

With the exception of severe pulmonary or neurological cases of acute decompression illness, one of the greatest problems a diving physician has to contend with is diver disbelief. The average macho male diver simply does not believe it possible that he has bent. Any number of reasons are given why symptoms such as joint pain, headache, numbness, weakness or excessive fatigue are due to a late night or two, falling off a horse or a bump on the dive boat. The presence of acute decompression illness is disregarded as unlikely because, of course, the dive profiles were impeccable in their performance …

The fact that said diver enthusiastically gambolled on the beach after the dive with a buxom young thing in a bikini is forgotten. So is the energetic post-dive game of beach volleyball or the squatting, with extreme bending of the knees, around the campfire telling jokes while a few beers numbed a progressively painful knee. It is only a few days later, when all the reasons and excuses run out, that the diver hesitantly apologises for disturbing the doctor, but …

If you develop any unexplained symptoms post-dive, even if they are seemingly minor, do not wait. Contact a dive doctor, explain the situation and let a medical professional handle the dilemma. A few words of advice may be all that is needed to sort out the problem but, if chamber therapy is required, it can then be arranged in good time before things really deteriorate.

FACTORS PREDISPOSING TO PULMONARY BAROTRAUMA OF ASCENT

Lung damage during ascent results from the lung tissue becoming overdistended due to the expansion of contained gas. The responsible factors are the same as those that can cause inadequate exhalation or obstruction to the airways (see also page 161):

1. PANIC, with an attempt at an emergency ascent.
2. Free ascents, especially uncontrolled free ascents, and submarine escape training.
3. Skip breathing, with a diver attempting to conserve air by breathholding and being unaware that he or she is ascending.
4. Buddy breathing at depth becoming uncoordinated and leading to panic.
5. Inability to gain comfortable and relaxed control of the regulator during ditch and recovery training, resulting in the exercise being abandoned in favour of a hurried return to the surface.
6. Apparatus difficulties, such as a high regulator resistance to inhalation because of an almost empty cylinder.
7. Water inhalation, causing choking, panic and laryngospasm, with frantic attempts to reach the surface.
8. Lung disorders, such as asthma and chest infections with a high resistance to outflow, or mucous plugs blocking bronchioles.

TIME OF ONSET OF ACUTE DECOMPRESSION ILLNESS

Acute decompression illness occurs during ascent or soon after the dive. About 60 per cent of incidents present within 30 minutes. Within six hours, about 90 per cent of incidents occur and by 12 hours up to 99 per cent of likely DCI incidents will have occurred. Occasionally, onset may be delayed by up to or over 24 hours.

The majority (about 60 per cent) of cases of DCI involve joints and skin. Of the remaining 40 per cent, the vast majority affect the brain and spinal cord.

However, as gas bubbles can appear anywhere, any presentation is possible, including irritability, confusion, weakness, paralysis, headache, coma, blindness, deafness, numbness, memory loss, chest pain, abdominal pain, etc. Consequently, **any** new symptom that appears after a dive must be regarded with extreme suspicion until proven unrelated to bubble formation.

TYPES OF DIVING

When it comes to decompression illness, the type of diving is important:

1. **Sport divers** usually perform deep air dives with rapid ascents, during which they beat their blood-alveolar degassing time and develop fast tissue bubbles. As blood is the fastest tissue, and veins are the transport network to the lungs, bubbles develop in venous blood and may then become widespread, with lung,

brain or spinal cord involvement. Spinal cord involvement frequently follows acute lung bubble overload (the 'chokes'). Massive bubble formation can lead to blood clotting throughout the entire vascular system (disseminated intravascular coagulation). This is fortunately rare, but invariably fatal.

2. **Saturation divers** and divers who undertake medium-depth long dives with slow ascents usually develop slow tissue bubbles, particularly in their joints and tendons. **Fast tissue bubbles are unpredictable and dangerous. Slow tissue bubbles are usually predictable.**

3. **Heliox divers** on very deep excursion dives frequently have inner ear bubbles at the beginning of their decompression or when changing their breathing mixes. Technical sport divers also commonly experience inner ear bubbles after they change their gas mix during the ascent.

PRESENTATION OF ACUTE DECOMPRESSION ILLNESS

As acute DCI is due to the presence of bubbles or trapped gas anywhere in the body, the way it presents will depend on the tissue or organ involved. For example, the formation of bubbles in a joint will present with joint pain after a dive; while features relating to loss of higher function, or motor or sensory function, will result from the formation of bubbles in the brain or a cerebral arterial gas embolism after pulmonary barotrauma of ascent (see page 161). Arterial gas embolism to the coronary arteries will present with chest pain, etc. Acute DCI is dynamic because bubbles may remain constant in size, or grow, shrink or move to a different area. Additional bubbles may develop in different tissues, or more gas may be vented into capillaries and be circulated throughout the body after lung damage.

Because the presentation is so variable, systematic recording by the diver or the attendant buddy of any untoward symptom after diving is very important. This will enable a diving doctor to make a clearer assessment of the case and provide proper definitive treatment.

The following six points must be carefully noted by the diver:

1. Evolution

Evolution refers to the development of acute DCI from onset to the present moment. It is a description of the dynamic quality of the illness before any recompression in a chamber. Evolution may be:

   (a) **Static** No change occurs. Any complaint remains constant – joint pain neither worsens nor improves; headache, dizziness, blurred vision persist.
   (b) **Progressive** The diver's condition worsens – pain increases; confusion develops, etc.

(c) **Spontaneously improving** The diver is getting better and any symptoms lessen.

(d) **Relapsing** After an initial improvement, symptoms recur.

2. Manifestations

This describes the details of the complaint. It could be:

- **musculoskeletal** (e.g. limb pain or aching),
- **neurological** (e.g. headache, unconsciousness, paralysis, ringing in the ears, vertigo); neurological assessments must be recorded as detailed on page 325,
- **cutaneous** (e.g. skin rashes or itching),
- **lymphatic** ('orange peel' appearance of the skin),
- **pulmonary** (e.g. breathlessness, coughing, husky voice, chest pain, 'chokes'),
- **constitutional** (e.g. loss of appetite, fatigue, nausea), or
- **other** (any other manifestation).

3. Time to onset

For each manifestation, the time that has elapsed between surfacing from the dive and the onset of the manifestation must be recorded. If a manifestation occurs during ascent, it must be recorded as such.

4. Gas burden

This is an estimate of the residual nitrogen overload present after a dive. It gives some indication of the degree of exposure. It could be described as minimal, moderate or substantial; or a no-decompression-stop dive, correctly completed decompression-stop dive, missed decompression-stop dive, or an emergency or uncontrolled ascent with missed decompression-stop dive. Accurate dive profiles of all dives performed during the last two to three days of the dive trip, including surface intervals, should be provided to the doctor, as well as details of all surface activities – exercise, exposure to heat, or any of the predisposing causes as described on pages 178–179.

5. Evidence of barotrauma

Be alert for possible pulmonary barotrauma (e.g. coughing up blood, tight chest, breathlessness, sudden unconsciousness). See page 160.

6. Response to treatment

Any treatment given (e.g. oxygen, painkillers) must be fully described, as well as the results achieved.

If the above points are noted and documented, the attending doctor will be presented with a clear and concise record of the event, without any assumptions, and an ideal matrix for database applications which will facilitate exchange of information between hyperbaric centres. A model report form follows:

ACUTE DECOMPRESSION ILLNESS REPORT

EVOLUTION		NAME:			
STATIC		AGE:	SEX:	DATE:	
PROGRESSIVE		ADDRESS:			
IMPROVING					
RELAPSING		TEL. WORK:		HOME:	

MANIFESTATIONS

MUSCULOSKELETAL:

NEUROLOGICAL:

CUTANEOUS:

LYMPHATIC:

PULMONARY:

CONSTITUTIONAL:

OTHER:

TIME TO ONSET		GAS BURDEN	
DURING ASCENT		NO DECO STOPS NEEDED	
ON SURFACING		COMPLETED DECO STOPS	
AFTER SURFACING	MINS	MISSED DECO STOPS	
EVIDENCE OF BAROTRAUMA		EMERGENGY ASCENT	
		UNCONTROLLED ASCENT	

RESPONSE TO TREATMENT

MANAGEMENT OF ACUTE DECOMPRESSION ILLNESS

It is essential for sport divers to have some knowledge of management of acute DCI; diving physicians or expert help are not always at hand and divers are often dependent on each other's knowledge and expertise. (Operating a therapeutic recompression chamber is beyond the scope of sport diving, but the relevant tables are mentioned here for completeness.)

All divers should complete a basic first-aid course as well as learn how to peform CPR. This training should be updated annually in order to provide intelligent and really effective support in an emergency.

Prevention
Learning how to avoid acute decompression illness is the basic objective of a diving course. Most people can swim and are reasonably drown-proof when they attend a diving school. They are then taught how not to bend or burst. Other underwater dangers come next in importance.

1. Preventing DCI requires strict avoidance of the factors that predispose to bubble formation and lung overdistension (see pages 178–179; page 161).
2. For divers, proper hydration is extremely important. Fluid keeps nitrogen in solution and good hydration can ensure gas solubility, even when a little latitude is taken with the predisposing factors for bubble formation. Drink a large glass of water or fruit juice 30 minutes before diving. With the exception of alcohol, drinking and diving is good!
3. Aerobic exercise, in the form of running, 24 hours beforehand and/or for 45 minutes just before a **non-repetitive dive**, has been demonstrated to reduce the number of venous gas emboli after the dive. The beneficial aspects of exercise for divers are still the focus of intensive research.
4. The use of a 2½ minute in-water stop at 15 msw, in addition to the usual five-minute stop at 6 msw, has been shown to reduce the risk of DCI in dives to 25 msw for 20–25 minutes.

Treatment
In the case of an episode of acute DCI, there are some things that fellow divers can do while waiting for the emergency services to arrive.

(a) Primary aid
This must commence as soon as the affected diver is out of the water, either on the boat or on land (in the case of shore entries or inland diving).

1. Send someone to contact the emergency rescue service and a dive physician.
2. Keep the diver relaxed, calm, quiet and lying flat.

3. Administer continuous 100 per cent oxygen via a demand valve.
4. Encourage oral fluid intake – 500 ml initially, then 150 ml per hour. Do not try to give oral fluids to an unconscious diver!
5. Keep the diver flat during transport to the recompression facility. If the diver is unconscious, placed him or her in the left lateral rescue position (see page 232).
6. If breathing or heartbeat fail, administer rescue breathing or CPR (see page 235). Remember AIDS awareness!

(b) Secondary aid
This requires at least paramedic training but has been included for completeness. Secondary aid should be implemented immediately a qualified person arrives.
1. Set up a Ringer's lactate intravenous lifeline.
2. Maintain continuous 100 per cent oxygen.
3. Maintain CPR if required. (AIDS awareness!)
4. Eliminating bubbles involves recompression, so it is necessary to reduce or eliminate any bubbles and then return the diver to 1 ATA in safety. It must be decided what depth is needed and at what rate return to surface pressure is required. The casualty should lie down during decompressions, as gas bubbles tend to rise towards the head and gravity tends to pool the blood in the veins of the legs when sitting or standing, thereby slowing the return of blood to the lungs for nitrogen elimination.

   On reaching the chamber, use the appropriate decompression tables, as outlined below (see Therapeutic Tables, pages 332–349). A dive doctor must be present during recompression:
   • If mild limb-only or just skin-related problems – Table 5 USN; 61 RN.
   • More severe symptoms as well as AGE – Table 6 USN; 62 RN.
   • If worsening – Table 67 RN **or else** Table 6A USN; 63 RN, **then** Table 4 USN; 64 RN.
   Do not recompress a pneumothorax with neurological manifestations until a non-return chest drain has been inserted!
5. If the situation with recompression is out of hand, compress to depth of pain relief **on air** and hold the casualty there until additional emergency specialist medical help can be obtained.
6. Give Vitamin C (1000 mg orally).
7. Give Valium (5 mg by mouth) if the casualty is very agitated.

Transporting divers with acute decompression illness
1. Follow the principles of managing acute DCI, as given above.
2. If the diver is in a remote place, there are two possibilities:
   (a) During transport, give the casualty 100 per cent oxygen via a demand valve. If it is essential to use an aircraft, it must fly as low as possible or be capable of being pressurised to 1 ATA.

(b) Bring a portable recompression chamber to the diver. Use Table 5 or 6 USN (61 or 62 RN). Do not place an unconscious casualty in a one-man chamber. You will have no control over any of the parameters of CPR and, if vomiting with inhalation occurs, the situation will become desperate. The emergency chamber should be able to couple under pressure to the multiplace chamber at the recompression facility. If it cannot, the diver must be returned from 18 msw in the chamber to surface pressure over two minutes, transferred with an assistant to the therapeutic chamber, and repressurised while breathing pure oxygen. (See Neurological Assessment Form, page 328.)

(c) In both (a) and (b), the recompression facility must be notified in advance and the case discussed before the casualty arrives.

CASE MANAGEMENT AFTER DECOMPRESSION

Even once the diver emerges from the chamber feeling well and symptom free, management is not over. Most cases of acute DCI recur to a lesser degree within a few hours. Some require further recompression therapy. Ample liquids, plus the use of 100 per cent surface oxygen by demand valve for 55 minutes, followed by air for five minutes, repeated for six hours, will help prevent a recurrence. This may be regarded as too much fuss or too time-consuming, but the results warrant the effort.

WHEN CAN I RETURN TO DIVING AFTER DCI?

The answer depends upon whether the episode of acute DCI was deserved or undeserved. If the episode was deserved (predictable) – that is, the cause was due to known breaches of decompression, and the diver is otherwise fully fit – diving can be resumed after the following intervals:

No danger of recurrence; pain only; fully resolved with recompression	7 days off
Unlikely to recur; pain only; partially resolved with recompression	4–6 weeks off
No danger of recurrence; serious DCI; completely resolved with recompression	6 weeks off
Unlikely to recur; serious DCI; resolved fully only after six weeks	6 months off

However, in an undeserved (unpredictable) episode – that is, no cause for the DCI was found or known and it remains unresolved and likely to recur, and/or the diver is physically unfit and/or any other risk factors are present – the diver must be declared permanently unfit to dive.

23

UNDERWATER MANAGEMENT OF ACUTE DECOMPRESSION ILLNESS

Despite advances in modern communication systems, divers in remote areas may find that they are unable to get a phone signal, make contact with an emergency rescue service or get to a hyperbaric facility in time to prevent the serious complications that can arise from acute DCI. In these circumstances, returning the affected diver to an elevated pressure under water (underwater recompression) may be the only alternative. There are two possibilities: underwater **air** recompression or underwater **oxygen** recompression.

IT MUST BE STRESSED THAT:
– Underwater recompression, followed by a timed decompression profile, is an emergency first-aid procedure for divers in remote areas only.
– It is not intended to replace hyperbaric chamber therapy.
– It must only be used for acute pain, or limb, joint or skin decompression illness when potentially life-threatening worsening is anticipated.
– It is not intended for severe decompression illness or arterial gas embolism. Placing an unconscious diver on a demand valve and returning him or her to the water **can never be accepted or condoned**.

UNDERWATER AIR RECOMPRESSION THERAPY

This must only be done by very experienced, highly trained divers. It involves taking the diver, plus an attendant, back into the water to a depth of 30 msw and ascending using Table 1A USN (+ 6 hours), see page 347, or Table 81 RN (± 5 hours). A vertical, calibrated shot line must be used and the ascent timed by surface tenders, using a signal line. There are **no advantages**, but plenty of disadvantages.

DISADVANTAGES
1. The diver must be taken to a depth of 30 msw. This usually means the open sea with swells, currents, wind, rain and, perhaps, the darkness of night.
2. An air supply for **two divers**, adequate for 6 hours each, must be available.

3. At 30 msw, wet suits are thin (Boyle's Law, see page 21), and prolonged exposure can cause hypothermia in both the diver and the attendant.
4. Boat difficulties, inclement weather, seasickness, fatigue, inadequate stocks of air, hypothermia and narcosis may force the therapeutic dive to be cancelled prematurely. In this situation, the diver will get worse from the increased nitrogen exposure and the attendant will bend too.

Underwater air recompression therapy is dangerous, and can only be considered when acute limb or skin decompression illness occurs very soon after diving and is likely to worsen, exposing the diver to the risk of life-threatening acute decompression illness. **Anticipating this requires knowledge, training and experience, and must only be considered when no other help is possible.**

UNDERWATER OXYGEN RECOMPRESSION THERAPY

This technique was developed in 1975 by the Royal Australian Navy School of Underwater Medicine, and reviewed by Dr Carl Edmonds in 1999 as a result of cases of acute decompression illness occurring in areas very remote from proper recompression facilities. It involves returning the diver, with an attendant, to the water at a depth of 9 msw, followed by an ascent programme.

ADVANTAGES
1. The shallow depth facilitates the selection of a protected area, possibly avoiding a return to the open seas and thereby reducing the potential for seasickness, narcosis and boat problems.
2. Less compression of wet suits occurs, with less likelihood of hypothermia.
3. There is no requirement for extended air supplies.
4. There is no risk of the attendant bending.
5. Terminating the treatment will not worsen the diver.

The principles are the same as those used in chamber oxygen recompression therapy tables, that is: bubbles are compressed and reduced in size; further nitrogen uptake is avoided; a large gradient is created for nitrogen from tissues to alveoli; oxygen availability to tissues is increased; and decompression time is shortened. (See page 332.)

DISADVANTAGES
1. Oxygen must be supplied from the surface. It should be supplied to a full face mask (e.g. Kirby Morgan or AGA), via a non-return valve on the mask. A full face mask reduces the risk of inhaling water, allows direct communication

between the diver and the surface crew, and permits breathing if consciousness becomes clouded or vomiting occurs in a dizzy or seasick diver.
3. Cerebral oxygen toxicity, although unlikely, must be borne in mind. The fire risk must also be noted and oil-contaminated fittings and hoses avoided.
4. This is an emergency regime and is not intended to replace chamber therapy. It is a remote-area option which requires pre-planning and careful preparation.

METHOD
1. **Preparation**
   (a) A large 'hospital-type' oxygen cylinder is needed. This is fitted to a two-stage regulator, the first stage gauge indicating cylinder pressure and the second stage indicating delivery pressure, which should be set to 550 kPa.
   (b) One end of a 12-metre length of clean hose is attached to the second stage outlet and the other end is attached to a non-return valve on the diver's mask inlet.
   (c) The diver must be **fully dressed** and negatively weighted, so that there is no difficulty in maintaining depth under water. A tendency to drift upward is contraindicated.
   (d) The attendant breathes **air** using conventional scuba. Adequate full spare cylinders plus attached demand valves must be available **on** the shot line.
   (e) A shot line clearly marked in metres and adequately weighted is suspended from a buoy large enough to support the two divers easily.
   (f) If the recompression cannot be done in a sheltered, quiet area, the buoy must be tethered close to the boat.
   (g) Hand and foot loops, and a seating system, must be fitted to the shot line to assist both the diver and the attendant.

2. **Recompression**
   (a) The diver and the attendant descend to 9 metres.
   (b) A timed stay of 30 minutes is done in mild cases, 60 minutes in worse cases, and 90 minutes if improvement does not occur.
   (c) Ascent is then commenced at **12 minutes per metre**. Ascent time between stops is included in each 12 minutes.

9 msw bottom time	Ascent at 12 min/metre	Total time
30 minutes	96 minutes	126 mins: 2 hr 6 mins
60 minutes	96 minutes	156 mins: 2 hr 36 mins
90 minutes	96 minutes	186 mins: 3 hr 6 mins

If necessary, this recompression may be repeated twice daily until the diver recovers fully or emergency assistance arrives.

24

PROBLEMS ASSOCIATED WITH DISSOLVED GASES

In the waterworld of 'fizz', Robert Boyle (1627–1691) is king. His theories reign over the physical properties of what happens when free gases expand and contract when out of solution. The results are dramatic, with burst lungs, squeezes and bends. But there is another world, where the laws devised by John Dalton (1766–1844) and William Henry (1774–1836) reign. It is a quiet, painless, soporific place, but no less dangerous, and with much more insidious difficulties awaiting a diver.

All the gases in any breathing mixture can cause trouble, even kill, while they are dissolved and in solution in the diver's body fluids. The trouble is due to high partial pressures in solution. Only oxygen can kill due to low partial pressures in solution. The gases involved are:

OXYGEN

Symbol O. It exists as two atoms linked together: O_2. Its molecular weight is 32. It makes up about 21 per cent of clean, dry air – the air that we breathe. Oxygen is the **only** essential requirement in any breathing mixture, but it is the amount in the mix that is important. If the concentration is too low, oxygen deficiency occurs; this is called hypoxia (see below). If the concentration is too high, oxygen toxicity occurs.

NITROGEN

Symbol N. It exists as two atoms linked together: N_2. Its molecular weight is 28. It makes up about 79 per cent of clean, dry air. For easy calculation, air is often taken to comprise 20 per cent oxygen and 80 per cent nitrogen. Under normal surface conditions, nitrogen is inert as far as most living organisms are concerned. For the diver, however, it can cause problems. At high partial pressures, nitrogen in solution exhibits the properties of an anaesthetic. This is called nitrogen narcosis (see page 202).

CARBON DIOXIDE

Symbol CO_2. It exists as a single atom of carbon bound to two atoms of oxygen. It is the end-product of oxygen-carbohydrate metabolism by the body, and an accumulation of carbon dioxide in the body is toxic. High partial pressures cause carbon dioxide narcosis (see page 204).

CARBON MONOXIDE

Symbol CO. It exists as one atom of carbon bound to one atom of oxygen. It is highly poisonous. It is sometimes found as a contaminant of breathing mixtures as a result of petrol or diesel exhaust fumes being drawn into the air intake of the supply compressor. High partial pressures cause carbon monoxide poisoning.

HELIUM

Symbol He. It exists as a single atom: He. Its atomic weight is 4. It is a totally inert gas, as no other chemical element can react with helium under any conditions. It is obtained from natural gas wells, such as those in Mexico and Russia. Helium is used to dilute oxygen at depths below 50 msw, where air or nitrogen cannot be used alone. This presents both advantages and disadvantages.

ADVANTAGES
1. It does not cause narcosis.
2. It is very light, making it easy to breathe.
3. Helium-oxygen (heliox) mixtures allow a shorter decompression time than an equivalent air-saturation dive, because helium diffuses very rapidly.

DISADVANTAGES
1. It is expensive.
2. Speech at depth is unintelligible – a descrambler is needed.
3. Helium has a very high thermal conductivity, rapidly transferring heat from or to a diver. This makes the diver very susceptible to hypothermia and hyperthermia.
4. At depths below 100 metres, helium can cause HPNS (see page 206).
5. As with nitrogen, acute decompression illness can occur.

HYDROGEN

Symbol H. It exists as two atoms linked together: H_2. Its molecular weight is 2, making hydrogen the lightest substance of all. After Zetterstrom's death in 1945 while breathing a hydrogen/oxygen mix (hydrox), work on hydrox as an alternative to heliox was confined almost entirely to animal experiments (see page 17). During the 1960s, the French company, Comex, revived experimental interest in hydrox but, on reaching depths of 300 msw in hyperbaric chambers, hydrogen narcosis appeared in the divers. This was relieved by adding helium to the hydrox mixtures and depths to 701 msw were then achieved in the Hydra programme. Nowadays, deep diving on hydrox is rare and the explosion risk makes it dangerous.

ADVANTAGES
1. It is cheap.
2. It is the lightest gas and the easiest to breathe.
3. HPNS is less likely to occur.

1. A hydrox mix is potentially violently explosive (e.g. the dirigible *Hindenberg*). This can be avoided by keeping the oxygen percentage in the mix below four per cent. Although such a mix will not explode, it can only be used for dives deeper than 30 metres (ppO$_2$ = 4% of 4 ATA = 0.16 ATA).
2. Speech requires a descrambler.
3. It has a high thermal conductivity.
4. Acute decompression illness can occur.
5. Hydrogen narcosis occurs below 300 msw.

NEON, ARGON, KRYPTON AND XENON

Like helium, these gases are all totally inert. Their use is limited to experimental diving and research. They are all expensive, denser and more narcotic than nitrogen (with the exception of neon), and require longer decompression schedules.

Attempting to memorise the various presentations of different problems associated with dissolved gas is confusing and difficult, as many of the signs overlap. It is vital, though, for rescuers to have a working approach to a diver who presents with confusion, convulsions or unconsciousness during or immediately after a dive. Without such an approach, no meaningful assistance can be given. An attempt has been made here to give a practical overview of the situation which requires only understanding and minimal memory effort.

The key to all these gas problems is **hypoxia** (lack of oxygen). Symptoms that are either due to or similar to hypoxia (see opposite), may be caused by any of the above-mentioned gases. Any other signs which may be present depend on the specific gas.

When determining the cause, the details of the dive are extremely important. An unconscious diver who has dived to 14 msw on air is unlikely to have nitrogen narcosis or oxygen toxicity. However, in the case of a diver on a pure oxygen rebreather at 14 msw, oxygen toxicity would be your first bet.

Similarly, a scuba diver who is not skip breathing[1] is unlikely to develop carbon dioxide toxicity, because all his or her exhaled air is being vented into the water. However, a Standard Diver on an open circuit freeflow system is in a different position because, if his ventilation flow rate is insufficient, carbon dioxide will build up.

The presentation of high gas partial pressures (or low oxygen) may be complicated by acute decompression illness (see page 178) but, even in such cases, the ultimate derangement is hypoxia. Inadequate oxygen is being absorbed or is reaching the affected site. As hypoxia is central to the story, it is dealt with first.

---

1. **Skip breathing** is a form of insanity affecting divers in love and newcomers to the sport. They need to impress and/or show their worth. For some peculiar reason, this means they must prove that they have low metabolic requirements and can breathe less than other mortals, so they hold each breath and exhale slowly while carbon dioxide steadily accumulates in their tissues. On returning to the surface, they proudly announce that their air cylinder is still half-full and quietly swallow a tablet for their splitting headache.

HYPOXIA

Hypo = too little, *oxia* = oxygen; therefore, **hypoxia** is a condition associated with a deficient supply of oxygen to the tissues.

Recall the petrol engine. Hypoxia is equivalent to decreasing the air supply to the engine. This drastically reduces engine's efficiency and may cause it to stall. Likewise, the tissue cells (our body's engines) suffer similarly from oxygen deprivation. Energy output is drastically reduced.

Hypoxia is often wrongly referred to as **anoxia**, which refers to no oxygen (*an* = without; *oxia* = oxygen), and is rapidly fatal. This would occur, for example, with strangulation, drowning, or breathing a tankful of pure helium or nitrogen. The closest a diver normally gets to anoxia is breathhold diving (see page 58).

CAUSES OF HYPOXIA The table below depicts the route followed by oxygen from gas supply to tissues. A breakdown anywhere along the route will cause hypoxia. (**Note**: this table is not a complete list of possibilities; it is simply intended to show that understanding, not memory, is the key to managing hypoxia.)

Failure of oxygen supply to tissues

Site of breakdown	Causes
Breathing source	Breathhold diving. Air supply exhausted. Wrong mix e.g. 2% oxygen instead of 20%. Equipment failure e.g. faulty regulator. Flow rate in a rebreather is too low.
Airway (mouth, larynx, trachea, bronchi, bronchioles)	Inhaled dentures. Laryngospasm. Inhaled foreign material e.g. vomiting under water.
Alveoli	Water in alveoli: drowning. Collapsed alveoli e.g. pneumothorax.
Lung capillaries	Obstruction with bubbles: 'chokes'. Compressed capillaries due to pulmonary barotrauma.
Arterial blood	Failure of circulation e.g. heart failure, hypothermia. Failure of oxygen carriage e.g. carbon monoxide. Lack of sufficient blood e.g. haemorrhage.
Tissue capillaries	Failure of capillary circulation e.g. inert gas bubbles or AGE in blood vessels.
Tissues	Poisoning of oxygen uptake e.g. carbon monoxide.

PRESENTATION OF HYPOXIA

The brain has a rich blood supply and is very sensitive to hypoxia. Not surprisingly, then, it is the brain that suffers first when hypoxia occurs. The degree of presentation depends on the degree of hypoxia.

With severe hypoxia: sudden unconsciousness can occur, for example, following ascent after breathhold diving.

With lesser hypoxia: any feature of a drop in brain oxygen may be evident, such as confusion, headache, fatigue, apathy, overconfidence, blurred vision, slurred speech, vertigo, stupor, etc.

So, with any change in:

– **higher cerebral function,**
– **the senses** (hearing, vision, touch, taste, smell), or
– **motor ability**

straight after diving, think of hypoxia, then consider the possible causes in the ladder from gas supply to tissues (see table on page 195).

Failure between gas supply and the lungs causes inadequate oxygenation of blood. The bright red arterial blood becomes darker and the diver becomes blue. This is called **cyanosis**. A cyanosed diver with blue lips and tongue **must** be considered to have hypoxia. **A blue diver is hypoxic.**

MANAGEMENT OF HYPOXIA

Just as the causes of hypoxia involve gas supply, airways and circulation, so does its management.

1. **ABC + Oxygen**

   A Airways – Ensure that these are clear by clearing the mouth of foreign material such as vomit, water, blood, etc. Do not forget to do this before beginning resuscitation (see page 231).

   B Breathing – Check that the diver is breathing. If not, begin mouth-to-mouth rescue breathing (see page 233).

   C Circulation – Is the heart beating? Listening with an ear on the left chest or feeling for the carotid artery will determine effective heartbeat. If not, begin CPR (see page 235). If the diver is bleeding, any haemorrhage must be stopped before starting CPR.

   Oxygen – When the ABC has been attained, give 100 per cent oxygen by demand valve or oronasal mask with a ventilation bag (see page 238).

2. **Summon medical assistance.**

Example

Mike and Jimmy decided to dive the wreck of *De Kelders*, which sank with a cargo of snooker balls. Mike, as usual, was meticulous in his preparation, but Jimmy wanted to try a twin-hose, two-stage set he had bought second-hand, complete with a full, but rusty, cylinder (he did not know that both the cylinder and the set were three years old). On descent, Jimmy began breathing and swimming erratically and rushed to the surface, where he gasped, spluttered and choked. The rusting in the cylinder had reduced his air to four per cent oxygen, causing hypoxia.

OXYGEN TOXICITY (HYPEROXIA)

Oxygen toxicity is a condition that caused by a high partial pressure of oxygen in the inspired gas supply. This relates to Dalton's Law (see page 24), which states that: Oxygen partial pressure = Percentage oxygen x Ambient pressure.
– Increasing the percentage of oxygen can cause toxicity.
– Increasing the pressure can cause toxicity.
– Increasing both percentage and pressure can cause toxicity.
– All of the above cause an increase in oxygen partial pressure.

CAUSES OF OXYGEN TOXICITY
1. Pure oxygen rebreathers.
2. High percentage oxygen mixes. Among sport divers, nitrox breathing to depths below 40 msw has resulted in a number of deaths.
3. Pure oxygen in decompression schedules.
4. Pure oxygen in therapeutic tables.
5. Prolonged exposure under pressure e.g. saturation diving.

Oxygen toxicity requires time to develop, and it is this time that permits the use of oxygen under pressure. Consider what happens: on exposure to pressure, oxygen is used to replace or reduce inhaled inert gas uptake and reduce or eliminate decompression time. A level of just below poisonous concentrations is set (i.e. 1.6 ATA when under water and 2.8 ATA in a chamber). When used in decompression, oxygen creates a large gradient from tissues to alveoli for inert gas.

Time is used to remove the inert gas before a diver becomes poisoned with oxygen. The length of time depends on the oxygen pressure used and on the diver. Some divers are sensitive to a high oxygen pressure and present with toxicity early. This is used as a selection test for naval divers in some countries.

FEATURES OF OXYGEN TOXICITY

As far as a diver is concerned, two tissues are primarily involved in oxygen toxicity: the brain and lungs.

BRAIN (CEREBRAL) OXYGEN TOXICITY The brain can tolerate an oxygen partial pressure of 2 ATA continuously in a chamber for about two hours, before toxicity becomes obvious. At this point, reducing oxygen pressure, for example, by breathing chamber air, rapidly reduces toxicity. In water, tolerance to oxygen is much less.

The US Navy oxygen in-water depth-time limits (expressed in msw) are given as:

Normal operations		Exceptional operations	
Depth (msw)	Time (mins)	Depth (msw)	Time (mins)
3	240	9	45
4.6	150	10.7	25
6	110	12	10
7.6	75		

In a chamber at 10 msw, 120 minutes is considered safe. In water at 9 msw, 45 minutes is considered safe under exceptional operations. Why should there be a difference? If ducks are ducks, and apples are apples, oxygen at 2 ATA should be oxygen at 2 ATA. There are two reasons why it is not: the first is that, in a chamber, divers are resting, whereas underwater they are swimming, working, fighting currents and controlling their depth in a swell. Effort reduces the time for the onset of oxygen toxicity, while rest increases it, allowing an oxygen partial pressure of 2.8 ATA in chambers. The second reason is that submerged divers are committed to their gas supply (oxygen), whereas men in chambers are not. They can remove their oxygen masks and take air breaks at regular intervals. This reduces the toxic effect of oxygen.

The effects of oxygen toxicity on the brain are very complex and incompletely understood. A number of metabolic processes are interfered with, including oxygen utilisation by the tissues. Famine in the midst of plenty occurs, and features **similar to hypoxia** appear (see page 195):
–   changes in higher cerebral function especially a feeling of terrible dread,
–   changes in the senses, and
–   changes in motor ability.
In addition:
–   **twitching**, especially of the face, is common,
–   **pallor** is evident. Pure oxygen causes intense constriction of blood vessels causing the skin to become very pale (a diver emerging from a chamber after an oxygen decompression schedule or an oxygen therapeutic table is always very pale),
–   **vertigo and nausea** are common (as with hypoxia), and
–   **tunnel vision, tinnitus and convulsions** can occur (as with hypoxia).

REMEMBER:
–   An unconscious **blue** diver is hypoxic.
–   An unconscious **white** diver could be oxygen toxic, depending on the gas supply being used. (Shock and hypothermia also cause **white** divers.)

MANAGEMENT OF CEREBRAL OXYGEN TOXICITY

The objective is the reduction of oxygen partial pressure in the inhaled gas.

PREVENTION

1. **Avoid very deep air dives.**

   Cerebral oxygen toxicity is rare among sport divers. It can occur during chamber oxygen therapy for acute decompression illness, but is also possible with very deep dives on air. Despite the risk of severe nitrogen narcosis, dives have been done to 90 msw, at which depth the oxygen partial pressure is 2.1 ATA. At shallower depths, or with strenuous underwater exercise, individual sensitivity to oxygen and carbon dioxide build-up may result in cerebral oxygen toxicity. Pure oxygen must be limited to 6 msw.

2. **Don't mess about with Dalton's Law.**

   The use of nitrox mixes in sport diving must always be very carefully controlled and the rig must be checked to be oxygen compatible. The objectives are:
   - to increase the dive time at a particular depth by decreasing equivalent nitrogen uptake at that depth, and
   - to reduce decompression and surface interval times.

Avoiding nitrogen narcosis must never be the objective for using nitrox mixes! Trying to reduce nitrogen narcosis below depths of 40 msw by diluting nitrogen in the breathing mix with oxygen can be, and has been, lethal.

If one considers a scale of concentrations – with pure nitrogen and narcosis at one end and pure oxygen and toxicity at the other – then clean, dry air lies on the 79 per cent nitrogen–21 per cent oxygen point. It is biased towards narcosis and deficient in toxicity. Adding oxygen to the mix slides the danger scale away from narcosis and towards oxygen toxicity. So air or nitrox breathing becomes a choice of potential dangers. Narcosis limits air diving, while oxygen toxicity determines safe nitrox depth. The first sign of oxygen toxicity may be a convulsion underwater. The diver can do absolutely nothing to save his or her life, and the emergency rescue of a convulsing diver by a buddy can easily cause added pulmonary barotrauma of ascent.

Air tables allow an advanced diver to descend to 40 msw without worrying about sudden unconsciousness underwater, but nitrogen narcosis will occur to some degree. The use of Nitrox 36 permits maximal depths to 34 msw, while Nitrox 32 permits dives to 40 msw without narcosis. No more than this is acceptable! If a diver wants to breathe nitrox beyond these limits he or she is, quite simply, messing about with Dalton's Law and will probably die.

TREATMENT

1. **In a recompression chamber**
   (a) Remove the diver's oxygen mask and allow him or her to breathe chamber air.

(b) Encourage hyperventilation of chamber air for about 30 seconds.

(c) If convulsions occur, immediately notify the chamber operator of the situation. It is essential to maintain the pressure constant in the chamber until the convulsions stop.

(d) Gently but firmly restrain a convulsing diver from incurring an injury due to forceful collision with surrounding hard objects. Try to keep the diver's head extended back. This ensures an airway when breathing recommences, and prevents the tongue from flopping back into the throat. Tongue depressors, although often recommended, are difficult to insert into a convulsing person's clenched mouth, and can break teeth or cause mouth bleeding with subsequent respiratory difficulty.

2. **Underwater (deep diver rescue)**

From a scuba-diving point of view, this refers almost entirely to sport divers who decide to use an oxygen-enriched breathing supply. A **deep diver rescue** must be performed (see also page 215).

(a) **Do not** bring a convulsing diver to the surface. The diver is not breathing, the jaws are clenched, and the risk of pulmonary barotrauma of ascent is very high. This requires extremely good nerves from a buddy, as natural instinct will prompt an immediate rescue ascent.

(b) Ditch the diver's weight belt. Wait until the convulsion stops (it always will).

(c) If the diver is breathing, commence a controlled ascent. If he or she has lost his or her regulator, turn the diver's head to one side and remove any foreign material (e.g. the bitten-off mouthpiece or vomit) by sweeping your forefinger around the mouth from cheek to cheek. Do not worry about water entering the mouth at this stage.

(d) Ascend steadily, holding the diver upright with the jaw well up and the mouth open. Keeping the diver's neck extended will allow expanding air to vent freely from the mouth during the ascent. Water will not enter the airway under these conditions. If air does not vent and the airway is clear, laryngospasm is present. **Wait for it to pass** before continuing the ascent – air will bubble freely from the mouth and blow any water out.

(e) Do not attempt buddy breathing with a semi-conscious diver. Perform a controlled emergency swimming ascent (see page 170). Breathe normally on your rig, and ensure free exhalation by the diver. Be careful that the ascent does not become an uncontrolled buoyant ascent.

(f) On reaching the surface, inflate the diver's BC and signal for help. Check whether the diver is breathing. If not, begin mouth-to-snorkel rescue breathing, see opposite. (This is easier than mouth-to-mouth in a choppy sea.)

(g) Continue rescue swimming until you get the diver out of the water, with frequent stops for rescue breathing.

(h) Once on land or on the boat, lay the diver flat and face-down. Straddle his or her hips and lift the pelvis to drain any water from the airway.

(i) If the diver is breathing, place him or her in the unconscious left lateral rescue position.

(j) If no breathing is evident, roll the diver on to his or her back and begin mouth-to-mouth rescue breathing or CPR (see page 235).

(k) Do not forget about any missed decompression stops!

Mouth-to-snorkel rescue breathing: Position yourself behind the diver. Ensure that the diver's snorkel is drained of water and that his or her mask is properly fitted on the face. With one hand, hold the snorkel mouthpiece in the diver's mouth, lift the jaw up and, using the thumb and forefinger, pinch off the diver's nostrils through the mask nosepiece. Tilt the diver's forehead back with the other hand. Blow slowly and deeply into the snorkel, then allow the diver to exhale passively. Repeat this 10 times.

PULMONARY OXYGEN TOXICITY (Also called the Lorraine-Smith effect.) The brain is rapidly sensitive to a partial pressure of oxygen exceeding 2 ATA. The lungs develop slow toxicity changes at oxygen partial pressures above 0.6 ATA for continuous long periods. Pulmonary oxygen toxicity is not seen in usual short-duration oxygen dives.

It requires long exposures as a result of:

– repetitive oxygen therapeutic tables, and

– saturation diving.

As with cerebral oxygen toxicity, the exact mechanism of pulmonary oxygen toxicity is incompletely understood. The alveolar-capillary system is affected, with loss of normal surfactant abilities and the collapse of alveoli, filling of the alveoli with secretions, and capillary breakdown. Eventually, extensive lung scarring may occur.

Presentation of pulmonary oxygen toxicity

1. 'Tickling' or 'scratching' feeling in the throat.

2. Coughing, which becomes uncontrollable.

3. Burning chest pain.

4. Breathlessness, becoming worse and worse.

Management of pulmonary oxygen toxicity

Reduce the oxygen partial pressure of inspired gas to between 0.2 and 0.5 ATA. If treated early, the pulmonary effects revert to normal.

NITROGEN NARCOSIS (Rapture of the Deep)

Nitrogen narcosis is a condition associated with a decrease in intellectual and physical ability due to a high partial pressure of nitrogen in the inhaled mix. It is equivalent to being stone-drunk underwater, and limits air diving to 50 msw.

Narcosis also occurs, and even more readily, with the heavier inert gases argon and krypton, but neon is less narcotic than nitrogen because it is less fat soluble. In addition, narcosis is caused by anaesthetic gases such as nitrous oxide, the 'laughing gas' used by dentists. Helium is the least narcotic inert gas, while xenon narcoses even at the surface.

NOTE: Narcosis is a 'nitrogen on descent' effect as the nitrogen is in solution in tissues. Acute decompression illness (see page 178) is a 'nitrogen on ascent' effect, as the nitrogen is out of solution as bubbles.

CAUSES OF NITROGEN NARCOSIS

At high partial pressures, nitrogen has an effect similar to that of an anaesthetic gas. The exact mechanism, as with oxygen toxicity, is not clear, but it is believed that nitrogen is rapidly absorbed into brain cells which:

- have a rich blood supply, and
- have a high fat content in their membranes.

The increased amount of dissolved gas may cause osmotic swelling of brain cells, interfering with membrane function and the delicate interrelationships between brain cells. No metabolism of nitrogen or any inert gas occurs. It appears to be a purely physical osmotic effect.

PRESENTATION OF NITROGEN NARCOSIS

As with hypoxia and cerebral oxygen toxicity, there are:

- changes in higher cerebral function
- changes in the senses, and
- changes in motor ability.

CHANGES IN HIGHER CEREBRAL FUNCTION This is usually the first presentation. From 30–50 msw there is a feeling of well-being and overconfidence, similar to the effects of alcohol. Learning, attention, memory and concentration are impaired (the diver may forget what was done or noted at depth). At greater depths, mental function gets worse, and hallucinations, sleepiness, stupor, coma and death can occur.

CHANGES IN THE SENSES Vision is most commonly affected, with sight becoming blurred or tunnel vision developing (the visual field becomes narrowed, rather like looking through a tube or tunnel).

CHANGES IN MOTOR ABILITY Movements first become awkward and automatic, then incoordinated and ineffectual.

Nitrogen narcosis occurs suddenly on reaching depth, but does not get worse with time. It occurs more intensely with very rapid descents (a very high gradient for the absorption of nitrogen is suddenly set up).

The depth at which narcosis occurs is variable. Some divers become narcosed at relatively shallow depths, while others are affected only beyond 50 msw. With regular diving, tolerance develops and the diver becomes less prone to narcosis, which can be aggravated by cold, alcohol, drugs, fatigue and anxiety.

The danger of nitrogen narcosis is usually not so much the narcosis itself, but the increased likelihood of incurring an injury or making a potentially fatal mistake while under water – the equivalent to driving a motor vehicle when drunk.

MANAGEMENT OF NITROGEN NARCOSIS

Nitrogen narcosis disappears rapidly during the ascent. It can be prevented from occuring by adding helium to the gas supply (trimix). This dilutes and reduces the partial pressure of nitrogen as well as the risk of oxygen toxicity.

Naturally, this discovery resulted in ad hoc groupings of trimix sport divers who began to confidently mix their own gases and gas switch-over depths, working purely on Dalton's Law of partial pressures (see page 24) to avoid narcosis and oxygen toxicity, and Haldane's exponential assumptions for upgassing and degassing (see page 174). They tended to ignore factors such as variable compressibility of gases, gas mixing and analysis equipment, variable tissue solubilities, diffusion and counter-diffusion rates and differing half times at different depths, and they often neglected to have emergency back-up support. They dived deeply, frequently suffered DCI and invariably knew someone who died underwater.

Nowadays, technical divers regularly use trimix in their deep dives, and more and more sport diving schools offer courses in trimix diving to over 100 msw to experienced and suitably advanced sport divers.

CARBON DIOXIDE TOXICITY

Carbon dioxide is a gaseous toxic waste product produced by metabolism and, unless a diver promptly removes it by effective exhalation, poisoning will occur.

1. Carbon dioxide is produced by the tissues in amounts proportional to oxygen used and work done. Production increases with exercise, including the work of breathing a dense mix at depth.
2. Carbon dioxide production is **independent** of depth alone.
3. Carbon dioxide is the **prime** stimulus for breathing. A rise in the carbon dioxide level in circulating blood stimulates breathing.
4. In a freeflow system, e.g. inside a decompression chamber, a submarine or when using a hard diving helmet, the maximum carbon dioxide partial pressure permitted in inspired gas is 0.02 ATA. This is:
   – 2 per cent at the surface (1 ATA),
   – 0.2 per cent at 90 msw (10 ATA), and
   – 0.07 per cent at 290 msw (30 ATA).

With increasing depth, carbon dioxide control becomes more and more exact and technically demanding. An increase in the amount of carbon dioxide in the body is called **hypercapnia** or **hypercarbia** and leads to carbon dioxide toxicity, then carbon dioxide narcosis.

CAUSES OF CARBON DIOXIDE TOXICITY

As with hypoxia, the causes are found from gas supply to tissues.

1. **Gas supply**
   (a) Contamination of the gas supply with carbon dioxide.
   (b) Failure of absorbent material used in scrubbers, the apparatus for eliminating exhaled carbon dioxide.
   (c) Poor ventilation flow in diving helmets and decompression chambers.
2. **Airways and lungs**
   (a) Breathhold diving.
   (b) Inhaled dentures.
   (c) Laryngospasm.
   (d) Inhaled foreign material, e.g. vomiting while underwater; or in cases of near-drowning.
   (e) Inadequate ventilation of alveoli. Breathing a dense mix at depth can be hard work in itself and becomes dangerous with any resistance to breathing due to tight suits, harnesses or floatation jackets. Not only does the diver have to work harder to breathe, but this increased work produces more carbon dioxide and demands more oxygen.
3. **Failure of carbon dioxide transport from tissues to lungs**
   (a) Failure of circulation due to shock, hypothermia or heart failure.
   (b) Failure of enough blood, e.g. haemorrhage.

4. **Excess tissue production of carbon dioxide.** Under normal circumstances, the blood and lungs can easily handle carbon dioxide production. However, under conditions of heavy work, if any of the foregoing causes are even moderately present, carbon dioxide will accumulate.

Note: In most cases, carbon dioxide toxicity and hypoxia develop concurrently. When using nitrox mixes, carbon dioxide toxicity enhances both oxygen toxicity and the development of narcosis. A convulsion is almost inevitable.

PRESENTATION OF CARBON DIOXIDE TOXICITY

1. Once again, features similar to those of hypoxia occur (see page 195):
   - changes in higher cerebral function,
   - changes in the senses, and
   - changes in motor activity.
2. Carbon dioxide is the most powerful respiratory stimulus of all. It activates the inspiratory centre in the brain stem, and the diver starts breathing rapidly and deeply.
3. Carbon dioxide causes **dilation** of blood vessels, so the diver becomes flushed and sweaty.
4. The blood vessels in the head also dilate, causing a throbbing headache.
5. If the carbon dioxide level rises too high, it no longer stimulates breathing, but **depresses** it. Unconsciousness or convulsions can occur – this is carbon dioxide narcosis.

Remember that flushing and sweating will not be noticed underwater and the diver may think that his or her increased depth and rate of breathing are due to the exertions of diving. He or she may then convulse, stop breathing or lose consciousness underwater **without any further warning**.

MANAGEMENT OF CARBON DIOXIDE TOXICITY

PREVENTION As always, this is the most important part of management. It involves:

1. Meticulous attention to scrubbers.
2. Constant care to ensure adequate freeflow volume.
3. Monitoring carbon dioxide levels in submarines, chambers, diving bells and other underwater habitats.
4. Ensuring there is no contamination of the air mix with carbon dioxide.
5. Avoiding restraining equipment and dense mixes.
6. Being aware of the problem. This can be difficult, as the first obvious signal may be sudden unconsciousness.

TREATMENT

1. If carbon dioxide toxicity underwater is suspected, stop swimming and relax (this results in less carbon dioxide production and oxygen use).

2. Signal to your buddy that something is wrong (unconsciousness may occur at any moment).
3. Begin the ascent.
4. At the surface hyperventilate atmospheric air.
5. If a diver sees an unconscious buddy, begin a deep diver rescue (see page 215).

Example

Pete Muckitt decided to make an air mix to go diving for abalone and crayfish at 8 msw in a protected marine reserve. Creeping into his neighbour's garage at night, he quietly filled his cylinder to 80 ATA from a Brunswick green bottle (containing carbon dioxide) which, in the dark, looked like a black (oxygen) bottle. Happily sneaking home, he topped up his cylinder to 200 ATA with air. Next day, he dived to 5 msw on his mix, promptly lost consciousness and convulsed. The local fisheries inspector, who had been watching from his boat, retrieved Pete from the water, resuscitated him and then arrested him.

HIGH PRESSURE NERVOUS SYNDROME

High Pressure Nervous Syndrome, or HPNS (also known as High Pressure Neurological Syndrome) is a condition caused by rapid compression, when using helium or hydrogen, to depths greater than 150 metres. It presents with fine tremors that progress to dizziness, nausea and vomiting, impaired consciousness and stupor at depths below 300 metres. Brain wave activity becomes abnormal. HPNS remains the limiting factor to the depths that humans can dive.

High pressure increases electrical activity and excitability in the brain. In animals, it progresses from tremors to drowsiness and convulsions to coma and, finally, death. Pressures well in excess of 200 ATA (over 2000 metres) have been used experimentally in animals.

The onset of the HPNS is delayed by:
1. narcosis-inducing gases, sedatives and anaesthetics, and
2. slow compression rates.

1. Narcotic gases

Narcotic gases, such as 5 per cent nitrogen, as well as anaesthetics and sedatives such as barbiturates, can delay or reverse HPNS. The opposite also occurs – very high partial pressures of helium can reverse anaesthesia.

The concept of a sedated, anaesthetised diver working alertly and efficiently at very great depths arises for the future. Nitrogen is commonly used for its narcotic effect. The mechanism is still unclear, but it appears that high-pressure helium tends to compress brain cell membranes. Nitrogen is believed to cause brain cell swelling.

Possibly the effects are mutually counteractive, but the precise mechanisms have yet to be elucidated. So, nitrogen the narcoser, the scourge of shallow diving, has a happier side in very deep diving:

(a) It is cheap and reduces the cost of the mix.
(b) It reduces heat loss by the diver in pure heliox atmospheres.
(c) It helps to reduce the garbled speech of helium.
(d) It prevents or delays the onset of HPNS.

2. Slow compression rates

As one dives deeper and deeper, it is necessary to implement ever-slower compression rates in order to avoid HPNS. For example, a diver can be taken to a depth of 100 msw at a rate of 30 metres per minute without causing HPNS. To safely reach 200 metres, the rate of descent must be slowed to less than 15 metres per minute, while to reach 300 msw, the rate of compression must be even less, with the diver slowing his descent to below one metre per minute.

It has been computed that if a compression rate of 10 metres per hour is used, the limit before HPNS convulsions occur in man would be about 84 ATA (855 metres). However, if sedatives, narcotic gases and anaesthetics are used, this limit will probably be exceeded.

HELIUM AND TECHNICAL DIVING

HPNS can occur in technical divers diving deeper than 190 msw on heliox mixes. At anything below this depth, 5 per cent nitrogen should be added. This trimix greatly reduces the onset of HPNS.

Bear in mind, however, that the slow descent rates undertaken by commercial divers are not used by technical divers because of gas and decompression restraints.

TABLE OF DIVING DISORDERS

	EFFECTS OF DESCENT		ASCENT
0 m	OXYGEN TOXICITY	SQUEEZE	ACUTE DECOMPRES-SION ILLNESS
O₂	**Cerebral:** Convulsions, pallor, twitching and FSH* **Pulmonary:** Scratchy throat, burning chest, cough, breathlessness	Lung, ear, sinus, mask, suit, diver.	OSTEO-NECROSIS
10 m	OXYGEN TOXIC FSH*	**FEATURES OF HYPOXIA**	BAROTRAUMA OF ASCENT
AIR	NITROX TOXIC NITROGEN NARCOSIS FSH*	1. **Higher cerebral function** Irritability, anger, fear, laughter, irresponsibility, hallucinations, hysteria, apathy, sullenness, stupor, uneasiness, illusions, confusion, automatism, amnesia, unconciousness.	AGE (arterial gas embolism); Pneumothorax; Mediastinal emphysema; Lung tissue damage; Sinus barotrau-ma of ascent; Ear barotrauma of ascent; Gut barotrauma of ascent; Suit blow-up.
50 m	SEVERE NARCOSIS Dense air → more work to breathe → CO₂ TOXICITY flushing, headache, breathlessness + FSH*		
AIR		2. **Changes in the senses** **Visual:** blurring, double vision, tunnel vision, blindness, dazzle. **Hearing:** deafness, ringing in the ears (tinnitus), loss of balance with nausea, vertigo, vomiting. **Touch:** Numbness, itching, pins and needles, burning. **Taste:** Loss of taste, or abnormal taste awareness. **Smell:** Loss of smell or abnormal smell awareness.	
90 m	Absolute limit to air dive: ppO₂ = 2 ATA CEREBRAL OXYGEN TOXICITY		
100 m	DIFFICULT TEMP REGULATION Hypothermia Hyperthermia Garbled speech Strict ppO₂ + ppCO₂ + gas purity control	3. **Changes in motor activity** Weakness, loss of balance, incoordination, tremor, abnormal gait, twitching, slurred speech, paralysis.	
He + O₂ mix			
150 m			
600 m ?? limit	HPNS Tremors and FSH* Deep saturation diving Liquid breathing ???		

* FSH = Features similar to those of hypoxia

25

INHALED GAS CONTAMINATION

Contamination of a diver's air supply is an insidious but potentially lethal hazard. It invariably occurs when compressors are used to fill scuba cylinders for air diving. Only rarely will commercially obtained gases, such as oxygen, nitrox, trimix and heliox, be contaminated.

Contamination comes from:
- the air,
- the compressor, and
- the storage tank or cylinder.

CONTAMINATION FROM THE AIR

Jimmy wants to go diving in Emmarentia Dam in Johannesburg. As it is winter, the glorious Highveld air contains the following pollutants, all of which must be filtered out during compression:
- Carbon monoxide from hundreds of home fires belching smoke, and from thousands of motor cars.
- Oxides of nitrogen and nitric acid from chemical factories.
- Oxides of sulphur and sulphuric acid from the same factories.
- Dashes of chlorine, bromine, lead, mine dust, pollen and other exotica.

CONTAMINATION FROM THE COMPRESSOR

Compressors have two possible points for contamination:
- from the engine driving the compressor, and
- from the oil used to lubricate the compressor.

FROM THE COMPRESSOR ENGINE

A very common method of driving a compressor is a petrol motor. If one visits a dive resort on a weekend, one can witness dozens of divers happily sucking their own and other people's engine exhaust fumes into their breathing mix, together with a little barbecue smoke for flavour. Using an electric motor to drive the compressor eliminates one's own petrol exhaust fumes, but not those of one's dive neighbours, nor the exhaust fumes from the diesel engine on the dive boat that is supplying the generated electricity. Remember that the air-inlet hose to a compressor must always be upwind of any contamination source.

FROM THE COMPRESSOR OIL

All compressors used to supply air for breathing should be in perfect running order, and should use a diving-approved vegetable oil as lubricant so that, if oil does enter the receiver or cylinder, it will be less toxic than mineral oil. Vegetable oils should also have a high resistance to breaking down when they are heated.

Unfortunately, compressors are expensive and divers are poor, so a 'make-do' is often the result, with a grossly overheating compressor labouring to fill a neglected and out-of-date cylinder. Overheating is the main reason for contamination.

Causes of overheating

1. Restriction of the air-inlet by a filthy filter or a kinked narrow-bore inlet hose.
2. Damaged cylinders, rings, pistons and valves, causing excessive friction.
3. Leaky valves, gaskets and fittings, causing a higher-than-designed final compression ratio to reach the required pressure.
4. Failure to cool the compressor.

Oil is not the most stable substance in the world. In the presence of high temperatures and pressures it can:
- vaporise, producing oil gas which reaches the receiver,
- 'crack' or break down into smaller, more volatile hydrocarbons, or
- 'flash', or burn like diesel fuel, releasing carbon monoxide.

For all these reasons, filters and traps are used. A filter is needed on the outer end of the air inlet hose (which should be wide-bore to reduce resistance). This eliminates leaves, dust, bits of braai *wors* and other large particles.

A high pressure compressor usually has three stages. Between the stages are finned cooling coils, which cool the air before it is further compressed by the next stage. This cooling causes moisture from the air to condense (rather like breathing on a cold mirror), and so water traps are used after each set of cooling coils between the stages, and they should be regularly vented.

After the third stage, the air is:
- at high pressure (say 200 ATA),
- fairly dry,
- contaminated with oil,
- contaminated with hydrocarbons and other gases, and
- generally unbreathable.

At this stage, filters are used, and there is a variety to choose from (see page 207). The controlling authorities in most countries set very strict standards of air purity, and these standards should be strictly adhered to, as they dictate the maximum amount of water, carbon monoxide, carbon dioxide, oxides of nitrogen, oil, odour and taste acceptable in a breathing air mix. Commonly used filters are:

1. Silica gel or activated alumina gel to remove water.
2. Activated charcoal to remove oil vapour and hydrocarbons.
3. Molecular ceramic sieves to remove oil and hydrocarbons.
4. Sodalime and baralyme to remove carbon dioxide.
5. Centrifugal filters to remove water and oil.
6. Cryogenic filters to freeze out carbon dioxide and water.

Oil-free compressors are also available, but they are very expensive and rarely used by sport divers.

TESTING FOR PURITY Ideally, the air drawn from a compressor should be checked after filtration. A number of simple test kits are available. For example, the Draeger Multi-Gas Detector is a simple gauging device which draws a sample of air through a small tube containing chemicals and indicator dyes specific for the gas being tested. Colour changes and tube markings indicate the degree of contamination for carbon monoxide, carbon dioxide, oxides of nitrogen, oil, hydrocarbons, chlorine, etc.

CONTAMINATION FROM THE STORAGE TANK OR CYLINDER

The diver's air cylinder could contain:
– oil from previous faulty fillings, or
– rust from water, either from the compressor or from a water cooling bath which has allowed water to enter the empty cylinder through an open valve.

EFFECTS OF BREATHING CONTAMINATED AIR

Divers are believers. They believe that they will be safe under water and they believe that the air in their scuba cylinders is always pure and breathable. However, there are several problems that relate to the inspiration of contaminated air:

OXYGEN
(Permissible range in air 20–22 per cent)

(a) Low oxygen content could occur with a long-forgotten filling, followed by the cylinder rusting and causing a reduction in the partial pressure of contained oxygen and subsequent hypoxia with diving.

(b) High concentrations of oxygen follow the addition of oxygen to air, for example, in the preparation of nitrox, while pure oxygen, as used in decompression chambers, can cause oxygen toxicity or pose a fire hazard.

CARBON DIOXIDE
(Maximum permissible 0.05 per cent or 500 ppm)
The presence of carbon dioxide and the effects of increasing its partial pressure have been discussed on page 204.

CARBON MONOXIDE
(Maximum permissible 0.001 per cent or 10 ppm)
Carbon monoxide is an extremely dangerous contaminant. It has three actions:
- it competes with oxygen for haemoglobin
- it delays or prevents the release of oxygen from haemoglobin to tissues
- it poisons tissue utilisation of oxygen.

Effects of carbon monoxide on the oxygen pathway

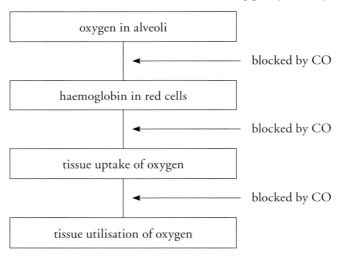

Carbon monoxide has an affinity for haemoglobin (the carrier pigment for oxygen in red blood cells) which is 200 times that of oxygen. The presence of carbon monoxide causes gross hypoxia in the presence of normal amounts of oxygen. If the carbon monoxide partial pressure is 1/200th that of oxygen, half of the haemoglobin will be bound to carbon monoxide, and half to oxygen. As the oxygen partial pressure in air is 0.21 ATA (21 per cent), a carbon monoxide concentration of 1/200 x 0.2 or 0.001 ATA (0.1 per cent) is enough to halve the available oxygen.

In addition, the presence of carbon monoxide interferes with the release of oxygen from the remaining oxygen-haemoglobin complex (oxyhaemoglobin) to tissues, further aggravating the hypoxia. Finally, carbon monoxide poisons the metabolism of oxygen once within the tissues.

The maximum carbon monoxide permissible is 0.001 per cent (10 ppm), which would reduce oxygen carriage by 0.5 per cent.

Divers on air are protected to some degree by increased pressure because, as the partial pressure of oxygen rises with depth (Dalton's Law, see page 24), more oxygen can be carried in free solution in plasma. This oxygen is not bound to haemoglobin and is more readily available to the tissues, but tissue utilisation will also be hampered by carbon monoxide which obeys Dalton's Law, too.

The problem really becomes critical in saturation diving, where the partial pressure of oxygen is kept between 0.2 and 0.5 ATA, to avoid pulmonary oxygen toxicity. With a saturation dive of 90 msw using mixed gas and an oxygen pressure of 0.21 ATA (the same as in air at sea level), if the amount of carbon monoxide was only one-hundredth of one per cent of the chamber atmosphere, half of the divers' available haemoglobin would be bound to carbon monoxide and they would die.

CAUSES OF CARBON MONOXIDE POISONING
1. Carbon monoxide in the air.
2. Carbon monoxide formed in the compressor by flashing of oil.

PRESENTATION OF CARBON MONOXIDE POISONING
1. The features of hypoxia are evident (see page 195):
    - changes in higher cerebral function,
    - changes in the senses, and
    - changes in motor ability.
2. In addition, carbon monoxide forms a bright red stable complex with haemoglobin. The poisoned diver may therefore have cherry red lips and 'healthy' red cheeks. This is not a reliable sign, however, and its absence need not mean the absence of carbon monoxide poisoning.

    Carbon monoxide poisoning can cause irreversible brain damage which persists after resuscitation and treatment.

MANAGEMENT OF CARBON MONOXIDE POISONING
Prevention Accidentally poisoning a sport diver with carbon monoxide can only mean sloppy 'housekeeping' techniques.
1. Ensure that the compressor air intake is upwind of petrol and diesel exhausts. Keep an eye on the direction of the wind. If it changes, move the intake hose.
2. If you have your own compressor, keep it serviceable. Have it maintained by someone who is knowledgeable and reliable.
3. Test the purity of the compressed air being pumped into your cylinder. It only takes a moment to draw a sample into a hand-held tester.

Treatment The principle involved is to induce a high oxygen gradient into the tissues and a high carbon monoxide gradient from the tissues via the blood to the lungs for exhalation. This is identical to the management of acute decompression illness. Pure oxygen is therefore used, either at surface pressure or, preferably via a short therapeutic oxygen table (such as Table 5 USN, see page 343).

Example

Jimmy was diving at 25 msw. During the dive he began to feel dizzy, felt his vision fading and became very breathless. He decided to ascend but, halfway to the surface, he became blind and had to fight to retain consciousness while hauling himself hand over hand up the shot line. Back on the dive boat he was flushed, confused and disorientated. As a chamber was not at hand, he was given pure oxygen by demand valve and, over the next two hours, his condition gradually improved. An examination of the air compressor showed that the wind had changed direction, and the diesel fumes from the boat's generator exhaust were blowing directly into the compressor's inlet filter. Jimmy had suffered carbon monoxide poisoning and resultant hypoxia.

OXIDES OF NITROGEN
(Maximum permissible less than 1 ppm)

Nitrogen reacts with oxygen to produce a variety of oxides:
- nitrous oxide – used in anaesthesia,
- nitric oxide – a pungent colourless gas, and
- nitrogen dioxide – a pungent brown gas.

Other oxides exist, but they are unstable and break down to nitric oxide and nitrogen dioxide, both of which are intensely irritating and very poisonous. They affect chiefly the eyes, nose, throat and lungs, producing coughing, wheezing and difficulty in breathing, and in severe cases, death.

OIL AND HYDROCARBONS
(Maximum permissible 1 mg/m³)

Contamination with oil-based products causes a characteristic oily taste. A chemical pneumonia may follow, especially if mineral oils are used. Oil and hydrocarbons are inflammable, and the risk of fire becomes great when hydrocarbon vapours are mixed with air under pressure. The air cylinder on a diver's back becomes a potential bomb, equivalent to the inside of a petrol engine during the compression stroke. All it needs is one bright spark...

26

DEEP DIVER RESCUE

Being faced with an unconscious diver at depth and safely returning him or her to the surface is one of the most responsible tasks any diver can undertake. If you do not clearly understand what you are about to do, then, unless luck plays a major hand, you will almost surely kill or maim the diver and suffer acute DCI yourself.

Worse, if the diver is already dead by drowning you could put yourself at serious risk of developing DCI by rescuing a corpse. For this reason, some authorities have suggested that if a diver is found on the seabed after an unobserved descent and the regulator is not in his or her mouth, he or she is invariably already beyond any hope of revival. Under these circumstances, and without risking the life or health of the rescuer, the victim's BC could be inflated causing a solo independent buoyant ascent to the surface where any possible chance of survival is slightly better. This approach obviously is fraught with huge ethical and moral arguments but it does ensure that the assisting diver's life is not compromised too.

All alive but unconscious divers, unless they fortuitously still have their regulators in their mouths and are actively exhaling gas bubbles, must be presumed to have attempted to breathe underwater and therefore to have inhaled water. The moment water is inhaled, the vocal cords in the larynx contract together, closing the larynx and sealing off the lungs. More water cannot enter, but lung air cannot leave either. This is called laryngospasm.

An unconscious scuba diver disconnected from his air supply must be presumed to have laryngospasm; i.e. his airway is totally obstructed.

Under these circumstances, the diver cannot inhale or exhale at all. Attempting to restore breathing by shoving a regulator into their mouth and pressing the purge button is totally futile. No air will reach the lungs; it will simply bubble from the mouth. If the diver is now rescued and brought to the surface, the air trapped in the chest will expand, causing the lungs to burst and shred, and he or she will die of massive pulmonary barotrauma of ascent (see page 161).

The same applies to a convulsing diver. During a convulsion, the diver is not breathing and his or her jaws are clenched. If the mouthpiece is bitten through or set free into the water, the first inhalation after the convulsion passes will cause water inhalation and immediate laryngospasm.

> If bubbles do not stream from the diver's mouth during the rescue ascent, the expanding air in the diver's chest is not escaping, and will cause massive pulmonary barotrauma of ascent and potentially fatal lung tearing, with all of its complications.

At this stage, a near-drowned diver may not even try to inhale during a rescue attempt. The rescuer must understand this and resist natural instinct, which will prompt an immediate and fatal rescue ascent. Always remember that the victim may already be dead and a hurried ascent to the surface will only result in serious DCI in the rescuer. The safety of the rescuer must always come first.

HOW TO RESCUE AN UNCONSCIOUS DIVER WHO IS DISCONNECTED FROM HIS OR HER AIR SUPPLY

1. Ditch the diver's weight belt.
2. Wait until any convulsions stop (they always will).
3. Turn the diver's head to one side. Clear the mouth of any foreign material by sweeping your forefinger around the diver's mouth from cheek to cheek. Do not worry about water entering the mouth – this has already happened, and caused laryngospasm when the diver tried to breathe under water.
4. Hold the diver upright, with the jaw well up and the mouth open, and ascend two to three metres. Keeping the diver's neck extended will allow expanding lung air to vent freely from the mouth during the ascent. Water will not enter the airways under these conditions. If air does not vent and the airway is clear, laryngospasm is present and the diver is still alive. **Stop and wait for the spasm to pass before continuing the ascent** – expanding air will then bubble freely from the mouth and drive most of the water in the mouth and throat out of the mouth.
5. Partially inflate the diver's BC.
6. Do not even attempt buddy breathing with an unconscious or semi-conscious diver. Perform a **controlled emergency ascent** (see page 170). At all times, breathe normally on your own rig, and ensure free exhalation by the diver. Be careful that any expanding air in your BC (or the casualty's BC) does not initiate an uncontrolled buoyant ascent. Vent BC air if necessary.
7. On reaching the surface, inflate the diver's BC and signal for help. Check whether the diver is breathing. If no breathing is evident, begin **rescue breathing** (see page 233). The most efficient method is via a plastic mouth-to-mouth airway fitted with a non-return valve to avoid contaminating the rescuer with the casualty's blood, fluids or vomit. These airways are relatively cheap, and small enough to be kept in a BC pocket. It is recommended that all divers have one in case of emergency, and become practiced in its use.
   If an airway is not available, **mouth-to-snorkel** rescue breathing should be done, as it is easier to do than mouth-to-mouth rescue breathing in a choppy

sea. Position yourself behind the diver. Ensure that the diver's snorkel is drained of water and that his or her mask is properly fitted on the face. With one hand, hold the snorkel mouthpiece in the diver's mouth, lift the jaw up and, using the thumb and forefinger, pinch off the diver's nostrils through the mask nosepiece. Tilt the diver's forehead back with your other hand. Blow slowly and deeply into the snorkel then allow the diver passively to exhale. Repeat this 10 times.

8. Rescue the diver from the water, with stops for rescue breathing every 15 seconds. If you can see that help is on the way, stay where you are and give continuous rescue breathing.

9. Once on land or on the boat, lay the diver flat and face down. Straddle the diver's hips. Turn the head to one side. Lift the pelvis to drain any water from the airway.

10. If the diver is breathing, place him or her in the unconscious left lateral rescue position (see page 232).

11. If no breathing is evident, roll the diver on to his or her back and begin **mouth-to-mouth rescue** breathing, or **commence CPR** if no heartbeat or carotid arterial pulse are found (see page 235).

12. Summon an emergency rescue service urgently.

13. Do not forget that **you** have missed all decompression stops and therefore have a very high probability of developing DCI following an untabled rapid ascent! Begin pure oxygen demand-valve breathing immediately and have someone urgently notify an emergency service, such as DAN, as well as the nearest recompression facility, about the incident.

27

ALTITUDE AND DIVING

Diving at altitude causes confusion. All the standard decompression tables are based on the assumption that a dive begins and ends at sea level (that is, 1 ATA; 760 mm Hg, 101 kPa; etc.). However, what is the position in Johannesburg, for example, which has an altitude of about 1830 metres (6000 ft) above sea level? Up here, a new set of special traps lurk for our gentle coastal sub-aquanaut. These traps are not immediately obvious and they make diving at altitude a constant grey area in the average sport diver's knowledge. When diving at altitude, the first thing a diver needs to know is the local atmospheric pressure at the dive site.

DETERMINING LOCAL ATMOSPHERIC PRESSURE

The air we breathe is not simply an even layer of gas surrounding the earth. The higher one goes on Earth, the lower the air pressure. Fortunately for diving calculations, the drop in pressure from sea level to 3600 metres (the altitude of Lake Titicaca in Peru, the highest lake in the world) is just about linear.

For every metre one rises, the atmospheric pressure drops about 10 pascals or 0.01 kPa; or, for every 1000 metres (one kilometre) one rises, the pressure drops about 10 kPa or 0.1 ATA. In other words, sea-level atmospheric pressure drops 10 per cent for every 1000 metre rise.

Represented as a formula it looks like this:

$$\text{Local atmospheric pressure (kPa)} = 100 - \frac{\text{altitude (metres)}}{100}$$

Or this:

$$\text{Local ambient pressure (ATA)} = 1 - \frac{\text{altitude (metres)}}{10\,000}$$

Therefore, in Johannesburg:

Altitude = 1830 metres

Local atmospheric pressure = 100 − 18.3 = 81.7 kPa

Local ambient pressure = 1 − 0.183 = 0.817 ATA

At the coast, Jimmy dives to 50 msw, where the pressure is 6 ATA. What's 0.183 ATA compared to 6 ATA? Now we have reached the trap. It is essential to realise that absolute pressures are not the point. Ratios are, and it is the ratio of change that will bend you.

Example

Pete Muckitt is on the run from the police for catching crayfish in berry on the West Coast. Taking refuge far inland, in Mafikeng, he decides to dive at the nearby Wondergat, a natural dolomite sinkhole at an altitude of ±1430 metres. He'd heard the rumour that a packet of diamonds was once thrown into the water there so, setting up a surface-supply system, he spends five hours searching a ledge for the fabled loot in 10 metres of fresh water (mfw), thinking he can spend an unlimited bottom time at 10 mfw and then surface without in-water decompression stops. Finally, cold and hungry, he surfaces in disgust and returns to Mafikeng to lose some money at the casino. Standing at the slot machines, Pete suddenly develops a terrible headache and blurred vision. Reluctantly, he calls a doctor, and ends up being rushed to Pretoria for a therapeutic recompression under the beady eye of the police. What happened?

Let's go back to John Haldane (see page 174). Many of the decompression tables are based on the fact that the majority of divers can tolerate a doubling of their tissue nitrogen without developing obvious bends. A coastal diver can ascend from a long dive at 30 msw (4 ATA) to 10 msw (2 ATA) for decompression; or from a long dive at 10 msw (2 ATA) to the surface (1 ATA) for decompression. A ratio of 2:1 between bottom depth pressure and ambient surface pressure is usually tolerated due to the 'oxygen window' (see page 176).

But look again at the figures for Pete Muckitt's dive. The surface of Wondergat is at an altitude of 1430 metres.

The local ambient surface pressure = 1 - $\frac{1\,430}{10\,000}$

$$= 1 - 0.143 \text{ ATA}$$
$$= 0.857 \text{ ATA}$$

But Wondergat contains fresh water:

33 feet (10 metres) of sea water = 1 ATA
34 feet (10.3 metres) of fresh water = 1 ATA
10 metres of fresh water = 0.97 ATA

At 10 mfw, the pressure is 0.857 (atmospheric) + 0.97 (water) = 1.827 ATA
The ratio therefore is 1.827 : 0.857 = 2.132, so Pete bent.

It is therefore obvious that a correction must be made for altitude diving. There are two ways to do this:

1. EASY WAY Use a specially prepared altitude table. This clearly defines depth, dive times and decompression stages. The tables on the following pages, which were compiled by the late Professor A.A Buehlmann of the University Hospital of Zurich, have been kindly made available for this section.

NO-DECOMPRESSION LIMITS
AIR DIVING DECOMPRESSION TABLE

Altitude 0 – 700 m above sea level

Ascent rate: 10 m/min — Safety stop: 1 min at 3 m

Depth m	BT min	Stops 6	Stops 3	RG
12	125		1	G
15	75		1	G
15	90		7	G
18	51		1	F
18	70		11	G
21	35		1	E
21	50		8	F
21	60		16	G
24	25		1	E
24	35		4	F
24	40		8	F
24	50		17	G
24	60	4	24	G
27	20		1	E
27	30		5	F
27	35		10	F
27	40	2	13	G
27	45	3	18	G
27	50	6	22	G
30	17		1	D
30	25		5	E
30	30	2	7	F
30	35	3	14	F
30	40	5	17	G
30	45	9	23	G

m	min	9	6	3	RG
33	14			1	D
33	20			4	E
33	25		2	7	F
33	30		4	11	G
33	35		6	17	G
33	40	2	8	23	G
36	12			1	D
36	20		2	5	E
36	25		4	9	F
36	30	2	5	15	G
36	35	2	8	23	G
39	10			1	D
39	15			4	E
39	20		3	7	F
39	25	2	4	12	G
39	30	3	7	18	G
39	35	5	9	28	G
42	9			1	D
42	12			4	D
42	15		1	5	E
42	18		4	6	F
42	21	2	4	10	F
42	24	3	6	16	G
42	27	4	7	19	G

m	min	12	9	6	3	RG
45	12				5	E
45	15			3	5	E
45	18		2	4	9	F
45	21		3	5	13	G
45	24		4	6	18	G
48	9				3	E
48	12			2	5	E
48	15			4	6	F
48	18		3	4	10	F
48	21		4	6	16	G
51	9				4	E
51	12			3	6	E
51	15		2	4	8	F
51	18		4	5	13	F
51	21	3	4	7	18	G
54	9			1	5	E
54	12		1	4	6	E
54	15		3	4	10	F
54	18	1	3	6	17	G
57	9			2	5	E
57	12		2	4	8	E
57	15	1	4	5	11	F
57	18	3	4	7	18	G

Altitude 701 – 2500 m above sea level

Ascent rate: 10 m/min — Safety stop: 1 min at 2 m

Depth m	BT min	Stops 6	Stops 4	Stops 2	RG
9	238			1	G
12	99			1	G
12	110			4	G
15	62			1	F
15	70			4	G
18	44			1	F
18	50			4	F
18	60			11	G
21	30			1	E
21	35			2	F
21	40			5	F
21	45			9	F
21	50		1	13	G
21	55		3	17	G
24	22			1	F
24	30			3	F
24	35			7	F
24	40		2	11	G
24	45		4	16	G
27	18			1	D
27	20			2	E
27	25			4	F
27	30		2	7	F
27	35		4	11	G
27	40	1	6	16	G

m	min	9	6	4	2	RG
30	15				1	D
30	20				3	E
30	25			2	6	F
30	30		1	4	11	G
30	35		2	7	15	G
30	40	1	5	10	20	G
33	12				1	D
33	15				2	E
33	20			2	4	F
33	25		2	3	9	G
33	30	1	3	6	14	G
33	35	2	4	9	20	G
36	10				1	D
36	15			1	3	E
36	20		1	3	6	F
36	25	1	3	5	12	G
36	30	3	3	8	19	G
39	9				1	D
39	12				3	E
39	15			2	4	E
39	18		2	3	7	F
39	21		3	3	10	G
39	24	2	3	6	15	G
39	27	4	4	8	18	G

m	min	9	6	4	2	RG
42	8				1	D
42	12			1	4	E
42	15		1	3	5	F
42	18		3	4	8	F
42	21	3	3	5	13	G
42	24	4	4	7	18	G
45	9				3	D
45	12			3	3	D
45	15		3	3	6	F
45	18	2	3	4	11	F
45	21	4	4	7	16	G
48	9			1	4	E
48	12		1	3	4	F
48	15	2	2	4	9	G
48	18	4	5	5	14	G
51	6				2	E
51	9		1	1	3	F
51	12	1	2	3	5	F
51	15	3	3	4	11	G
54	6				2	D
54	9		1	3	3	F
54	12	2	3	3	7	F
54	15	4	4	6	13	G

© A.A. Beuhlmann, University of Zurich/Switzerland 1986

REPETITIVE DIVE TIME-TABLE – 2 500 m above sea level

BUEHLMANN TABLE

Surface Interval Times

RG at start of surface interval (left column); RG at end of surface interval (column headers). The last two columns correspond to '0' and → (flying).

RG	G	F	E	D	C	B	A	'0' hrs	→ hrs
A								2	2
B							20	2	2
C						10	25	3	3
D					10	15	30	3	3
E				10	15	25	45	4	3
F			20	30	45	75	90	8	4
G		25	45	60	75	100	130	12	5
G	F	E	D	C	B	A		hrs	hrs

Example:
Previous dive: 24 m, 35 min =
Repetitive Group (**RG**) = **F**
– after 45 min at surface: RG = C
– after 90 min at surface: RG = A
(intermediate time: use next **shorter** interval time)
– after 4 hrs: flying is permitted
– after 8 hrs: **RG** = '0', no more Residual Nitrogen Time (**RNT**)

RG for No-Decompression Dives and RNT for Repetitive Dives
Repetitive dive depth m (intermediate depths: use next **shallower** depth)

RG	9	12	15	18	21	24	27	30	33	36	39	42	45	48	51	54	57
A	25	19	16	14	12	11	10	9	8	7	7	6	6	6	5	5	5
B	37	25	20	17	15	13	12	11	10	9	8	7	7	6	5	5	5
C	55	37	29	25	22	20	18	16	14	12	11	10	9	8	7	7	6
D	81	57	41	33	28	24	21	19	17	15	14	13	11	10	9	9	8
E	105	82	59	44	37	30	26	23	21	19	17	16	14	13	12	11	10
F	130	111	88	68	53	42	35	30	27	24	21	19	17	16	15	14	13

Example: RG = C at end of surface interval. Planned depth of repetitive dive = 27 m.
RNT = 18 min, to be added to Bottom Time (BT) of repetitive dive.

2. HARD WAY Use standard dive tables to calculate the correction required for a particular altitude. This will be necessary if altitude tables are not available, if the bottom times exceed the altitude tables, or if special decompression techniques are used e.g. surface recompression and decompression using oxygen. The calculation is actually very simple. One just has to think in **local atmospheres**.

    At sea level, the local atmosphere is at 100 kPa or 1 ATA. At 10 msw the pressure doubles, at 20 msw it triples, etc. At Wondergat, the local atmosphere is 0.86 ATA or 86 kPa. Therefore at 8.6 msw (if it contained sea water) the pressure doubles, at 17.2 msw it triples, at 25.8 msw it quadruples, etc.

NOTE: As fresh water is less dense than sea water, allowance must be made for the difference. (The calculated depth must be multiplied by a factor of 1.03.) This means that at 8.9 mfw the pressure doubles, at 17.7 mfw it triples, at 26.6 mfw it quadruples, etc.

To put it another way, in the fresh water of Wondergat, an 8.9-metre dive is equivalent to a 10-metre sea dive; a 17.7-metre dive is equivalent to a 20-metre sea dive; and a 26.6-metre dive is equivalent to a 30-metre sea dive.

Example

Martin Martin is enjoying 'second honeymoon' at Lake Titicaca with his wife Dulcinea. Here, in the Peruvian Andes, the altitude is 3600 metres. Martin decides to dive to 36 metres. The local atmospheric pressure is:

$$100 - \frac{3600}{100} = 100 - 36 = 64 \text{ kPa}$$

Or

$$1 - \frac{3600}{10\,000} = 1 - 0.36 = 0.64 \text{ ATA}$$

Every 6.4 x 1.03 metres of fresh water depth is equivalent to 10 metres of sea water. So 36 metres of actual fresh water depth at an altitude of 3600 metres is equivalent to:

$$\frac{36 \times 10}{6.4 \times 1.03} = 54.6 \text{ msw}$$

Using RN Tables, Martin Martin must plan the dive on a 57-metre schedule. If no in-water decompression time is needed, there is no further problem. But, on a 57-msw apparent dive there will be decompression stops. Martin Martin decides to dive for 20 minutes at 36 metres.

He calculates that his apparent depth is 57 metres and, looking at the applicable Royal Navy table, sees that he must spend:

5 minutes at 9 msw,
10 minutes at 6 msw, and
20 minutes at 3 msw.

Now trap number two opens. At an altitude of 3600 metres, water depths of 3, 6 and 9 metres are not the same as sea level. The total pressure (ambient atmospheric + water pressure) is less. Therefore, the water stop depths must be **reduced** in depth. Just as the actual depth was 36 metres although a 57-metre table was used, so the decompression stops are equivalently shallower.

In this case:

The 9-metre stop is done at $\dfrac{6.4 \times 1.03 \times 9}{10} = 5.9$ metres

The 6-metre stop is done at $\dfrac{6.4 \times 1.03 \times 6}{10} = 4$ metres

The 3-metre stop is done at $\dfrac{6.4 \times 1.03 \times 3}{10} = 2$ metres

These reduced stops give the same ratio of pressure change as the tabled 9, 6 and 3 metre stops at sea level. The time spent at the bottom and on decompression stops remains the same.

To summarise:

$$\text{Apparent depth (metres)} = \frac{\text{Actual depth x 1 ATA}}{\text{Local ATA}}$$

$$\text{Or, even more simply} = \frac{\text{Actual depth}}{\text{Local ATA}}$$

$$\text{Using kPa : apparent depth} = \frac{\text{Actual depth x 100 kPa}}{\text{Local pressure in kPa}}$$

The depth of the decompression stops is exactly the same calculation, except with the sea level and local pressures transposed.

$$\text{Decompression stop (metres)} = \text{Tabled stop x Local ATA}$$
$$= \frac{\text{Tabled stop x Local kPa}}{100}$$

Finally, when diving at altitude:
1. Remember that fresh water is involved and an actual chosen **fresh water** depth must be divided by 1.03 to convert it into density equivalence of sea water.
2. A chosen table sea water depth must be multiplied by 1.03 to obtain fresh water equivalence.
3. Remember to think in terms of local atmospheric pressures.
4. Remember that all depth corrections are only ratios of sea level tables.

FLYING AFTER DIVING

The issue of flying home after a diving holiday often worries sport divers. Moving rapidly to altitude after diving at depth can precipitate acute decompression illness (DCI) due to both reduced ambient pressure and a reduced partial pressure of oxygen (which then decreases tissue tolerance to a nitrogen load).

Bear in mind that pressurised aircraft are not pressurised to sea level values. They are commonly pressurised to 6000–8000 feet above sea level (0.81 to 0.76 ATA).

There are two very important variables concerning flying after diving:
- the inert gas load of the diver, and
- the imposed physical conditions in an aircraft.

THE INERT GAS LOAD OF THE DIVER

The higher the inert gas load a scuba diver has dissolved in his or her tissues before a flight, the higher the risk of acute decompression illness. It takes any saturated tissue six half times to degas (see page 174). Blood, which has a 5-minute half time, takes 30 minutes to degas. Therefore, the 120-minute tissue requires 12 hours to degas. For safety, this is the minimum time permitted between surfacing after short underwater exposures and flying in a pressurised aircraft. Longer exposure to diving requires more surface time.

Minimum time to allow between diving and flying

Daily exposure to diving	Accumulated bottom time	Any tabled deco stops in last 48 hrs	Minimum time before flying
48 hours or less	Under 2 hrs	No	12 hrs
48 hours or less	Under 2 hrs	Yes	24 hrs
48 hours or less	Over 2 hrs	No	24 hrs
Multi-day	Unlimited	No	24 hrs
Multi-day	Unlimited	Yes	24–48 hrs

THE IMPOSED PHYSICAL CONDITIONS IN AN AIRCRAFT

If the diver has an inert gas load, it is the venous system that transports this load from the tissues to the lungs for degassing. Platelet clumping, which leads to blood sludging and clotting, occurs much more readily in nitrogen-loaded venous blood. Flying aggravates sludging in the venous system by inducing dehydration and by limiting movement.
- The cabin humidity in a commercial aircraft is only eight per cent. Breathing dry air rapidly depletes tissue fluids, including blood.

- Alcohol and caffeine (found in tea, coffee, cola, some energy drinks) stimulate urine production without adequately replacing the resultant fluid loss.
- Eating large, fatty meals causes shunting of peripheral blood to the gut. Peripheral venous blood flow becomes sluggish and slow.
- Sitting for extended periods in an aircraft seat drastically reduces venous blood flow in the lower limbs. This is especially dangerous in divers. Acute decompression illness may occur, with numbness or pain in the legs. In addition, swelling of the feet and pooling of the blood in the calf veins, leading to deep vein thrombosis (DVT), is not uncommon.

Flying also exposes one to infection. Forty to sixty per cent of the air in an aircraft is recirculated. This means enforced sampling of a pot-pourri of perspiration, human body odours and a polyculture of bacteria and viruses. Behind the plasticised décor and piped background music lurks an airborne bacterial colony nearly 30 times greater than that found in an average sleazy bar. Upper respiratory tract infections, presenting two to three days after a flight, are very common.

WHAT SHOULD DIVERS DO BEFORE, DURING AND AFTER A FLIGHT?

If you are travelling by air, the last dive of the holiday should preferably be a short, deep dive. If you are planning a deep dive (25–30 msw), save it for last, but keep it well within no-decompression time limits. This primarily loads the fast tissues which then have ample time to degas while you wait out the required surface interval before flying home.

If you are at a remote dive destination and must take a short flight in an unpressurised aircraft from your outlying resort to the main island in order to catch a long-haul flight, it is best to allow 24 hours to elapse before getting on to the plane.

If you have been diving and experience any untoward symptoms before a flight, which you think may be related to acute decompression illness, do not fly. Reducing altitude could be disastrous. Contact a diving doctor immediately.

During flights, eat frugally and drink copious amounts of water, fruit juice and non-carbonated beverages. These prevent dehydration and also induce the desire to urinate, which then means a walk down the aisle, facilitating circulation in the legs. Try to move about regularly during the journey.

At the start of your holiday, particularly if you have had a long international flight to your diving destination, drink lots of fluids, spend the first day swimming and snorkelling, and go to bed early, especially if you have crossed time zones. Don't do any dives on day one – let your body recover from the insults of travelling in a cramped, stuffy, potentially air-polluted aircraft.

28

DROWNING AND NEAR-DROWNING

Drowning is death due to the inhalation of fluid. If a person survives immersion, drowning did not occur. The victim **nearly** drowned, so survival after fluid inhalation is called **near-drowning**. There are three basic causes to drowning or near-drowning: accident, suicide or homicide. Only accidental drowning is relevant to divers. While anyone can drown anywhere, there is a pattern to how drownings occur:
- swimming pools: mostly babies and very young children,
- rivers, dams and the seaside: mostly teenagers and young adults,
- boatsmen and fishermen at sea: mostly adults, and
- bathtubs: mostly babies and the aged.

PREDISPOSING FACTORS FOR ACCIDENTAL DROWNING

Drowning is usually preventable, but accidents do happen, and you can never be too careful around water. In addition, conditions such as heart disease, epilepsy, high blood pressure and diabetes can place even a strong swimmer in a drowning situation.

In the home, a major cause of accidental drowning in children is lack of supervision. Never leave an unattended child in a bathtub or near a swimming pool while chatting on the phone or answering the door. Proper pool fencing, 'drown-proofing' lessons, and learning to swim come next as safety measures.

ALCOHOL AND DRUG ABUSE
It is a sad fact that about 80 per cent of adults who drown used alcohol and/or drugs before entering the water. Alcohol, drugs and water **never** mix. Look at some of the reasons. Alcohol causes:
- overconfidence; risks are taken beyond training, fitness and ability,
- inability to react adequately to the situation, resulting in panic,
- hypothermia due to skin flushing and rapid heat loss,
- increased likelihood of vomiting, with inhalation of vomit and water, and
- possible suicidal tendencies.

DIVING

Divers dive in water, so the spectre of drowning always lurks. The causes of drowning in scuba divers are wide-ranging, covering everything from panic to falling victim to an unexpected underwater explosion. The most common causes include:

- gas problems, including hypoxia,
- oxygen toxicity; carbon dioxide toxicity; carbon monoxide poisoning,
- nitrogen narcosis,
- HPNS (Nuno Gomes almost died underwater from this in his world record dive),
- pulmonary barotrauma (ascent and descent),
- hypothermia,
- seasickness (with vomiting and inhalation),
- marine animal stings and bites,
- underwater injuries or entrapment, and
- medical problems, both known and unanticipated.

MECHANISM OF DROWNING

Much of the early research on drowning was done by experimenting on animals, by introducing sea water or fresh water into the lungs of the anaesthetised animals. Large quantities of water were poured into their lungs – up to 20 ml/kg body weight. Two types of drowning were then described: freshwater drowning and saltwater drowning. The following applies to the experimental drowning of animals only. It does not happen in cases of human drowning.

1. FRESHWATER DROWNING

Blood contains a great assortment of salts, proteins, glucose, hormones and other chemicals. These concentrate the blood, making it more dense than water. The presence of fresh water in the alveoli results in the water moving from an area of low concentration (the alveoli) to an area of higher concentration (the blood in the lung capillaries). This dilutes the blood and increases blood volume. In addition, the red blood cells within the blood absorb water from the diluted blood, swell and then burst, releasing free haemoglobin into the blood. The increased blood volume causes heart overload, while the rupture of red blood cells means reduced oxygen-carrying capacity and hypoxia. Heart failure then causes lung congestion and more hypoxia. Death results from cardiac arrest or ventricular fibrillation (incoordinated rippling of the ventricles of the heart without any effective pumping action).

2. SALTWATER DROWNING

Sea (or salt) water contains many dissolved salts which make it even more concentrated than blood. Salt water in the alveoli causes water movement in the opposite direction to fresh water, with water moving from the blood in the lung capillaries to the alveoli. This causes marked lung congestion with water and decreases blood volume. The red cells lose water to the concentrated plasma and shrink.

NOTE: Lung congestion occurs in both saltwater and freshwater drowning. In freshwater drowning, this is because of heart overload with damming back of blood in the lungs due to pump failure; in sea water, drowning occurs through movement of water from the blood into the alveoli. Both cause boggy, fluid-filled lungs. Movement of oxygen through the flooded alveoli is impeded and there is interference with circulation through the lungs – both factors cause more hypoxia.

WHAT HAPPENS IN HUMANS?

Ethics and morals do not permit the deliberate drowning of anaesthetised people by pouring 20 ml/kg of fresh or sea water into the lungs! In a 70 kg man this would amount to the introduction of 70 x 20 ml or 1.4 litres of water! In accidental human drowning, only about 2 ml/kg is usually inhaled. This is too little to cause the clear picture that is obtained by the experimental drowning of animals.

Therefore, in accidental human drowning:
–   there is very little change in blood volume,
–   rupture or shrinkage of red blood cells is very uncommon,
–   dilution or concentration of blood is rare, and
–   ventricular fibrillation does not occur.

Why are humans different from animal experiments?

1.   DIVING REFLEX Immersing the face in water causes reflex breathholding and slowing of the heart, especially in babies.
2.   LARYNGOSPASM Inhaling water causes immediate spasmodic closure of the vocal cords, shutting off the larynx so water (or air) cannot enter. The casualty is no longer attempting to breathe, so water will not enter unless the person is head-up and face-up in the water. Most drowned casualties are face-down.
3.   HYPOTHERMIA In cold water, cooling protects the brain and heart by reducing oxygen requirements. Because babies have a relatively large surface area compared with adults, hypothermia occurs more rapidly in infants.

These three factors – diving reflex, laryngospasm and hypothermia – decrease the likelihood of inhaling water and prolong possible survival time under water. There have been reports of people who, after vigorous resuscitation, have revived after being submerged for up to 40 minutes in cold water, and suffered no apparent damage.

PRESENTATION OF DROWNING

The following is the sequence of events in drowning:

1. When the casualty submerges, the diving reflex operates and breathholding occurs. How long the breath can be held depends on the individual's degree of fitness, fatigue and fear.
2. Meanwhile, oxygen is being used and carbon dioxide produced within the body. Two things can now happen:
   (a) Hypoxia and the rising carbon dioxide levels can cause cardiac arrest, so no further oxygen circulates to the brain and the larynx relaxes. Water can now passively enter the lungs. This is **wet drowning** and occurs in 80–90 per cent of casualties.
   (b) Hypoxia and rising carbon dioxide levels force the casualty to inhale.
3. Water is inhaled and laryngospasm occurs, keeping the casualty's lungs more or less dry. This is **dry drowning**.
4. Oxygen is still being used and hypoxia worsens. Consciousness is lost. The heart begins to fail, causing lung congestion.
5. Still more hypoxia occurs. Breathing attempts stop and the laryngospasm relaxes. Passive flooding of the lungs may now occur if the casualty is head-up and face-up in the water. Death occurs.

Depending on the water temperature, the person's age, weight, how much clothing is being worn (insulation), plus any injuries related to the incident, hypothermia will protect the casualty to some degree. Theoretically, a skinny, naked casualty should do better than a fat, dressed casualty.

Rescue before death in a near-drowned casualty reveals the following:

1. The casualty is unconscious and limp.
2. The skin is pale or blue, and cold to the touch.
3. No breathing is evident and there is no pulse or heartbeat.
4. The pupils do not react to light.
5. Copious frothy blood-stained foam may be flowing from the mouth due to lung congestion – secondary to heart (pump) failure from hypoxia.

Management of near-drowning

The aim is to restore spontaneous breathing and an effective heartbeat – this is CPR (see page 235). Most people who die after immersion do so because resuscitation was started too late or stopped too soon. If a casualty is not breathing, he or she should be assisted while still in the water, even while being brought to shore or to the boat. Supporting the head in the water and giving mouth-to-mouth or mouth-to-snorkel resuscitation may make all the difference to the outcome. **Continue resuscitation until a doctor calls off the attempt because of definite death.**

29

CARDIOPULMONARY RESUSCITATION

Cardiopulmonary resuscitation (CPR) is an emergency procedure used in the management of cardiac arrest and/or respiratory arrest. Since the 1950s, CPR has comprised both artificial blood circulation (chest compressions) and artificial respiration (lung ventilation), the latter also being known as mouth-to-mouth ventilation or expired air resuscitation (EAR).

In March 2008, the American Heart Association and European Resuscitation Council surprised the medical world by officially approving the effectiveness of chest compressions alone – without artificial respiration – for adults who collapse suddenly with cardiac arrest or ventricular fibrillation. This is called Hands-Only CPR. The rationale is that chest compressions, in addition to compressing the ventricles to maintain blood circulation, also compress and empty the lungs. The subsequent elastic recoil of the chest between compressions automatically draws fresh air into the lungs.

CPR must be continued until the patient regains a heartbeat or is declared dead. It should be understood that CPR rarely restarts an arrested heart, its purpose being the maintenance of a flow of oxygenated blood to the brain and heart, until electrical defibrillation and advanced life support become available to restart the heart and provide successful resuscitation.

This compression-only technique of CPR has not yet received official endorsement by the international diving medical fraternity as divers tend to only require CPR after an in-water rescue following a variably prolonged period of submersion. However, they might possibly benefit from assisted ventilation as well as cardiac compressions. At this stage, this author recommends a combination of chest compressions and artificial respiration when administering CPR to diver casualties.

Do not rush blindly into administering CPR. A 20-second initial assessment of the situation is vital. Six essential questions must first be answered; using the mnemonic HHHABC will help you to remember them.

Assessment prior to administering CPR:

1.	Are casualty and rescuer in a safe place?	H	HAZARDS
2.	Is the casualty rousable?	H	HELLO
3.	Is anyone on hand to help?	H	HELP
4.	Is the airway clear?	A	AIRWAY
5.	Is the casualty breathing?	B	BREATHING
6.	Can a pulse be felt?	C	CIRCULATION

1. ARE THE CASUALTY AND THE RESCUER IN A SAFE PLACE?

Both must be in a safe place – out of the water and on the beach beyond any tidal action of the sea, or on the deck of the dive boat. If on land, ensure that you are out of the way of oncoming traffic and well clear of any hazards.

2. IS THE CASUALTY ROUSABLE?

Assess whether the casualty is rousable by **gently** shaking his or her shoulder and yelling 'Are you OK?' Use your shouting voice, not forceful shaking, to gain their attention. Violent shaking may aggravate spinal, neck or internal injuries.

(a) If the casualty responds, check for injuries, render assistance, summon help if required, then wait with the casualty until trained aid comes.

(b) If the casualty does not respond, call for help **before** clearing the airways.

3. IS ANYONE ON HAND TO HELP?

You need two kinds of help: someone to summon trained emergency assistance and someone to assist with resuscitation of the casualty.

(a) Send someone else to make the emergency call. If you are alone, make the call yourself **before** starting CPR. It is essential to ensure that advanced life support is rushing to help you. Quickly telephone DAN, your private rescue service or an appropriate emergency number.

(b) Tell the rescue service that CPR is about to be performed or is being done. Do not waste time explaining the case. Just say 'CPR in progress'.

(c) Be calm and relay all asked-for information clearly.

(d) Go back to the casualty immediately after the rescue service hangs up.

4. IS THE AIRWAY CLEAR?

Quickly partially unzip the casualty's wet suit or slacken any tight neckwear. Perform the **'head tilt–chin lift' manoeuvre** as follows:

(a) Place one hand on the casualty's forehead and tilt his or her head well back. This straightens the windpipe and provides a good airway. This is essential, as it is impossible to breathe properly with the head flexed forward on the neck.

(b) Use the fingers of your other hand to lift up the front of the casualty's jaw – this pulls the tongue forward and prevents it from flopping backwards and blocking the airway.

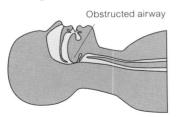
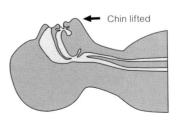

Head tilt–chin lift position

(c)   Look inside the mouth. Quickly remove any foreign material. Clear any vomit, blood or water by wiping the mouth from cheek to cheek with a forefinger wrapped in a piece of cloth. In near-drowning there is often copious pink froth swelling up from the lungs. This must continuously be wiped away. Dentures, unless very loose or ill-fitting, must be left in place as they will support a proper lip seal with mouth-to-mouth resuscitation.

5. IS THE CASUALTY BREATHING?

While maintaining the head tilt–chin lift position, use the next five seconds:
−   to listen for breathing next to casualty's mouth and nose,
−   to feel for any movement of breath with your cheek, and
−   to watch the casualty's chest for movement.

(a)   If the casualty is unconscious and breathing: turn him or her as a unit (head and body together to avoid worsening possible neck trauma) into the **left lateral recovery** position (see below):
  −   casualty lying on the left side with the left leg extended,
  −   head resting on the left arm extended in line with the body,
  −   right knee flexed and resting on the ground in front of the casualty, and
  −   right elbow flexed and resting on the ground in front of the casualty.

This position ensures that the tongue cannot obstruct the airway and allows water, blood or vomit to drain away. Summon emergency help, then wait with the casualty until professional aid comes, constantly monitoring satisfactory pulse and breathing.
(b)   If the casualty is not breathing: feel for a carotid pulse.

Left lateral recovery position

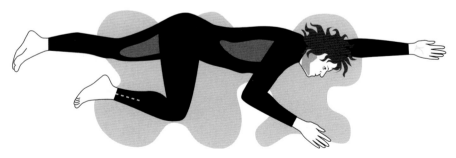

6. CAN A PULSE BE FELT?

The carotid arteries are the large arteries in the neck supplying blood to the head. They are easily found by placing the fingertips on the larynx and then moving them round to either side into the hollow next to the neck muscles and gently pressing back. It is essential to spend 5–10 seconds in finding a pulse.

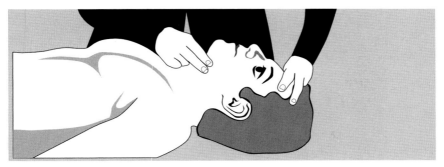
Locating the carotid pulse

A pulse is normally easily felt, but a very slow or weak pulse will not be found with a too rapid or cursory feel. **Do not:**
- try to find a wrist pulse – it is invariably impalpable,
- use a thumb to find a carotid pulse – you will feel your own pulse, or
- press too hard – you will not feel a weakly pulsating artery.

(a) If the casualty is not breathing but a pulse can be felt, perform mouth-to-mouth rescue breathing immediately.

(b) If, after performing rescue breathing, the casualty is still not breathing and no pulse can be felt: summon emergency assistance, as CPR and defibrillation are required.

MOUTH-TO-MOUTH RESCUE BREATHING

This is also known as mouth-to-mouth ventilation, artificial ventilation and expired air resuscitation (EAR).

1. Prepare the casualty to receive EAR:
   - Ensure that he or she is on a firm, flat surface.
   - Roll the casualty as a unit on to his or her back, protecting the neck and spine.
   - Ensure the head tilt–chin lift position (see page 231).
   - If available, and especially if the casualty is a stranger, place a disposable non-return airway between the casualty's lips, with the thin plastic skirt of the airway covering the casualty's face.
   - Pinch off the nostrils, using the thumb and forefinger of the head-tilt hand. (Remember to pinch off the nose. It is pointless to blow air into the casualty's mouth and have it vent through his nostrils!)

2. Take a normal breath, then place your mouth firmly over the casualty's mouth or the non-return airway.

3. Blow into the casualty's mouth or the non-return airway. Take one second (no longer) to do this.

4. Allow the casualty to exhale passively while you take another normal breath.
5. Repeat this ventilation twice. There should be very little resistance.
6. Watch the casualty's chest. It should rise when you blow. Be sure it is not the casualty's stomach that is rising. If this happens, you are filling the stomach with air which will predispose to vomiting. If the casualty's chest does not move, it means there is an obstruction or leakage. If this is the case, then:
   - ensure that the head is tilted well back,
   - ensure that the jaw is well lifted,
   - ensure that the nostrils are pinched closed,
   - ensure that the casualty's mouth is partially open, and
   - ensure a good mouth-to-mouth or mouth-to-airway seal.
7. If the chest still does not rise when you blow, there is foreign material in the airway. With the casualty flat on his or her back, straddle their upper legs.
   - Place the palm of one hand on the back of the other and link your fingers.
   - Place the heel of the lower hand on the casualty's abdomen just above the navel and well below the breastbone.
   - Push sharply upwards and inwards. Repeat this thrust up to five times. This will force inhaled foreign material from the airway. Clear this away by sweeping your forefinger around the inside of the cheek and behind the material.
   - Listen, feel and watch for breathing. If no breathing is evident, recommence rescue breathing.
8. When the casualty is being ventilated properly, there will be passive exhalations between breaths.

Mouth-to-mouth ventilation must be done at a rate of 10–12 breaths per minute in an adult (about one breath every 5–6 seconds), checking the carotid pulse after each cycle of 10 breaths.

AIDS WARNING!
AIDS has made CPR a potentially dangerous procedure for the rescuer. If any bleeding is present, rescuers must protect themselves by using a non-return airway, gloves, goggles and a plastic apron, unless the casualty is known to be HIV-negative.

CARDIOPULMONARY RESUSCITATION

Until 2004, the protocols for CPR were clearly defined; circulation of the blood and ventilation of the lungs were two distinct procedures. If one person was performing CPR, the rate was 15 chest compressions to two breaths, while two-rescuer CPR was done at a rate of five compressions to one breath. After 2004, a ratio of 30 compressions (at two per second, or twice the previous speed) to two breaths, became the norm, irrespective of the number of rescuers. In 2008, Hands-Only CPR (dispensing altogether with artificial ventilation) at a rate of 100 chest compressions per minute was endorsed by the American Heart Association for adults with cardiac arrest.

Until clear confirmation is presented that oxygen-deprived divers who require CPR will not benefit from additional artificial ventilation, this author recommends retaining the '30 compressions to two breaths' protocol.

In order to maintain the proper sequence in what are often extremely emotional and confusing circumstances, it is essential to call out each step.

A = AIRWAY – Call 'A' and perform the **head tilt–chin lift manoeuvre**.

B = BREATHING – Call 'B' and **deliver two normal breaths** to the casualty at a rate of one breath per second. Watch that chest movement occurs.

C = CIRCULATION – Call 'C' and perform **chest compressions**.

CHEST COMPRESSIONS

1. Prepare for chest compressions:
    - Place the heel of one hand on the centre of the chest two fingerbreadths above the lower end of the breastbone. Now place the other hand on top of the first with your fingers off the chest and facing away from you.
    - Keep your elbows straight.
    - Keep your shoulders directly above the casualty's breastbone.
    - Keep your fingers off the casualty's chest. You must press on the breastbone, not on the ribs.

Chest compressions

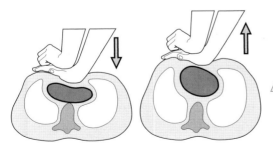
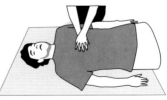

Position the hands two fingerbreadths above the lower end of the breastbone.

2. Press smoothly downward, using the weight of your upper body to push the breastbone down 4–5 cm. Do not jerk downwards – you will break ribs and damage internal organs.

3. Release the pressure, allowing the chest wall to spring back, but without losing your hand position on the breastbone. This process compresses the heart between the front of the chest and the spine, forcing blood from the ventricles. On releasing the pressure, the chest will spring back and the ventricles will refill from the venous system. If done properly, a pulse will be felt in the neck with each compression.

4. Repeat the compression 30 times at a rate of two compressions per second (push hard and push fast), while loudly reciting 'one, two, three, four etc...' Compress with each number and release before the next one. You will achieve a rate of about 100–120 compressions per minute.

CPR is hard and desperate work, but persistence is vital. When you have done a full sequence of two rescue breaths followed by 30 chest compressions (as described above), you have completed one cycle of 'A–B–C'.

Repeat the cycle of two breaths and 30 compressions (2:30) until help arrives, or the victim breathes or moves. (If you are alone, do not waste time trying to find a carotid pulse again – it will break your rhythm and timing.)
   – Call A and return to the airway.
   – Call B and give two mouth-to-mouth breaths at a rate of one per second.
   – Call C and commence counting 'one, two, three …'

If the casualty shows no sign of life after about two minutes of CPR, and an automatic external defibrillator (AED) is available, it should be applied and the prompts followed. Administer one shock, then immediately recommence CPR for two minutes before providing a second shock. The use of an AED requires some training, but staff at DAN or an emergency call centre may be able to assist telephonically if you are untrained.

If spontaneous breathing recurs, place the casualty in the left lateral position (see page 232), give 100 per cent oxygen by mask if it is available, and stop CPR.

NOTES ON ADMINISTERING CPR
1. If two-rescuer CPR is being performed, the rescuer in charge of circulation must wait after each cycle of 30 compressions while the first rescuer administers two rescue breaths. If the chest is compressed during a rescue breath, most of the delivered air will not enter the casualty's lungs – it will be blown back into the first rescuer's mouth or diverted into the casualty's stomach and predispose to vomiting and aspiration.

2. If too much air is delivered during rescue breathing, it increases the casualty's chest pressure and reduces the volume of blood returning to the heart and then

leaving the heart with subsequent chest compressions. The air volume should just be sufficient to produce a visible chest rise (500–600 ml); a normal breath will suffice.

3. If two rescuers are present they should change roles after every five cycles of CPR (one cycle = two rescue breaths and 30 compressions). The switch-over must be completed in less than five seconds.

SIGNS OF IMPROVEMENT

CPR is a dire measure for someone who performs it for the first time. Any sign that it is working will give courage and strength to aching arms and back. Signs include:
– The casualty's lips become pinker.
– The pupils start to react to light. They become smaller when a torch or other light is shone into them.
– Spontaneous heartbeat starts. Stop chest compressions straight away.
– Spontaneous breathing starts. Stop rescue breathing and give oxygen by mask.

SECONDARY EFFECTS OF NEAR-DROWNING

Bear in mind that a near-drowned diver may also have substantial decompression requirements, an arterial gas embolism, or both. In this case, administer CPR until expert help takes over and then transport the casualty to the nearest recompression facility. Remember to notify the facility so that qualified help is waiting and the chamber can be prepared in advance.

Even if a near-drowned person appears to have fully recovered, in that he or she is breathing, the heart is beating and consciousness has returned, medical help must be obtained and the casualty admitted to hospital for observation. The secondary effects of near-drowning and hypoxia can kill a recovered casualty hours later (this is called secondary drowning). A further complication is the development of an infected pneumonia due to bacteria inhaled along with water. Inhaling micronised salt water can cause a pneumonia called salt water aspiration syndrome, an inflammatory response of the lungs to hypertonic seawater.

RESUSCITATION KITS

Divers Alert Network (DAN) provides a complete resuscitation kit comprising a face mask, ventilation bag, oxygen cylinder and all the required valves and attached tubing for use with CPR. Resuscitation kits and supplementary oxygen should also be available from reputable medical equipment suppliers.

DAN also offers a course in how to administer emergency oxygen, which is highly recommended for all divers; and provides training in how to use an Automatic External Defibrillator (AED).

30

ADMINISTERING EMERGENCY OXYGEN

Oxygen is the only vital gas in any breathing mix. Administered pure at surface pressure, it is also the single most important primary treatment in the management of all serious diving injuries. Not only can oxygen reduce the severity of symptoms and help prevent permanent damage, including paralysis, but it can also be life-saving after near-drowning, lung overpressurisation, acute decompression injuries and many marine animal stings or bites.

ALL divers, no matter where they are, what sort of dive they are doing, or the size of the boat or vessel, must ensure that at least one person in the group has oxygen to hand and knows how to use it. Remember, you don't have to be able to diagnose the dive problem or even have a clue as to what it might be. You only have to be competent in providing pure oxygen to the casualty at the surface, and that requires some formal training. The only exception would be oxygen toxicity – which does not occur in sport diving unless an idiotic, very deep nitrox dive occurred.

There are two critical aspects to providing oxygen:
- the time to onset of pure oxygen breathing, and
- the method of administration.

Time is everything. The sooner oxygen is provided, the greater the potential for recovery and the less the chance of progressive damage. This means that oxygen must be instantly available on the dive boat or at the banks of a dam or lake. To have to wait hours, or even days, while the diver is transported from a dive boat, a liveaboard or a remote site truly is courting disaster.

The method of administration is just as important. Ideally, pure oxygen must be provided to the diver. This means a demand valve or, in the case of a non-breathing diver, a full oronasal mask with attached ventilation bag.

Using a normal hospital-type oxygen administration mask and tubing does not provide 100 per cent oxygen – it only provides oxygen-enriched air and this not what a diver with arterial gas embolism or acute decompression illness really needs. Pure oxygen means zero nitrogen. This allows rapid exhalation of a high tissue nitrogen overload and no further nitrogen in gas emboli, even at surface pressure and before later chamber treatment.

The biggest practical problem is that oxygen cylinders are often big and bulky. As divers already have lots of heavy equipment to lug onto a cramped dive boat, they may opt for the 'it won't happen to me' approach and choose a token small cylinder in the hope that it will suffice if they eke out the oxygen by reducing the flow rates. It won't. Life support isn't chicken soup and can't be eked out!

Even worse, space-constrained divers may opt for no oxygen at all. Remember that DCI and AGE are merciless and can occur anytime. A burst O-ring or a jellyfish sting can send a diver rushing for the surface to bend or burst and die in minutes.

All divers, no matter where they are, what sort of dive they are doing or the size of the vessel, **must** ensure that at least one person in the group has oxygen to hand.

HOW MUCH OXYGEN IS ENOUGH?

As the objective is to get the diver to professional help, enough oxygen is needed to achieve just that. DAN provides an aluminium alloy Jumbo-D oxygen cylinder that is available worldwide, although the cylinder size may vary from country to country.

In South Africa, the cylinder weighs just under 4 kg and it contains 647 litres of oxygen at 153 bar. Using a demand valve, this will provide nearly an hour of pure oxygen. In comparison, using a free flow supply to a mask will only provide about 40 minutes of oxygen. Reducing the flow to the mask to try and gain time will only decrease effectiveness. Demand valve oxygen breathing is the only way to go if the attempt to help the diver is serious and, when it happens, it had better be!

If your dive site is within an hour of professional help, a DAN Jumbo-D oxygen unit, equipped with a demand valve, mask and all the required attachments, and a waterproof case, is enough. But divers are often not within an hour of trained help. So what does one do? Realistically, work out how long it will take you to reach help and then do the sums. Assume that about 600 litres of cylinder oxygen will give an hour of surface oxygen on a demand valve. A two-hour delay is provided for by DAN with their dual-pack oxygen cylinders.

If the dive site is still further away from professional assistance, you probably need a large oxygen cylinder, as supplied by gas companies to hospitals. Ideally, enough oxygen should be available to supply a conscious, breathing diver for eight hours.

It takes proper training to be able to provide effective, life-saving oxygen assistance. I would strongly recommend that every serious diver has a formal course in the administration of oxygen. A list of trained oxygen administrator instructors for each country is available on the country-specific DAN websites.

It is vital that every dive boat, liveaboard, dive school and diving club has a dedicated oxygen unit especially designed for divers, as well as personnel trained to use it. If remote diving is done, the availability of a prolonged oxygen supply must become a necessity too.

Providing oxygen via a freeflow silicone hospital mask is just not good enough. Demand valve administration is essential. The whole set-up costs less than a decent dive rig; it is not worth losing a life for that price.

31

VERTIGO UNDER WATER

Vertigo is a subjective illusion of directional movement – left or right, upwards, downwards, or round and round like a merry-go-round. A diver may feel that he or she is spinning or falling in a particular direction or, conversely, that he or she is quite still but that the environment is suddenly moving or turning topsy-turvy.

Vertigo is extremely disorientating. It is frequently accompanied by intense nausea and vomiting and, when it occurs underwater, can become a rapidly life-threatening condition. Vertigo is **not** the same as dizziness, faintness, light-headedness or giddiness. There is always a profound hallucination of movement which can render a diver totally incapable of any safe, or even life-saving, reaction.

Several conditions cause vertigo on land. Their importance in divers relates to the fact that they all prohibit safe diving. They include:

1. **Benign positional vertigo (BPV)** This illness results in short episodes of vertigo caused by moving the head either left or right. It most commonly occurs when turning over in bed, lasts less than one minute, then passes. There is no associated hearing loss or tinnitus. The cause involves microscopic crystals in the fluid-filled balance organs. These loosen (possibly following previous trauma) and float inside the fluid of the inner ear. Turning the head causes the crystals to move and create a rippling effect (like a stone thrown into water). The ripples initiate a sensation of motion in the inner ear, which causes vertigo. The spinning stops as the crystals settle and fluid movements stop.

2. **Meniere's Disease** This is a recurring episodic vertigo that is associated with fluctuating hearing loss, tinnitus and a feeling of pressure in the ear. Symptoms are provoked by stress, a high salt intake, caffeine and alcohol. The spinning lasts at least 30 minutes but may last up to 24 hours. The cause is unknown. Meniere's disease can often be controlled by reducing stress and salt intake, and avoiding caffeine and alcohol. (See also page 103.)

3. **Acoustic neuroma** This benign tumour of the acoustic (hearing) nerve most commonly presents with sudden one-sided hearing loss (total or partial) and ringing in the ear. Vertigo and, infrequently, numbness of the face may be present. The vertigo may be short-lived, recurrent, or ongoing. Treatment may require surgical removal of the tumour.

4. **Labyrinthitis** This viral infection of the inner ear results in severe vertigo, nausea and vomiting. It starts suddenly, lasts 2–3 weeks, and is often associated with hearing loss and ringing in one ear. Treatment involves medication to reduce the vertigo and nausea, as well as oral cortisone.

5. **Vestibular neuronitis** This believed to be caused by a viral infection of the balance nerve. It is associated with severe vertigo, imbalance, nausea and vomiting, commences suddenly and lasts 2–3 weeks. No hearing loss occurs. Any movement of the head aggravates the vertigo. Cortisone is used to alleviate the symptoms.

For scuba divers, vertigo is invariably caused by:
- sensory deprivation,
- disorders of the ear, or
- inhaled gas toxicity, including hypoxia and hypocapnia.

SENSORY DEPRIVATION

Under conditions of poor visibility, such as occurs in turbid water or on night dives, disorientation is very common. In inexperienced divers, such disorientation may proceed to true vertigo, as a result of any combination of hyperventilation, loss of visual reference or anxiety, all of which reduce the inner ear threshold for the onset of vertigo.

When a diver is suspended in water with neither the surface nor the bottom visible, he or she may ignore the ongoing orientating messages of the vestibular apparatus in the inner ear and choose to orientate on things in the immediate vicinity. For instance, the diver may swim down a shot line instead of up, or adopt the orientation of his or her buddy regardless of direction. If one loses sight of one's buddies while diving, disorientation can even progress to true agoraphobia with a terrifying feeling of unending and featureless isolation. Thankfully, returning to the surface or being able to see the bottom restores equilibrium.

Experienced divers will find that a cool head and trained sensitivity will give them plenty of underwater clues when visual and gravity deprivation occur.

Although a diver may be neutrally buoyant, gravity is a fact, and non-buoyant equipment will dangle underwater. A weight belt or contents gauge will drop downwards – home and safety are obviously in the opposite direction. Buoyant equipment is even more user-friendly, for example, a dive torch attached by a cord to the diver's wrist will tug upwards. The body itself also provides orientation. If a disorientated diver lies absolutely still, the air in his or her lungs will cause the chest to rise while the denser legs sink (ankle weights or negatively buoyant fins will increase this bias).

An experienced diver, finely tuned to his or her gas spaces, is able to orientate on these clues. Exhaled gas bubbles will rise but, even if these cannot be seen, such as in conditions of absolutely zero visibility, they can certainly be felt by a hand placed near the exhaust port of the regulator. Ascent is then confirmed by clicking sounds as the expanding air vents from the middle ears through the Eustachian tubes. In contrast, descent can be verified by an awareness of an increase in ear pressure.

However, all these pointers require a calm and sensitive assessment and will be missed or disregarded by an inexperienced, anxious or panicky diver.

DISORDERS OF THE EAR

Ear disorders are the most common cause of underwater vertigo and can involve all three aural compartments – the external, middle and inner ears.

EXTERNAL EAR

Vertigo can result from disorders of the external ear, such as an obstruction in one of the external ear canals (see page 151).

CALORIC VERTIGO Vertigo can be induced if the temperature of the water entering the external ears varies. The temperature of the water in each external ear affects its respective inner ear. If one external ear canal is blocked by wax, a foreign body such as an ear plug, bony thickening (exostoses), or obstruction by swelling due to swimmer's ear, then cold water cannot easily enter that ear canal and the information relayed to its semicircular canal in the inner ear (vestibular apparatus) will differ from the much colder news delivered to the other ear. It is the horizontal semicircular canals that are especially relevant.

On land, when we are in the upright position, the horizontal semicircular canals relay information to the brain about sideways movements of the head. But, if a diver is descending head-down with the angle of the head at 30 degrees to horizontal, the horizontal semicircular canals become vertical. Under these conditions, any partial obstruction to an external ear can induce profound temperature-induced or **caloric** vertigo. Vertical information from one ear is interpreted by the brain as horizontal, and intense disorientation results. The solution is simple: once the diver assumes an upright, vertical position under water, the vertigo disappears.

EXTERNAL EAR BAROTRAUMA OF DESCENT Total obstruction of one external ear canal by wax, a foreign body or inflammation prevents water from filling the canal during descent. The air space trapped between the obstruction and the eardrum contracts and the eardrum bulges outwards, pulling the bony chain of the middle ear with it. Pulling on the stirrup reduces the pressure of the footplate in the oval window on the affected side. A difference in pressure in the inner ears results and vertigo can occur. (See also page 93.) In this case, the diver is often in a vertical position underwater and changing position does not relieve the vertigo. Ascent is required.

MIDDLE EAR

MIDDLE EAR BAROTRAUMA OF DESCENT If a diver fails to equalise but persists with descent, the shrinking air volume in the middle ear sucks the eardrum inwards. Haemorrhage into the middle ear may occur to equalise pressure, and vertigo can result. (This is also known as ear squeeze, see also page 152.)

EARDRUM PERFORATION   If haemorrhage does not occur into the middle ear to compensate for failed equalisation during continued descent, the eardrum will burst inwards. The diver hears a sudden noise, then experiences intense vertigo as cold water gushes into the middle ear. This is the second cause of **caloric vertigo** (see above). The cold water rapidly warms to body temperature and the vertigo passes. On returning to the surface, the diver notices deafness in the ear, often accompanied by bloody fluid leaking from the affected ear.

MIDDLE EAR BAROTRAUMA OF ASCENT   During ascent, air in the middle ear expands with reducing ambient pressure. If there is an unequal release of excess volume through the Eustachian tubes, the resulting pressure variation in the two middle ears can cause unequal inner ear stimulation and vertigo. This is called **alternobaric vertigo** (literally, 'vertigo due to two kinds of pressure'). It can occur with descent too, if there is a variance in Eustachian tube equalisation between the two ears.

If one Eustachian tube is blocked by blood or mucus from a previous middle ear squeeze, nasal allergy or infection, the eardrum may rupture outwards during ascent. In this case the diver clearly hears gas bubbling out of the ear as he ascends; water does not enter the middle ear because of the vigorous passage of expanding gas through the external ear; and vertigo may not occur. (See also page 154.)

INNER EAR

INNER EAR BAROTRAUMA   Trauma to the inner ear, including round window rupture, can follow a very forceful equalising attempt (see page 155). Vertigo may be immediate or, if the leak of inner ear fluid is slight, delayed for days.

SEASICKNESS   With unequal or aberrant stimulation of the vestibular apparatus, intense seasickness with vertigo can occur above and below water (see page 103).

ACUTE INNER EAR DECOMPRESSION ILLNESS   Acute decompression illness that involves only the inner ear is very rare in sport divers. Invariably, any vertigo is only part of a more widespread and serious neurological involvement. Pure inner ear decompression illness is far more common in deep heliox or trimix diving, especially on changing the gas mix.

CALORIC STIMULATION   Some divers have different caloric responses to the same cold temperature from the vestibular apparatus in each ear. This third type of cold-induced vertigo occurs without any equalising difficulty, external ear obstruction or eardrum injury. The diver equalises easily, reaches his or her bottom depth effortlessly and then develops disabling vertigo about five to ten minutes after starting the dive. This type of caloric vertigo can usually be prevented by wearing a hood.

GAS TOXICITY

A sport diver depends for his life on the purity and safety of his breathing mix. Several gas-induced disorders can present with vertigo. It is essential that a diver recognises vertigo for what it is, signals his buddy for help, and commences an assisted ascent.

NITROGEN NARCOSIS At depths below ±40 msw, nitrogen narcosis can present with giddiness. True vertigo is uncommon, and a sense of rotation will be relieved on ascent.

OXYGEN TOXICITY Breathing pure oxygen or nitrox mixtures rapidly induces toxicity when the oxygen partial pressure exceeds 2 ATA. The onset of vertigo is indicative of an incipient convulsion underwater.

HYPOXIA In sport diving, hypoxia (insufficient oxygen reaching the tissues) occurs most commonly with breathhold diving. Other causes are considered on page 195. Vertigo is one of the usual presenting features.

CARBON DIOXIDE TOXICITY Skip breathing, breathing dense nitrox mixtures, a contaminated air supply, or a faulty rebreather can result in vertigo as a result of inner ear and cerebral carbon dioxide build-up due to a build up of CO_2 in the inner ear and brain.

HYPOCAPNIA Hyperventilation at the surface by breathhold divers, or underwater by anxious scuba divers, causes the alveolar and arterial carbon dioxide levels to drop. An increase in the alkalinity of the blood occurs and vertigo is frequent.

CARBON MONOXIDE POISONING Divers who inhale CO as a result of their air supply being contaminated with exhaust fumes, frequently present with vertigo.

MANAGEMENT OF UNDERWATER VERTIGO

Vertigo that occurs underwater can be life-threatening. It is virtually impossible for an affected diver to react rationally to a sudden and spinning loss of orientation; all that can be done is to rely on a vigilant buddy. The onset of nausea, vomiting, disorientation, panic and frantic attempts to reach a non-discernible surface make the assisting buddy's task very difficult. Firmness is essential. The affected diver must be returned to the surface. It is impossible to perform required in-water decompression stops under conditions of severe vertigo. In most cases, ascending will reduce vertigo.

However, in cases with profound vertigo and uncontrollable disorientation, it may be necessary to initiate a controlled buoyant ascent. The consequences of missed decompression stops and possible pulmonary barotrauma of ascent must then be considered and acted on; this applies to both the affected diver and the assisting buddy.

32

COMMON INFECTIONS
IN SCUBA DIVERS

It is axiomatic that divers expose themselves to water, so any water that harbours bacteria, viruses, fungi, yeasts and parasites can cause problems in divers. Infection can occur whenever contaminated water gains entry into a diver's body by any means – through the skin, via the mouth, ears or eyes, or into the lungs. Infection can also occur when an intermediate host harbours a developmental stage of an infecting organism and then directly or indirectly infects the diver.

Divers should consult their doctors for expert advice before leaving on a diving holiday or expedition. **All divers should maintain their immunity to tetanus by having tetanus toxoid booster injections every three years, and should also be immunised against hepatitis A and B.**

SKIN INFECTIONS

Skin infections are common in divers. They usually occur following injury, e.g. coral cuts or fin blisters, or by allowing the skin to become excessively soggy, predisposing to yeast and fungal invasion. It is important that divers care for their skin. Using an antiseptic soap is wise. Tea tree oil is also a very effective antibacterial product.

TINEA PEDIS (Athlete's foot)

This fungal infection of the skin of the feet follows barefoot exposure to contaminated wet areas such as showers and decks, or sharing rubber diving bootees. The skin, most often between the toes and on the soles of the feet, becomes very white, itchy and cracked. Small blisters appear which later burst and are followed by skin ulcers and peeling. Pain is not usually a feature unless secondary bacterial infection occurs in the broken skin.

TREATMENT
1. Keep the skin dry. Exposure to sunlight dries out the blisters.
2. Bathe the feet in 0.05 per cent potassium permanganate solution (about one-third teaspoon in 5 litres of water) twice a day when the blisters are first noticed. Dry carefully with paper towels.

3. Apply topical antifungals such as ketoconazole, zinc undecanoate with undecanoic acid, tolnaftate or miconazole for three to four weeks.
4. In severe cases, oral fluconazole, at a dose of 150 mg once a week, may be needed.

TINEA VERSICOLOR

This superficial fungal infection of the skin is caused by the fungus *Malassezia furfur*. It presents with many brownish spots over the body, especially the chest and back. It is usually very mild and is only noticed after sunbathing, when the skin becomes tanned everywhere except for the untanned paler spots affected by the fungus.

TREATMENT

Applying half-strength Whitfield's ointment, 15 per cent sodium thiosulphate solution, or 5 per cent salicylic acid in alcohol, for three to four weeks cures the condition. The conazole group of antifungal creams is also effective.

CORAL ABRASIONS AND CUTS

Inadvertent contact with the hard corals frequently results in skin nicks and grazes which are only noticed after returning to the surface. Infection is almost invariable if calcific fragments, nematocysts and contaminating bacteria are not thoroughly removed from the wound. Infection becomes apparent after a few days with heat, swelling and redness in the area, then spreads to surrounding normal tissues. Skin wounds sustained by divers do not heal well if diving is continued. Repeated wetting removes antiseptic or antibiotic creams, reinfects the wound and causes bogginess of the skin. Under these conditions healing can be very delayed.

TREATMENT

If possible, consult a doctor.
1. Avoid direct contact with coral. This usually occurs due to excessive negative buoyancy in inexpert divers and dive students.
2. Wash any coral injury thoroughly with antiseptic solution such as cetrimide and chlorhexidine. Ensure that all foreign debris has been removed.
3. Apply an antiseptic cream, e.g. povidone iodine, or an antibiotic cream such as neomycin, mupirocin or fusidate.
4. If infection spreads, as evidenced by increasing pain, swelling and redness, consult a doctor. An oral antibiotic, such as broad-spectrum penicillin or tetracycline, is necessary.
5. Treat any non diving-related cut or blister with frequent applications of antibiotic or antiseptic cream. Diving and immersion in water may aggravate these injuries too.

INFECTIONS VIA THE MOUTH, EARS, EYES AND LUNGS

Infection can occur when contaminated water gains access to the mouth, the ears, the eyes and the airways.

MOUTH INFECTIONS

Swallowing water that has been contaminated by sewage can cause a host of illnesses, including bacterial gastroenteritis, amoebic dysentery, cholera, typhoid and paratyphoid. If the measures described on pages 132–134 are ineffectual in controlling any episode of diarrhoea and vomiting, expert medical advice becomes essential. Avoid sewage-contaminated water like the plague – it can cause it!

EAR INFECTIONS

External and middle ear infections are discussed on pages 98–102.

EYE INFECTIONS

Exposing the eyes to chlorinated or sea water may result in chemical irritation or infective conjunctivitis. Chemical or allergic irritation presents with red, burning or itchy eyes, but is rapidly relieved by the use of 0.9 per cent saline eye baths followed by antihistaminic drops containing antazoline, oxymetazoline or phenylephrine.

Bacterial conjunctivitis (pink eye) requires antibiotic therapy. Numerous preparations are available, containing antibiotics such as neomycin, chloromycetin, fusidic acid, gentamycin, polymixin and sulphacetamide; consult a doctor before any of these are used. (Never use eye preparations containing cortisone derivatives without medical opinion, as corneal ulceration and scarring can occur with viral eye infections.)

LUNG INFECTIONS

Inadvertent inhalation of water, or a near-drowning episode, may be followed by secondary infection of the lower respiratory tract, such as pneumonia or abscesses in the lungs. This is one of the reasons for seeking urgent medical attention after a near-drowning experience. In addition, a delayed chemical pneumonia due to irritation of the lungs by small volumes of sea water can place the victim in dire straits hours after an apparent full recovery from near-drowning. Hospitalisation, oxygen therapy and antibiotics become essential.

Contaminated regulators are another source of respiratory infection. Caused by failure to clean regulators after diving, the condition has been labelled **scuba disease.** Bacteria, commonly *Pseudomonas* and *Moraxella*, as well as other marine bacteria, can survive inside the regulator and are inhaled with the next dive. Thoroughly cleaning and drying your scuba regulators and cylinder HP outlets after use is an essential part of safe diving practice.

INFECTIONS VIA AN INTERMEDIATE HOST

Aside from being directly infected by contaminating organisms found in water, divers are often exposed to diseases which possess a more complex infective pattern. These are carried in intermediate hosts – other creatures that harbour the disease and pass it on to man. The route of the infection may be oral, such as contracting paralytic shellfish poisoning (PSP) after eating contaminated molluscs, or via penetration of the skin by the organism or the intermediate host.

TICK-BITE FEVER

Not all ticks carry tick-bite fever, but divers camping in African and Mediterranean countries may be bitten by ticks harbouring *Rickettsia conori*, the causative organism of tick-bite fever. Most tick bites simply heal but, if the tick harboured the organism, a black sore will develop after a few days at the site of the bite, followed by painful enlargement of nearby lymph glands. Fever, severe headache and a spotted rash will appear. The disease is self-limiting, even without treatment, and is rarely fatal.

TREATMENT
1. Prevention is always the first step, so take adequate precautions to avoid being bitten, including the use of insect repellents.
2. Remove any ticks found on the skin. Do not pull off a tick, as it usually breaks in two, leaving the head embedded in the skin. Apply a drop of petrol, paraffin or diesel to the tick. This will induce it to let go and it can then be removed using tweezers.
3. Tetracyclines cure tick-bite fever, but should not be given to children under eight years, as they can cause staining and damage to unerupted teeth.

MALARIA

Malaria is carried by the female *Anopheles* mosquito. Infection follows a mosquito bite and the injection of the insect's saliva, containing the malaria parasite, into the wound. The disease, which occurs in many parts of the world, is caused by a parasite called *Plasmodium*, of which there are four species: *P. vivax*, *P. ovale*, *P. malariae* and *P. falciparum*. Of these, the most dangerous is *Plasmodium falciparum* as it has become resistant to chloroquine and can have lethal complications. In Africa, about one million people die of malaria annually.

Once in the blood, the parasite multiplies inside red blood cells, which swell and burst to release more parasites. These attack other red blood cells and multiply. In severe cases, the urine becomes blood-stained due to the excretion of clumps of released haemoglobin from billions of destroyed red cells.

Obstruction to microscopic kidney tubules disrupts their filtering capacity and can lead to kidney failure; this occurs in the serious complication of malaria called blackwater fever.

Alternatively, the red cell debris may clog and obstruct the capillary networks in the brain, leading to very dangerous cerebral malaria, with confusion, convulsions, coma and even death.

PRESENTATION Malaria generally presents initially with flu-like symptoms – headache, muscle and joint aches, and fever. Severe shivering attacks (rigors) and high fever then occur, and recur in a cyclic pattern every third or fourth day. It can, however, present under a multitude of disguises such as fatigue, sore throat, nausea, vomiting and diarrhoea, making the diagnosis difficult. Diagnosis is made on the basis of a blood test, and repeated blood tests may have to be done over several days until a positive test occurs. It is safest to regard every flu-like illness that occurs within three months after visiting an endemic area as malaria until another illness is positively proven or the diver recovers from actual influenza.

PREVENTION There is no drug on the market that gives 100 per cent protection against malarial infection. Prophylaxis must involve both avoiding mosquitos and taking antimalarial drugs.

Avoiding mosquitos involves:
–   meticulous application of insect repellent to exposed skin **and** clothing – the repellent of choice is N, N-diethyltoluamide spray (DEET),
–   wearing long-sleeved shirts or blouses, slacks and socks between sunset and sunrise (the feeding time of the *Anopheles* mosquito),
–   moving continuously when outdoors at night (mosquitoes prefer a static meal),
–   mosquito screening on all doors and windows, or air-conditioned rooms;
–   spraying insecticide inside living quarters every day at dusk,
–   burning insecticide coils in the sleeping quarters at night, and
–   sleeping under insecticide-impregnated mosquito nets that are tucked in under the mattress.

ANTIMALARIAL DRUGS The drug of choice depends on the area visited, the presence or absence of chloroquine-resistant *P. falciparum* malaria, personal allergies and idiosyncrasies to antimalarial medication, drug interaction with any maintenance medication a diver may be using, pregnancy, age, health, and the availability of the drug. Consult your doctor to determine the best choice of medication and to ensure that no untoward side-effects or contraindications are present. (See table on page 250.)

An utterly incorrect and very dangerous myth exists. Many people believe that antimalarial drugs should not be taken because they 'mask' the disease and make the diagnosis difficult. This is absolute rubbish and the sooner this myth disappears the better. If you don't take antimalarial medication you may die! Malaria is diagnosed on blood tests (smear and antibodies). Medication does not make the diagnosis more difficult but it does slow the development of serious malaria and offers protection against blackwater fever and cerebral malaria. Any side-effects, although unpleasant in some people, are preferable to death.

Drugs recommended in the prevention of chloroquine-resistant *P. falciparum* malaria

Preventative drug	Dose in adults	Dose in children
Mefloquine Trade names: – Lariam – Mefliam	250 mg each week on the same day. Start 24 hours before entering the area and continue for four weeks after leaving the area. *Mefloquine can cause vertigo, drowsiness and tremors, and divers are advised not to use it if at all possible.* About 90% effective.	Do not use in children under 15 kg. Take 5 mg/kg body mass per week, at the same time intervals as adults. *Contraindicated in first trimester of pregnancy and while breastfeeding babies under 5 kg.*
Chloroquine Trade names: – Nivaquine – Daramal – Plasmaquine	400 mg each week on the same day. Start one week before entering the area and continue for six weeks after leaving the area. Must be taken in combination with proguanil. The combination is about 65% effective.	5 mg/kg body mass per week, at the same time intervals as adults. *Safe in pregnancy.*
Proguanil Trade name: – Paludrine	200 mg daily. Start two hours before entering the area and continue on a daily basis for six weeks after leaving the area. *Must only be taken together with chloroquine.* Interacts with Warfarin. About 65% effective.	Under 1 year: 25 mg/day. 1–4 years: 50 mg/day. 5–8 years: 100 mg/day. 9–14 years: 150 mg/day. *Safe in pregnancy, but take folic acid supplements. Can cause heartburn, so don't lie down after a dose.*
Doxycycline Trade names: – Cyclidox – Doxyclin – Doxylets – Doxymycin – Vibramycin, etc.	100 mg daily after food. Drink a full glass of water with it. Start 48 hours before entering the area; continue on a daily basis for four weeks after leaving the area. *Skin sensitisation and severe sunburn may occur; use a block-out cream!* About 95% effective.	*Do not use in children under 8 years. From 8–15 years: 3 mg/kg daily as for adults. Contraindicated in pregnancy and breastfeeding. Side effects include nausea, vomiting, diarrhoea, vaginal thrush and possible decreased effect of oral contraceptives.*
Atovaquone/ Proguanil Trade names: – Malanil – Malarone	One tablet daily with food. Start two days before entering the area and for seven days after leaving. Probably safe for divers. Side-effects include headache and heartburn; don't lie down after a dose. About 98% effective.	Safety in children not proven.

SELF-TREATMENT OF MALARIA

Divers in remote malarial areas, who are without any possible access to immediate medical treatment, may be faced with the problem of unexplained fever, headache, body aching and rigors. If malaria is strongly suspected and you have absolutely no way of obtaining help, then Coartem, a combination drug comprising Artemether (the 'Chinese drug') and Lumifantrine, may help. However, it is not recommended for malaria with complications, such as cerebral malaria or blackwater fever. Medical assistance is then mandatory. Coartem must be taken with foods high in fat. Take a repeat dose if vomiting occurs within one hour.

Dosage for Coartem:

- Children 10–15 kg: 1 tablet to start; repeat after 8 hours; then 1 tablet twice a day for 2 days. Total 6 tablets.
- Children 15–25 kg: 2 tablets to start; repeat after 8 hours; then 2 tablets twice a day for 2 days. Total 12 tablets.
- Children 25–35 kg: 3 tablets to start; repeat after 8 hours; then 3 tablets twice a day for 2 days. Total 18 tablets.
- Persons 35–65+ kg: 4 tablets to start; repeat after 8 hours; then 4 tablets twice a day for 2 days. Total 24 tablets.

Think carefully before undertaking treatment with this medication. It is not a recommended procedure and you are taking total responsibility upon yourself for the life of a patient, as serious side-effects have been reported! Safety has not yet been established in pregnancy and lactation. Contact a doctor as soon as possible.

BILHARZIA

Named after Theodor Bilharz, a German physician, this disease occurs in both tropical and subtropical areas. It is contracted by swimming near the banks of dams and rivers infested with the cercarial larval form of one of the human blood flukes belonging to the *Schistosoma* genus.

Their life cycle is amazingly complex. Cercariae in the water burrow through the diver's skin and capillaries and enter the bloodstream to reach the veins of the liver. Here they mature into adult worms and then migrate to veins in the membranes of the gut or to the pelvic veins where they live for several years. The female worm begins to produce eggs (over 1000 per day) which are excreted in the urine or stool, depending on the species involved. The eggs must now reach a dam or sluggishly flowing water where they hatch within a few minutes into an intermediate larval form (miracidium). However, to achieve this, the water must to be contaminated by urine or stools. Once hatched, the miracidia have less than 24 hours to find and penetrate the skin of a specific species of water snail; if they fail to find a snail, they die. Inside the snail, the miracidium makes its way to the digestive gland and begins to produce thousands of cercariae.

A single miracidium can produce over 200 000 cercariae. Burrowing out of the snail, the cercariae are released in puffs into the water to complete the life cycle. They now have only two to three days to find a swimmer to invade, or they will die.

Divers in bilharzia-infested inland water are obviously at risk. Their wet suits afford protection, but any exposed skin may be a target site for cercarial penetration.

PRESENTATION Bilharzia eggs have sharp spines, exude digestive enzymes, and work their way through blood vessels and tissues in the bladder and bowel to reach the inside of the organ involved. Blood in the urine (frequently the last few drops) or stool may be a presenting sign, and diarrhoea or difficulty with urination may occur. Generalised fatigue and loss of appetite and energy reserves may develop due to anaemia. If untreated, severe scarring occurs later on as a result of the passage of millions of spiked eggs through the involved organs, with ulceration, obstruction and interference with the function and venous drainage of the abdominal organs. Cancer of the bladder is not uncommon in late cases.

Management of bilharzia

PREVENTION Avoid bilharzial areas! Divers who do swim in water suspected of harbouring bilharzia should wear full wet suits, hoods, gloves and bootees. They should have their blood tested twice a year to exclude undiagnosed bilharzia. Unexplained fatigue should also be checked to exclude possible bilharzia.

TREATMENT The drug of choice for proven bilharzia is praziquantel (Biltricide). It is a single-dose oral treatment but must only be given with a proven diagnosis of bilharzia. This requires finding schistosome eggs in urine or stool specimens, or in the tissues of the rectum or bladder on biopsy.

SCHISTOSOME DERMATITIS (Swimmer's itch)

If non-human schistosome larvae (whose hosts are normally migratory water birds or muskrats) penetrate human skin, an itchy inflammation can occur. These cercariae invade man by accident and cannot survive in the wrong host. They are destroyed by the human inflammatory response.

TREATMENT Soothing creams or lotions, such as calamine lotion, or zinc oxide with salicylic acid and ichthammol, are all that is required.

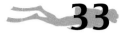

BURNS

When it comes to skin damage, in addition to fungal or bacterial skin infections, divers can suffer as a result of excessive sun exposure, as well as from burns or scalds received at camp fires.

SUNBURN

Exposure to excessive ultraviolet radiation causes sunburn – an inflammation of the skin presenting with redness, pain and swelling. In tropical and subtropical areas, 30 minutes of sun exposure can be enough to cause sunburn. Symptoms only appear after several hours – excessive morning exposure presents with pain and redness the same night. With extreme exposures, the skin becomes very red and painful, with blistering occurring over the next 24 hours, and skin peeling follows.

Depletion of the ozone layer by the worldwide use of chlorofluorocarbons (CFCs) has resulted in much harder and intensely active ultraviolet light reaching the earth's surface. Radiation induces cancerous changes in skin, and the incidence of basal cell carcinoma, squamous cell carcinoma and malignant melanoma, a highly malignant tumour of the skin, has risen in recent times. These cancers need dematological excision and, in the case of melanoma, radical surgery may be required.

PREDISPOSING FACTORS TO SUNBURN

Retinoids Divers are generally young and acne, with all of its cosmetic and social implications, is common among them. Medicine has addressed the problem of acne and several oral and topical medications, based on vitamin-A retinoid precursors, are available, which achieve very gratifying results in acne management. The problem is that the use of retinoids – such as topical tretinoin and oral isotretinoin – sensitises the skin to sunlight and predisposes it to severe sunburn and all its complications.

An additional problem with oral isotretinoin is its effects on the membranes of the nose and throat. Severe drying of nasal membranes is a common side-effect, predisposing to nose bleeds, Eustachian tube dysfunction, and middle ear barotrauma of descent and ascent (see pages 152–154). The use of oral isotretinoin is usually contraindicated with diving.

Antibiotics Other antibiotics commonly used in acne management, such as tetracyclines and sulphonamides, also sensitise the skin to sun damage.

MANAGEMENT OF SUNBURN

PREVENTION

1. Divers unaccustomed to sun exposure must take steps to protect their skin. Many barrier creams offer partial to total protection from ultraviolet light. These must be reapplied after diving, as water exposure tends to wash off the protective screening layer. The use of creams or moisturising preparations can lead to problems with masks underwater. The mask may slip and slide over oiled skin, and wiping the glass surface of the mask with greasy hands can result in blurring under water.
2. Avoid skin-sensitising medications.

TREATMENT

1. Moist bandages offer relief to areas of painful sunburn.
2. The use of half-strength cortisone creams in a moisturising base increases the soothing effect of moist bandages.
3. In severe cases of sunburn, with generalised symptoms such as fever, nausea, vomiting and malaise, a doctor must be called. Oral cortisone may be indicated.
4. Antihistamines, whether by mouth or in cream form, do not help sunburn.
5. Oral painkillers will afford some relief.

BURNS AND SCALDS

Burns are skin damage caused by fire or hot solids such as hot coals, or by touching a hot surface. Scalds are damage caused by hot liquids, such as boiling water or steam. Chemical burns result from skin contact with toxic substances in liquid or solid form. Electrical, or thermal, burns are usually accompanied by shock.

Incidents involving burns and scalds are common in a camping and boating environment. The depth and extent of the injury are very important in determining the management of burns and scalds.

First-degree burns cause the skin to redden and swell, and peeling occurs after a few days. **Second-degree** burns result in blistering under the epidermis (the outer layer of skin), often with bleeding into the blisters. **Third-degree** burns cause full-depth destruction of the skin and permanent scarring is inevitable.

If second-degree burns involve more than nine per cent of the skin (equivalent to a whole arm, half a leg, or half of the back or front of the torso), hospitalisation and intensive local and intravenous treatment are essential. The same applies to third-degree burns affecting more than two per cent of the skin area.

TREATMENT

1. Move the casualty to a safe area.
2. Drench the burnt body-area immediately with copious cold water and continue water cooling for 30 minutes. Speed is essential, so do not waste time first removing bits of burnt clothing. Hot skin continues to suffer more damage until the temperature of the skin and underlying tissues cools down.
3. Rinse off loose bits of burnt clothing and dead skin with very dilute antiseptic solution. Do not remove adherent charred skin or clothing.
4. Leave blisters alone – do not deroof or remove blisters.
5. **Do not apply sugar, honey, flour, powder, etc. to a burn!**
6. Seek medical help if the burn is more than first-degree.
7. If medical help is not available, leave small blisters alone and use a sterile syringe and needle to drain large blisters. Once drained, blisters flatten and will form a 'biological bandage' over the area.
8. Apply synthetic dressings such as OpSite Flexigrid, Granuflex or Omniderm if they are available. These maintain a humid environment under the dressing, allow oxygen and carbon dioxide transfer, are effective bacterial barriers and, being transparent, permit visual examination of the burn. Change the dressings every five to seven days.
9. If synthetic dressings are unavailable, cover the burnt area with a non-adhesive dressing impregnated with silver sulphadiazine or furacin cream; or apply Vaseline gauze, or cover the area with an antibiotic-impregnated gauze such as Sofratulle or Fucidin tulle.
10. Cover the dressing with layers of gauze, then cotton wool, and bind gently in place with a crepe bandage. Change the dressing daily.
11. Before changing any dressing, thoroughly soak the area with dilute antiseptic solution to loosen any dressing that might be sticking to the wound.
12. Oral painkillers should be given.
13. If the wound becomes septic, broad-spectrum antibiotics are needed.
14. In severe cases of second- and third-degree burns, and if paramedically trained:
    (a) Set up a Ringer's lactate drip. The volume (in millilitres) required is determined by the formula weight (kg) x % burn x 4. Half must be given in the first eight hours and the rest in the next 16 hours.
    (b) The casualty must be catheterised as soon as feasible. Urine output must be 30–50 ml/hour (1 ml/kg/hour in children), so increase the administration of fluids, if required.
    (c) Give intravenous morphine 0.1 mg/kg as a single dose, then titrate as required.
    (d) Use mask oxygen if flame or smoke inhalation has occurred.
    (e) Transfer the casualty urgently to hospital.

34

THERMAL PROBLEMS IN DIVERS

Divers may be exposed to very hot as well as very cold conditions, so variations in both extremes of temperature are relevant to them. On land, particularly in tropical and subtropical conditions, heat exhaustion and heatstroke can occur. In cold water, hypothermia awaits an incautious diver.

HEAT EXHAUSTION

Heat exhaustion may range from mild heat cramps to overt heat exhaustion and can progress to life-threatening heatstroke. It is uncommon in divers unless they engage in strenuous surface physical activity in torrid environments. Signs and symptoms usually begin slowly after excessive exercise in hot, humid conditions with heavy sweating, loss of fluids and salts (electrolytes), and inadequate fluid intake. The body temperature rises up to 39°C. It usually occurs in people unaccustomed to humid environments. Evaporation of sweat is the prime cooling mechanism of the skin, but with increased humidity this evaporation may be impaired. If fluid replacement is also inadequate, circulatory disturbances similar to those of shock appear.

PRESENTATION
- heavy sweating,
- cool, moist, pale skin,
- muscle cramps,
- headache, weakness, fatigue,
- thirst,
- nausea and vomiting,
- feeling faint or dizzy ,
- rapid, weak pulse,
- low blood pressure,
- fever with an elevated core rectal temperature up to 39°C, and
- dark-colored urine.

Management of heat exhaustion
- Get the person out of the sun and into a cool or air-conditioned area.
- Lay the casualty down and elevate the legs and feet slightly.

- Loosen or remove any excess clothing.
- Encourage the casualty to drink cool water or cool sports drinks containing electrolytes with six per cent or less glucose.
- Do not give any beverages containing alcohol or caffeine.
- Cool the casualty by spraying or sponging them with cool water and fanning.
- Monitor them carefully. Heat exhaustion can quickly become heatstroke.
- Intravenous fluid may be needed if the casualty cannot tolerate oral replacement because of vomiting.
- The casualty should stay in a cool environment and avoid strenuous activity for several days.
- If the fever is greater than 39°C or fainting, confusion or seizures occur, call for emergency medical assistance.

HEATSTROKE

Heatstroke is the most dangerous of the heat-related problems, because the primary mechanisms for dealing with heat stress (sweating and the temperature control centre in the brain) become deranged. It often develops rapidly and there is an extremely elevated body temperature (usually above 40°C), associated with severe changes in mental status ranging from minor personality changes to confusion and coma. The skin is usually hot and dry, but if heatstroke is caused by physical effort, the skin may be moist.

It is commonest in young children, the elderly and obese individuals, and can be precipitated by dehydration, alcohol abuse, cardiovascular disease and medications that may affect the ability to sweat – some antihistamines and certain anti-hypertensives and antidepressants. The condition is life-threatening, as the body temperature can increase to the point where brain damage or damage to other internal organs occur. Two forms of heatstroke have been described:

- The classic form, occurring in people whose cooling mechanisms are impaired. This includes divers wearing a wet suit while exposed to hot environmental surface conditions. Resistance to sweating within the very humid confines of a sun-heated wet suit, accompanied by the total absence of any possible skin cooling by evaporation, can result in a speedy rise in body temperature and lead to depression of cerebral temperature control and heatstroke.
- The exertional form, occurring in healthy people performing strenuous activity in a hot environment without adequate fluid and electrolyte intake.

PRESENTATION
- cessation of sweating with a flushed, hot and dry skin,
- dizziness,
- irritability, confusion, hallucinations or coma,

- headache,
- vomiting,
- rapid heartbeat (160 beats/min or more) with rapid, shallow breathing or frank hyperventilation,
- elevated or lowered blood pressure, and
- rectal (core) temperature of 40°C or more.

Management of heatstroke

Treatment is aimed at bringing the casualty's core temperature to normal as quickly as possible while ensuring hydration and normal blood flow. Immersion, evaporative and invasive cooling techniques are used.

- Call for emergency medical assistance.
- Move the casualty out of the sun and into a cool or air-conditioned space.
- Encourage oral cold water if the casualty is aware and able to swallow. Confused persons will choke on orally administered fluids.
- Place ice packs in the neck, armpits and groin. These are areas of high heat loss. (Wrap ice packs in cloths to prevent ice-burn on the skin.)
- If the casualty is conscious, cool him or her in a cold bath of water.
- Keep the skin moist with cold cloths or allow fans to blow across wet sheets over the casualty's body if the victim is unconscious.
- If a doctor is present, commence rapid intravenous fluid therapy and monitor urine output.
- When the casualty's body core temperature is 39°C, stop active cooling and admit to hospital for further management.

HYPOTHERMIA

Hypothermia is the process that occurs when a warm diver gets into cold water. The normal central body temperature – the core (or rectal) temperature is 37°C (98.6°F). Within the body, there is a fine balance between heat production from metabolism and heat loss to the environment. If heat production equals heat loss, a stable temperature exists. If heat production is less than heat loss, the body temperature falls and hypothermia occurs. If heat production exceeds heat loss, the body temperature rises and hyperthermia occurs.

Hypothermia is a drop in core temperature below 37°C as a result of heat loss being greater than heat production.

The process is comparable to the elimination of inert gas after a dive, where **gas** is exhaled as a result of a gradient between a high tissue concentration and a lower environmental concentration. With hypothermia, **heat** is lost along a gradient from a higher core temperature to a lower environmental temperature.

THE IMPACT OF ENVIRONMENTAL TEMPERATURE

Temperature is the degree of hotness or coldness of a body or environment. The sea has an extreme range of temperatures, from -2°C in the polar oceans to 25°C in shallow tropical waters. A diver therefore has a possible heat loss gradient ranging from 39°C to 12°C between the body's core temperature and the ambient water temperature. As water conducts heat about 25 times more efficiently than air, cold water causes a diver's body temperature to cool rapidly.

HOW IS HEAT LOST?

When the body loses heat, several processes occur:

1. **Conduction** Direct mass transfer of heat occurs along a gradient from a warm diver to the colder surrounding water. As the diver cools down, the water in the immediate vicinity warms up.

2. **Convection** Water warmed by conduction is less dense and rises, so more cold water moves in to take its place. This puts our poor diver in the unfortunate position of trying to warm up the sea! Convection is increased by movement, especially swimming. When measured by thermograms (infra-red photographs that depict hotter and colder areas), certain areas of the body show a higher heat loss. The greatest sites of heat loss are:
   - the head and neck (up to 50 per cent of heat loss occurs here),
   - the axillae (armpits) and sides of the body, and
   - the groin.

   The amount of heat lost can be reduced by flexing the head onto the chest, folding the arms across the chest and drawing the knees up to the body. This diminishes the exposure of these key sites to the water. It is a position similar to that of an unborn baby in its mother's womb – the foetal or spheroidal position.

   Swimming exposes the areas that are most vulnerable to heat loss, increasing conduction, while movement increases convection. The use of alcohol and/ or marijuana decreases skin arteriolar constriction and promotes flushing, so further increasing heat loss.

3. **Breathing** Every inhaled breath of air is warmed by the respiratory passages and the lungs. Every exhaled breath means heat lost from the body. As helium and hydrogen have a high thermal conductivity, being much more efficient in conducting heat than nitrogen, the use of these gases in the breathing mix will cause much greater respiratory heat loss.

4. **Urine output** Exposure to cold causes blood vessels in the skin to constrict, and the skin becomes pale. When blood vessels constrict, the blood volume within them decreases. This blood must go somewhere and it is to the warmth of the core that it goes. This increases the core blood volume. As the kidneys are in the body's core, blood flow increases through the kidneys, which means increased urine production. This, in turn, causes heat loss when the warm urine is voided, as well as a decrease in the diver's total fluid content, including his blood volume.

Suppose a diver, clad in a swimming costume only, falls into water at 2°C:

1. Sudden exposure to cold can cause a **gasping response** with abnormal heart rhythm or even cardiac arrest. So, sudden death can occur.

2. In mammals that dive, such as whales and seals, exposing the face to cold water causes a diving reflex, which manifests as breathholding and a slowing of the heart rate. This is also associated with intense constriction of arterioles throughout the body, except those of the heart and brain. Virtually the entire blood supply becomes an oxygen store for these two organs alone. Shunting of the blood from the skin also means less heat loss to the water.

   In man, however, the diving reflex is very poorly developed. Sudden exposure to cold can cause **an acceleration in heart rate**, with the development of an irritable and excitable heart muscle. This can result in the development of abnormal heart rhythms and death (see page 42).

   In infants, the diving reflex appears to be more efficient. If an infant's face is immersed in cold water the following occurs:
   - breathholding,
   - slowing of the heart rate, and
   - oxygen conservation, due to shunting of blood to the heart and brain.

   This is of immense importance in cold-water drowning.

WHAT HAPPENS WITH HYPOTHERMIA?

Humans can tolerate a maximum drop of 12 degrees in core body temperature before death occurs, that is, a fall from 37–25°C. Think about what happens: the longer the diver spends in cold water, the more heat from the warm central core is transferred by the bloodstream to the periphery, where it is lost to the water. Cold peripheral blood is then returned to the core, causing core cooling. With each repeat cycle, further cooling occurs.

As the body temperature falls, the diver experiences three phases of cooling:
1. reaction to the cold,
2. increasing passivity, and
3. loss of consciousness.

1. At a core temperature of 37–34°C, the diver feels cold, begins shivering and becomes pale. Shivering is the body's attempt to produce more heat by muscle contraction. In the sea this is obviously a futile exercise. At about 34°C, shivering is replaced by muscle rigidity. Movements become difficult and awkward, power decreases and swimming ability falls.

2. Between 34°C and 30°C, the effects of cold begin to impact on the brain. The blood becomes more viscous or 'thicker'; transfer of oxygen from haemoglobin to tissues decreases; and hypoxia begins. Confusion, disorientation, lack of judgement and amnesia occur. In the absence of some form of flotation device, the diver will now drown. Human heart muscle becomes

very irritable with the onset of hypothermia and irregular rhythms develop. Breathing becomes shallow and slow.

3. Between 30°C and 25°C, consciousness is lost, going on to deep coma and death by ventricular fibrillation (uncoordinated 'rippling' contractions of the muscles of the ventricles, without any pumping effect – similar to muscle shivering).

PROTECTION AGAINST HYPOTHERMIA

The effects of hypothermia are very bad for business in the diving industry, and an immense amount of research and expense has gone into solving some of the problems. As mentioned above, heat is lost by conduction and convection (see page 259).

Choice of protective clothing

Reducing the amount of heat conducted by a diver to the surrounding water requires **insulation**. Fat is a good insulator, and fat people exposed to very cold water generally survive for longer than thin people. Fatties also have a body shape closer to that of a sphere, giving a maximum volume to minimum surface area for heat loss. Lanky divers have small volumes and large surface areas. Long-distance swimmers use the insulating properties of fat by covering their bodies with mineral grease before entering the water.

In order to reduce the amount of heat they lose, scuba divers use protective suits, which also have the advantage of offering protection against contact with stinging marine life and rough surfaces.

There are several types of protective suit; the choice depends upon the water temperature, as well as the depth and duration of the dive:

— wet suits,
— dry suits (these can be constant volume or variable volume), or
— heated suits (thermochemical, electrical or hot-water).

1. Wet suits

Wet suits are made of closed-cell expanded neoprene that varies in thickness from 3–8 mm or more. The bubbles in the neoprene sponge are poor heat conductors but good insulators. As their name implies, wet suits allow water to enter through the neck, the cuffs and the zippers. Once inside the wet suit, this water soon warms up, forming a warm layer between the diver's body and the neoprene sponge suit.

Wet suits are effective at shallow depths, but lose their efficiency with increasing depth. This is because the bubbles in the neoprene sponge obey Boyle's Law (see page 21), which states that as pressure increases, bubble volume decreases. Accordingly, at depth, a wet suit becomes thinner and thinner while the water gets colder and colder. This also reduces buoyancy, and so the diver becomes more negatively buoyant at depth (Archimedes' Principle applies, see page 26).

2. Dry suits

There are two types of dry suit: constant volume and variable volume. Dry suits rely on warm underwear and a layer of insulating air to provide warmth. Water must not be allowed to enter the suit.

(a) **Constant-volume dry suits** Made of incompressible rubber or neoprene-impregnated fabric, no trapped bubbles are present in the material so they do not change thickness with depth. The suit material has constant volume. Alone, they have very little insulating capacity against cold, but they are made large and baggy, allowing very warm polyamide-nylon fleecy undergarments, known as 'woolly bears', to be worn.

These suits, being large and loose, are liable to cause suit squeeze on descent. Adding an inflation device powered by a suit-bottle or the LP stage removes the 'wrinkles' and provides a layer of insulating air. As care must then be taken to avoid an uncontrolled ascent, a dump valve is fitted. Any holes or leaks in the suit will allow water to enter, converting it into a bulky, negatively buoyant, waterlogged and soggy bag containing one miserably cold diver!

(b) **Variable-volume dry suits** These are foam neoprene suits, usually double-lined with nylon. The presence of the foam neoprene adds insulation and buoyancy. As with the constant-volume suits, warm undergarments are worn, and inflation and dump devices are fitted. Inflating the suit provides a water seal at the cuffs and neck. The variable-volume dry suit is superior in insulation to wet suits and constant-volume dry suits. Air is a good insulator, while the foam neoprene adds the advantage of further insulation. Warm undergarments result in a warm, dry and happy diver who looks and feels like a contented teddy bear. Again, a leak guarantees misery.

3. Heated suits

Instead of trying to prevent the diver's body warmth from seeping into the sea, heated suits dispense with baggy and bulky insulation and provide external heat to the diver. They are the ultimate in diving suits, but require energy input.

(a) **Thermochemical** The simplest method involves a chemical reaction with water. A wet suit is used and porous bags containing iron filings and magnesium are placed inside the suit. Contact with water starts a heat-evolving reaction, which provides body warmth to the diver. Placing small bags within the gloves provides hand warmth. Exiting the water causes the chemical reaction to stop.

(b) **Electrical** Electrical suits have built-in heating elements, much like an electric blanket. Their power source may be carried by the diver (but this means the extra burden of a bulky power pack), or supplied from the surface or via a diving bell. Repeated kinking with movement, for example at the elbows and knees, can cause the wires to break and interrupt the electrical flow.

(c) **Hot-water suits** These are the most efficient type of heated suits, but also the most expensive to power, and so are used mainly by commercial divers.

Sea water is heated at the surface and then pumped down a hose to the diver. A bypass valve fitted to the suit allows the diver to select whether the water enters the suit or is dumped into the sea. Within the suit are perforated tubes supplying hot water to the neck, arms, hands, body, legs and feet. The water exits the suit through the cuffs into the sea and is constantly replaced by more hot sea water from the surface. The water temperature is adjusted at the surface to provide optimal diver comfort but, as this is a very subjective means of temperature control, care must be taken to avoid over-heating and hyperthermia. Local 'hot spots' of water entry can cause scalding and, if the hot-water supply fails, a very cold and angry diver soon results.

REDUCING HEAT LOST THROUGH BREATHING

With each exhaled breath, a diver loses heat. In addition, when gas passes from a higher to a lower pressure (e.g. from a high-pressure scuba cylinder to a low pressure regulator), it cools down. The diver therefore inhales gas which is even colder than the sea. Prewarmers have been devised to warm the inhaled air, while countercurrent insulating devices limit exhaled heat loss. The problem is fitting a bulky prewarmer to a diver's face, which is already overloaded with high-precision contraptions.

MANAGEMENT OF HYPOTHERMIA

The most important message in the management of hypothermia (low body temperature) is to understand that a diver in deep hypothermia may **appear to be dead**. Never assume that a cold diver **is** dead. True stories abound of hypothermic and comatose people regaining consciousness in a mortuary. 'Dead' children, presumed to have drowned, have recovered spontaneously, being protected by their hypothermia. **Only a warm dead diver is a dead diver.**

1. Management of mild hypothermia

This is rarely a problem, and has relatively simple solutions:
(a) Remove the diver from the cold water.
(b) Place him or her in a protected place, lying flat.
(c) Cover the diver; use a space blanket, normal blankets, sleeping bags, warm clothes and/or body-to-body contact.
(d) Encourage the diver to drink warm fluids.

2. Management of deep hypothermia

Understanding how to actively manage a case of deep hypothermia requires an initial explanation of **afterdrop** – a phenomenon whereby a casualty's core temperature (as measured rectally) continues to drop, even during a period of actively rewarming a hypothermic victim in a bath of water heated to 43°C.

It has long been presumed that the heat of the bath water caused the blood vessels in the arms and legs to dilate, sending a flush of cold peripheral blood back to the core, causing further central cooling and precipitating **ventricular fibrillation** and death. For this reason, the casualty's arms and legs were kept out of the warm bath and were just covered. However, afterdrop is a rectal fact only and does not reflect true core temperature, as core mixing of venous blood is poor in a passive, hypothermic diver. Rectal afterdrop is due to continuing mass tissue conduction of heat from a relatively warmer lower part of the torso to colder upper legs during the initial minutes of rewarming.

As the diver's heart and brain are of greater concern to us than his or her rectum, we need to ask what causes the ventricular fibrillation that kills up to 20 per cent of hypothermic divers after rescue and during rewarming. If it is not a surge of cold blood to the heart, what is it?

There are several causes. The cardiovascular system involves the blood, the heart and the blood vessels. With exposure to severe cold, the increased output of urine decreases the total body water. When tissue cells lose water, their contents become more concentrated. As water moves from the blood into tissue cells and into the spaces between tissue cells, the blood becomes more viscous and the total volume of blood decreases.

A **hypothermic heart** contracts slowly. The heart rate is low and each contraction (systole) of the ventricles takes longer, but the filling time of the ventricles as they relax between beats (diastole) is short. The coronary arteries, which supply blood to the heart muscle itself, are the only arteries in the body that depend on ventricular relaxation for filling. As their filling time decreases, the heart muscle is supplied with less blood and oxygen, and that blood is also thicker and its flow more sluggish.

When the diver is immersed, the water supports the blood vessels in his or her limbs. There is no gravity-inducing pooling of blood in the limbs. Once the diver is rescued from the water, gravity suddenly causes blood to pool in dangling legs and arms. His or her heart rate increases to circulate these columns of blood, but the time taken to fill the coronary arteries, which is already reduced, becomes border-line for the adequate supply of oxygen to the heart muscle. As the rescuers rush the diver to safety, they are likely to move his or her arms and legs. This causes a further reflex acceleration of the heart rate. The blood supply to the heart, with its increased workload, becomes inadequate, and ventricular fibrillation and death can occur.

In addition, movement or exercise can promote the return of cold venous blood from the limbs, and this can cause sudden further cooling of the core. Intensely cold, but conscious, divers must be discouraged from making any unnecessary voluntary movements, and extreme care must be taken to keep the limbs of unconscious hypothermic divers immobile and horizontal.

REMEMBER TWO THINGS:

1. **A cold diver may appear to be dead:**
   - there may be no discernible heartbeat,
   - there may be no obvious breathing,
   - the pupils may be fixed and unreactive, and
   - no blood pressure may be measurable.

2. **Do not move or handle the diver too much.** Even in an emergency situation, grabbing a diver by the arms and legs, handling the neck roughly, pounding the chest and frantically giving mouth-to-mouth resuscitation can precipitate ventricular fibrillation which will **kill** the diver.

   (a) Be gentle. Do not move the limbs unduly.

   (b) Check the airways – if they are obstructed, clear very gently.

   (c) Check breathing – if the diver is breathing, even very shallowly and slowly, **leave the diver's chest alone**.

   (d) Check the heartbeat – if a heartbeat is present, even if very indistinct or slow, **leave the diver's chest alone**. Do not try to improve circulation by thumping the chest.[1]

   (e) If a low-reading clinical thermometer is available, gently check the diver's rectal temperature. If the temperature is above 34°C, the diver is not in hypothermic coma. Treat as for an unconscious diver (see page 308) plus offer passive rewarming by applying blankets etc.

   (f) **Rapid rewarming** Leave the diver in his or her wet suit if one is being worn. This limits excessive manipulation of the limbs, protects against scalding (from being immersed in a too hot bath), and the rubber support retards pooling of blood in the limbs. Circumstances will dictate the method chosen. Generally, active rewarming is done in water. If a bath is unavailable, a hole in the sand or ground lined with a tarpaulin will do. A bath of water provides hydrostatic support for the limbs, reduces gravity-pooling and decreases the forward load on the heart. If the diver is wearing a hot-water suit, reconnect it to a warm water supply and circulate the water through it.

   NOTE: While the bath is being prepared, cover the diver with blankets or sleeping bags and hot-water bottles, or even body-to-body contact in a sheltered place out of the wind. The bath should be as hot as possible without causing scalding – i.e. hot enough for the helpers to tolerate without flinching; this should be about 43°C. Place the diver in the bath for 20–30 minutes, making sure his or her limbs are **included** in the bath water. Disturb the diver as little as possible.

---

1. Active cardiac massage and mouth-to-mouth ventilation may cause ventricular fibrillation. If no breathing is discernible when using a mirror in front of the mouth to look for condensation, and no carotid pulse is felt, or heartbeat heard by an ear to the left chest, then CPR could be given at a rate of one chest compression per two seconds (30 beats per minute) and one chest inflation after every fifth compression (six breaths per minute). The use of CPR in hypothermic coma is dangerous.

Do not perform CPR in a bath of hot water as you will drown the diver as well. Maintain the water temperature by adding more hot water as required.

(g) **Monitor the pulse rate continuously.** Placing a hypothermic diver in a warm bath **does** cause dilation of arterioles in the periphery and can cause a drop in blood pressure. This, in turn, causes the heart rate to accelerate in an attempt to maintain the blood pressure. This does not occur immediately, but over a period of 15–20 minutes after immersion. If the pulse starts to accelerate, **quickly cool the water down again until the pulse rate settles**. Then continue with the hot water bath. If the diver is conscious, keep him or her in the bath until sweating starts. After the bath, the diver must lie flat in a warm place, covered liberally with blankets, and should be encouraged to take warm drinks.

ACCIDENTAL EXPOSURE TO COLD WATER

This could occur by falling overboard or as a result of a boat capsizing. **Swimming** is the danger here. Exercise exposes the body to increased conduction and convection, with a greatly increased speed of heat loss. In cold water (below 10°C), an uninsulated man of normal build, without any flotation device or the protection of a wet suit, will not manage a one-kilometre swim.

If you find yourself in cold water as a result of an accident or unexpected incident, and are not able to get out of the water immediately, take steps to reduce hypothermia by adopting the foetal position to conserve body heat. If there are several people in the water, everyone should link elbows to form a 'hot-tub' and adopt the foetal position. Remember to stay with the boat or any other floating material.

35

NITROX SPORT DIVING

In 1985, Dick Rutkowski, director of diver training at the US-based National Oceanic and Atmospheric Administration (NOAA), formed the International Association of Nitrox Divers (IAND) to teach nitrox diving to sport divers. Since then, dive schools worldwide have introduced specialised nitrox and trimix courses into their training schedules, in addition to teaching traditional air scuba diving.

Two nitrox mixes are commonly used by sport divers:
- Nitrox I (oxygen 32 per cent, nitrogen 68 per cent), and
- Nitrox II (oxygen 36 per cent, nitrogen 64 per cent).

The use of nitrox in sport diving followed the publication, in 1970, by Dr Morgan Wells of NOAA, of guidelines for the use of nitrox in NOAA divers. The original concept for the use of nitrox instead of air was aimed at **preventing** pulmonary oxygen toxicity (see page 201) at shallow saturation depths. The maximum permissible oxygen partial pressure for prolonged periods is 0.5 ATA. This would allow air saturation at a depth of only 13.8 msw. At deeper depths, the amount of oxygen must be **reduced** and the amount of nitrogen **increased**. This reduces the depth at which nitrogen narcosis occurs and makes nitrox saturation diving safe only in a very limited and shallow depth range. Air, with a higher oxygen pressure, is then used on shallow downward excursions from saturation depth.

In its original sense, nitrox was a nitrogen-enriched gas with a reduced oxygen partial pressure. Since 1985, however, in sport diving terms, nitrox has come to mean 'oxygen-enriched air'. Despite objections by purists that the word 'nitrox' should be reserved for its original sense of reduced oxygen, and that the term 'oxygen-enriched air' should be used for nitrox as a sport-diving gas, common usage has prevailed and **nitrox now means oxygen-enriched air**. In 2000, NOAA published its Nitrox 32 and Nitrox 36 dive tables for sport divers.

The rationale for using nitrox in sport diving is that pulmonary oxygen toxicity takes days of continuous high exposure to develop, so it cannot occur in sport diving. Increasing the oxygen in the breathing mix means an equivalent drop in the nitrogen in the mix. This then reduces the risk of acute decompression illness and can nearly double maximum bottom time. But it increases the risk of cerebral oxygen toxicity which takes minutes, not days, to develop at depth.

Among sport divers, the maximum safe oxygen partial pressure is set at 1.6 ATA. Air then has a maximum safe oxygen depth of 66 msw, but nitrogen narcosis prohibits its reasonable use beyond 40 msw (the maximum depth for sport divers using air). Nitrox I has a maximum safe depth of 40 msw, and Nitrox II 34 msw. This would seem to make nitrox the ideal breathing mix for the shallow diving depths of up to about 12–24 msw found on most reefs, because nitrogen uptake and the chances of bends would be substantially reduced.

However, while the theory seems fine, the reality is that, over the years, nitrox divers have died. There will always be cowboys, and instead of aiming to increase the duration of shallow dives, some divers changed the objectives, targeting nitrogen narcosis on the basis that, if the mix had a lower nitrogen content, it stood to reason that nitrogen narcosis would occur at deeper than air-breathing depths. This resulted in deep nitrox divers who had no nitrogen narcosis, but experienced sudden cerebral oxygen toxicity and underwater convulsions, and drowned.

TECHNICAL REQUIREMENTS FOR SAFE NITROX MIXING

The safe use of nitrox requires knowledge and training, as well as an awareness of the problems that may occur.

Accurate mixtures

Making a nitrox mix by using Dalton's Law of Partial Pressures (see page 24) is dangerous. Oxygen is the problem, as it does not quite obey Dalton's Law. Oxygen is physically more compressible than nitrogen and, if compressed air is mixed with oxygen until the calculated pressures are reached, the mix will not be the required one. It will contain too much oxygen. This means that oxygen analysers are necessary, and these are expensive and require precise calibration with known standard mixes. In commercial use, mixes are made by precise flow (not pressure) mixers with continuous analysis facilities.

Oil-free compressors

Increasing the oxygen content increases the risk of fire and explosion. Standard sport diving air compressors are not oil-free, and using them to top up a cylinder containing pressurised oxygen is hazardous.

NITROX AND CARBON DIOXIDE BUILD-UP

Nitrox is denser than air, so the work of breathing nitrox causes the lungs to produce more carbon dioxide than air breathing does. The problem with any build-up of carbon dioxide due to exercise, tight gear, skip breathing, etc, is that it dilates blood vessels in the brain and increases the supply of blood to the brain. If the blood is also loaded with a high concentration of oxygen in solution, unconsciousness and convulsions can occur without warning.

SHOULD SPORT DIVERS USE NITROX?

It is essential to understand that the only reason sport divers use nitrox is to decrease their tissue nitrogen loading during diving.

This has several advantages:

- bottom time at depth can be extended to that of an equivalently shallower air dive,
- the same bottom time and depth as an air dive results in far less tissue nitrogen loading,
- decompression times are shorter,
- the surface interval between dives can be equivalently reduced, and
- repetitive dives can be longer and/or more frequent.

All this sounds terrific. So what's the catch? The catch is that a diver breathing oxygen partial pressures above 1.6 ATA can suddenly, and without any warning, lose consciousness, convulse and drown.

IS NITROX SAFE?

Nitrox diving is certainly 'safer' than air at **shallow depths** because the amount of inert gas in the breathing mix is less, so nitrogen loading by body tissues is proportionally reduced. Nitrogen loading is substantially less than that of an equally deep air dive. It is equal to an equivalently shallower air dive. This is fine and true as far as nitrogen loading and the risk of acute decompression illness go.

HOW DO I CALCULATE AN EQUIVALENT AIR DEPTH?

The equivalent air depth (EAD) is the calculated depth, breathing air, at which a diver is exposed to the same nitrogen partial pressure, absorbs the same amount of nitrogen, and has the same decompression commitments as a given depth on nitrox. As the gas concerned is nitrogen, in order to calculate the EAD, one has to know the **fraction of nitrogen** in the mix.

- Nitrox I (oxygen 32 per cent, nitrogen 68 per cent) contains 0.68 nitrogen
- Nitrox II (oxygen 36 per cent, nitrogen 64 per cent) contains 0.64 nitrogen

The equivalent air depth (EAD) is then calculated using the formula:

$$EAD = \left\{ \frac{FN_2}{0.79} \times (d + x) \right\} - x$$

Where:

- FN_2 is the fraction of nitrogen in the nitrogen mix (commonly 0.64 or 0.68)
- 0.79 is the fraction of nitrogen in air (including other trace gases)
- d is the actual depth in fsw or msw
- x is the depth of water equivalent to 1 ATA (33 fsw or 10 msw)

Example:

Pete wants to dive to 30 msw using Nitrox II. What is his EAD?

$$EAD = \frac{0.64}{0.79} \times (30 + 10) - 10 = 0.81 \times 40 - 10 = 32.4 - 10 = \textbf{22.4 msw}$$

This means Pete can dive to 30 msw on Nitrox II, but only incur a nitrogen loading equal to a dive of 22.4 msw using air as a breathing source.

Calculating the EAD enables dives on nitrox to be planned using standard air tables. When diving on air, the EAD is the actual tabled depth. If the nitrox mix contains less oxygen than air (less than 21 per cent oxygen), the EAD will be deeper than the tabled air depth. If using a mix containing more oxygen than air (more than 21 per cent oxygen), the EAD will be shallower than the tabled air depth.

For a particular nitrox mix and a planned maximum actual depth, calculating the EAD provides the bottom time, subsequent in-water decompression obligations (if any), the surface interval, and any repetitive dive penalties.

WHEN SHOULD SPORT DIVERS USE NITROX?

This depends on what you want to do. It is true that it is safe to use nitrox at shallow depths. Therefore, if you want to increase your bottom time at depths shallower than 40 msw, the answer is that it is fine to use nitrox, but care and knowledge are needed to ensure that the correct mix is chosen. Breathing Nitrox II when you are deeper than 34 msw is dangerous! You will reduce your equivalent nitrogen uptake and convert your dive to a proportionately shallower air dive. This questions whether your bottom time warrants a reduced nitrogen load.

Breathing nitrox does not reduce your breathing gas volume requirements. It does not increase available gas supply. Whether air or nitrox are breathed, the volume and pressure demands of Boyle's Law must still be met to avoid squeeze. Nitrox only reduces your nitrogen loading for the same air-breathing time and increases safe permissible dive duration. This means that the diver must carry a larger, heavier cylinder, or use twin cylinders for longer than would the case for dives planned with air tables.

The diver must also ensure that the breathing mix is correct; that the correct tables are being used; or that the dive computer is calibrated to the nitrox mix. There is usually no surface back-up in case of trouble.

If your ambition is to spend the same time at depth as with a tabled air dive, nitrox will allow you longer or more frequent repetitive dives or shorter surface intervals.

However, if your aim is to avoid nitrogen narcosis at depths greater than 40 msw, make sure your buddy is breathing air, because you are going to lose consciousness, convulse and die unless he or she is able to provide really expert assistance!

NITROX COURSES

Most major sport diving training centres offer basic and advanced nitrox courses. It is essential that a diver thinking of using nitrox takes these courses and fully understands the use of mixed gas in scuba diving. If the advantages of nitrox are correctly applied, the diver will certainly benefit, but if the disadvantages are abused, death can occur.

I believe that nitrox should not be supplied to anyone who has not had formal training in its use and can prove it by producing a nitrox diver certification.

36

DIVING GAS SYSTEMS

There are two ways of delivering a supply of fresh gas to a diver:
- **freeflow system**: the gas flow to the diver is continuous, and
- **demand system**: the gas flow to the diver is triggered by inhaling.

There are three ways of handling exhaled gases produced by the diver:
1. **Open circuit** – all of the diver's exhaled gases are dumped into the surrounding water.
2. **Semi-closed circuit** – some of the diver's exhaled gases are dumped into the water while the rest are purified and recirculated for rebreathing.
3. **Closed circuit** – all the diver's exhaled gases are purified and recirculated for rebreathing, none are dumped into the water and no bubbles occur in the water.

There are therefore a number of possible combinations of supply and exhaust systems. Some are in common use, for example, the demand valve–open circuit system of sport scuba diving. Some are in commercial use, such as the freeflow–closed circuit system using expensive helium and oxygen in decompression chambers and diving bells. Others, such as the demand valve–closed circuit systems of oxygen rebreathing sets, are used by the military when no telltale bubbles are wanted in the water during clandestine operations, such as planting limpet mines.

FREEFLOW SYSTEMS

A freeflow system delivers a continuous fresh supply of breathing gas to the diver. A very simple freeflow system would be an inverted weighted bucket placed over the diver's head with a hose supplying a continuous flow of air from a surface compressor into the bucket. The diver breathes from the air space in the bucket and excess air, together with the diver's exhaled gases, is vented as a continuous flow of bubbles from the open bottom of the bucket. This is a freeflow–open circuit system.

Modifying the material and shape of the bucket in order to completely surround the diver originally resulted in a copper diving helmet with glass viewing ports, coupled to a rubberised and weighted suit – the classic Standard Diving Equipment (SDE). A continuous flow of air is pumped into the helmet and excess air is vented through a valve in the helmet, but the diving helmet is basically no different from the bucket system. Extending the size of the 'bucket' then resulted in diving bells and underwater habitats where the 'bucket' is so large that the diver can walk, eat, sleep and move around in it.

All freeflow systems have the diver breathing freely from the atmosphere within the system, while simultaneously contaminating it with his exhaled carbon dioxide. The accumulation of carbon dioxide is the basic underlying problem of the freeflow system. Sufficient air must continuously be supplied to the system to dilute and flush out carbon dioxide to acceptable levels. This is obviously very wasteful of air or a gas mix. The greatest danger in the freeflow system is helmet squeeze. If a Standard Diver's hoses rupture or if he descends too quickly, the surrounding water pressure rapidly exceeds the pressure in his suit. In a worst-case scenario, his whole body will then be squeezed up into his copper helmet. A non-return valve on the helmet prevents this disaster in case of hose rupture, and a controlled descent is mandatory when using this equipment.

CARBON DIOXIDE LEVELS The maximum acceptable level of carbon dioxide within any diving system is 0.02 ATA. At first sight, this may not appear too much of a problem; it is two per cent at the surface. But at 10 msw (2 ATA) this shrinks to one per cent, and at 90 msw (10 ATA) a level of only 0.2 per cent of carbon dioxide will cause carbon dioxide toxicity. This means that, with increasing depth, more and more air or gas mix is needed to dilute and purge exhaled carbon dioxide.

In general, divers on a freeflow system are working divers – they are doing some sort of physical activity under water. This means they are exercising and, with effort, the amount of carbon dioxide they produce and exhale rapidly increases. Their breathing gas requirements drastically increase. A few examples illustrate the point:
–   At rest, a diver produces about 0.25 litres of carbon dioxide per minute. At the surface, a maximum permissible concentration of carbon dioxide is two per cent. This means that the carbon dioxide exhaled must be diluted 50 times, so the air supply requirement would be 50 x 0.25 litres, or 12.5 litres of air at the surface.
–   At hard work, a diver produces about 2 litres of carbon dioxide per minute, so a flow rate of 50 x 2 litres, or 100 litres of air per minute must be supplied while working at the surface.
–   Underwater, when working hard at 30 msw (4 ATA), the diver's air supply requirement increases to 4 x 50 x 2 litres, or 400 litres per minute!

In situations where a very large and expensive supply of fresh gas would be needed to eliminate the accumulation of carbon dioxide, the solution is to introduce a carbon dioxide scrubber into the system. This chemically removes exhaled carbon dioxide from the gas mix, allows exhaled gases to be rebreathed and greatly reduces ventilation requirements. However, it does convert a freeflow–open circuit system into a freeflow–semi-closed one with its inherent properties and difficulties.

REBREATHING SYSTEMS

The primary reason for the development of rebreathing systems is to conserve the gas supply. Helium, nitrogen and oxygen mixes (heliox, nitrox and trimix) are expensive and time-consuming to produce, and it is wasteful simply to dump them into the sea with each exhaled breath. When diving continues for prolonged periods (which can be weeks or months in the case of major expeditions), even air becomes expensive in terms of the fuel costs needed to run the compressors and generators.

A diver using a rebreathing system has **three** life-support needs, all of which **must** be fulfilled:
1. Availability of adequate oxygen supplies.
2. Efficient removal of carbon dioxide.
3. Sufficient gas volume to allow the lungs to fill and empty readily.

1. Availability of adequate oxygen

Since rebreathing systems dump little or no unused exhaled oxygen into the sea, an adequate oxygen supply is the simplest need to fulfil.

An average man gardening fairly hard at the surface uses about one litre of oxygen per minute. He breathes about 20 litres of air per minute. As air comprises roughly 20 per cent oxygen, this means he inhales about four litres of oxygen (20 per cent of 20 litres) and exhales three litres of oxygen per minute. Seventy-five percent of the available oxygen is 'wasted'.

Oxygen requirements do not increase with depth for the same work. Oxygen usage is a metabolic requirement and is independent of depth. More **air** is required, however, to maintain the same lung volume with increased depth.

Suppose the same man dives to 40 msw (5 ATA) on scuba and exerts the same amount of effort at that depth. He still only needs one litre of oxygen per minute (excluding the work of breathing a denser mix), but his regulator has to deliver 20 x 5 litres, or 100 litres per minute in order to avoid lung compression by the surrounding water pressure. This 100 litres of air contains 20 per cent of oxygen, or 20 litres. Of this oxygen, 19 litres (95 per cent) will be exhaled into the sea. If he could reuse his exhaled air, he could use 16 of the 19 litres of oxygen before he ran any risk of hypoxia. That is, he could dive 16 times longer using the same air source.

2. Efficient removal of carbon dioxide

Removing carbon dioxide requires venting the diver's exhaled air into a suitable reservoir or bag underwater, passing it through a scrubbing apparatus, and then recirculating it via a suitably valved hose system for rebreathing at the mouthpiece. This bag is commonly called a counterlung or breathing bag.

Carbon dioxide is generally removed by the use of soda lime – a mixture of calcium hydroxide (slaked lime) and a small amount of sodium hydroxide (caustic soda).

There are three reactions and they work as follows:

(a) Carbon dioxide first reacts with moisture to form a weak acid, carbonic acid (soda water): $CO_2 + H_2O \rightarrow H_2CO_3$.

Although acidic, it does not react very readily with such a weak base as calcium hydroxide, so a very strong base, such as sodium hydroxide, is added as a catalyst. The carbonic acid readily reacts with sodium hydroxide which removes the carbon dioxide and is converted to sodium carbonate:
$H_2CO_3 + 2\ NaOH \rightarrow Na_2CO_3 + 2\ H_2O$

(b) Sodium carbonate then transfers the carbon dioxide to the calcium hydroxide, forming calcium carbonate and regenerating the caustic soda which is now free to react with more carbon dioxide: $Na_2CO_3 + Ca(OH)_2 \rightarrow CaCO_3 + 2\ NaOH$.

(c) The reaction stops when all the calcium hydroxide has been converted to calcium carbonate.

Because carbon dioxide scrubbers are prone to failure, they pose an immediate hazard to divers. There are two main dangers:

− The chemical mixture has to be correctly granulated and carefully packed into the canister through which the exhaled gases are directed. Special care must be taken to avoid channels of loosely-packed material, as these would provide a direct passage through the container for exhaled gas without removing the carbon dioxide. Toxic levels of carbon dioxide in the recycled gas then result.

− Care must be taken to avoid extraneous water contamination. A highly corrosive and poisonous sludge containing caustic soda then results, which can easily result in the inhalation or swallowing of a 'caustic cocktail' under water.

3. Sufficient gas volume to allow the lungs to fill

As the diver breathes from a breathing bag (counterlung), it follows that the bag must first be filled before any descent (the diver would have nothing to breathe if this was not done). During descent, the volume of gas in the bag and in the diver's lungs, tends to diminish due to increasing pressure (Boyle's Law, see page 21), so additional gas volumes have to be released constantly into the bag during descent in order to maintain surface lung volumes. This requires divers to calculate the pressure–volume conditions at bottom depth, as well as the composition of the gas mix to be used.

REBREATHING SETS

Rebreathing sets use two common patterns: pendulum and circuit breathing systems.

1. Pendulum breathing system

In this system, the diver breathes through a breathing tube (that is directly connected to a carbon dioxide scrubber canister) into and from a breathing bag, and no one-way valves are needed. This has a number of advantages. The apparatus is simple and small as it only needs one breathing tube, and carbon dioxide scrubbing is more efficient, as both inspired and expired gases pass through the scrubber.

The disadvantages are that it requires more breathing effort as both inhaled and exhaled gases are forced through the scrubber unit, and inhalation or swallowing of caustic material in solution can occur if water inadvertently enters the system – the so-called soda or caustic cocktail. In addition, carbon dioxide left in the breathing tube at the end of each exhalation is re-inhaled with the next breath.

PENDULUM REBREATHER

compressed breathing gas from a storage cylinder
↓
flow regulator valve
↓
breathing bag (counterlung)
↓ ↑
scrubber
↓ ↑
diver

2. Circuit breathing system

In the circuit breathing system, the movement of gas is controlled by one-way valves and the gas moves around in a circuit. The advantages are that it is easier to inhale, there is less chance of a caustic cocktail, and there is no initial inhalation of carbon dioxide-rich gas. The disadvantages are that it is bulkier, requires two hoses, non-return valves, and a larger canister than a pendulum set (with the same endurance).

CIRCUIT REBREATHER

compressed breathing gas from a storage cylinder
↓
flow-regulator valve
↓
breathing bag (counterlung)
↓ ↑
diver → scrubber

THE FLOW-REGULATOR VALVE This valve may be manual or automatic (usually both). With automatic control, the flow of gas into the breathing bag may be continuous or intermittent, being triggered, for example, by a volume drop in the bag beyond a set point. The manual control allows the diver to control gas flow if the automatic valve fails, permits flushing of the bag to remove gas from a previous dive (this is very important), and allows buoyancy control by adjusting the bag volume.

THE BREATHING BAG (COUNTERLUNG) The counterlung is a gas storage bag from which the diver breathes. It is equipped with a relief valve which releases excess gas into the water so preventing an excessive volume build up, for example, on ascent. Gas is released continuously in semi-closed sets, because the flow-regulator supplies a little more gas than the diver actually needs.

USING A SEMI-CLOSED-CIRCUIT MIXED-GAS REBREATHER SYSTEM

Before using a semi-closed system, two things must be decided:

1. The composition of the gas to be breathed.
2. The flow rate of the gas into the breathing bag.

The highest safe partial pressure of oxygen must be chosen for the particular maximum depth of the dive (1.4–1.6 ATA, depending on the duration of exposure). The flow rate must be set to provide the maximum anticipated volume of oxygen required. This rate is calculated in surface volumes, and the diver **will not** need more oxygen at depth. Oxygen need is a metabolic requirement and is independent of depth.

An example will illustrate the situation: a diver wanting to dive to 40 msw (5 ATA) chooses 40 per cent oxygen in nitrogen, which will provide an initial maximum of 2 ATA of oxygen at 40 msw. He anticipates working very hard and decides he will need three litres of oxygen per minute. As his mix contains 40 per cent oxygen, he sets his flow rate to 10 litres per minute, which will provide him with four litres of oxygen per minute, so guaranteeing an adequate oxygen supply.

At 40 msw, the mix in the bag is dependent on:

- flow of gas into the system (i.e. 10 litres per minute),
- his consumption, and
- loss through the relief valve.

If the diver lies quietly on the bottom, the mix in the bag would be approximately that of the supply tank. However, because rebreathers are freeflow systems supplying only small volumes of fresh gas per minute as the diver breathes from the breathing bag, most of the contained oxygen is removed, resulting in a steady drop in the total percentage of oxygen in the mix. Excess gas is steadily vented through the release valve. Exposure to very high oxygen partial pressures does not occur. At maximum work, the diver would be absorbing nearly all of the calculated available oxygen and the mix in the bag would be approximately 20 per cent oxygen.

In this example, there is a steady flow of 10 litres per minute (surface volume) of breathing gas into the bag. Compare the saving of a flow rate of 10 litres per minute to the 100 litres per minute of air required while working at 40 msw on a scuba demand-valve–open-circuit system.

It is absolutely essential to understand that the nitrogen–oxygen gas mix used in semi-closed diving rigs **is not equivalent to nitrox diving on scuba!** Semi-closed and closed diving systems are designed and intended to provide only a small excess of oxygen above the metabolic needs of body tissue. Only enough oxygen is provided to cover the diver's needs. The body and brain are not exposed to high oxygen partial pressures. The diver's breathing continually lowers the oxygen partial pressure in the breathing bag until a steady state of about 20 per cent oxygen is reached. Demand valves, on the other hand, provide a constant large excess of oxygen.

as solo divers are a prime target. A dive buddy may also be able to warn you of a shark's presence in time to take avoiding action. During the day, and with good visibility, meeting one or two sharks should present no immediate peril, but if three or more sharks appear, look for some type of underwater back-up shelter. Sharks very rarely attack submerged divers, but they are curious creatures and will circle, disappear, and then guardedly return, giving the divers ample time to decide calmly whether to continue the dive or return to the boat.

Spear fisherman should avoid 'baiting' themselves by tying their catch to their weight belts. At all times, avoid provoking a shark by touching it, pulling its tail or prodding it with any object. If you have been fishing from a boat, and have just cleaned your catch, wash yourself thoroughly with soap and water before diving, to remove any lingering aroma that might attract a hungry shark.

Some sharks, notably Great White and Blue sharks, will naturally and fearlessly attack any floating object – even outboard motors have been attacked. Despite being small, young or juvenile sharks of many species are often audacious and can inflict savage wounds; they are best avoided too.

3. THE ENVIRONMENT

Shark attacks tend to follow a fairly predictable pattern: most attacks occur during the day, in warm weather and during holiday periods, simply because this is when bathers enter the sea in large numbers. Most attacks on swimmers take place in water that is about chest deep, while surfers are usually within 30 metres of the shore. Almost invariably, the victim is swimming or surfing on the surface, not snorkelling or scuba diving, there is only one shark, and the attack occurs without any warning.

Some larger sharks feed towards evening and at night, favouring murky (turbid) water, and lurking in drop-offs and deeper offshore water – areas that are often the favourite habitat of divers.

WHAT TO DO WHEN CONFRONTED BY ONE OR TWO SHARKS WHILE DIVING

The majority of sharks do not attack people, but they are inquisitive and may approach divers for a 'look see'. Divers should learn something of shark behaviour, so that they know how to behave in the presence of a non-threatening shark, as well as how to react to a potential threat or actual attack.

1. Remain submerged, if possible.
2. Use slow, soft, purposeful movements; panicky and erratic movements can excite a shark. Avoid any sudden positional changes.
3. Do not attempt to swim away. Stay calm – sharks can somehow sense fear. Keep facing the shark and try to get a reef or wreck at your back. This at least ensures a frontal attack.
4. Ensure that the shark has an escape route. Putting it in the position where the only escape is past yourself is unwise.

5. If the shark starts showing signs of aggression, try to fend it off with something in your hand – a rock, your camera, a piece of wreckage or your spear. A shark billy (equipped with points or short nails at its end to avoid sliding off the shark's skin) is best if diving in known areas for sharks, but use it only to fend off the animal and ensure a distance between you. Do not strike at the shark.
6. Try not to wound the shark – it may become angry.
7. If the shark becomes openly aggressive and attacks, all your defensive options disappear. Try to hit the shark as hard as you can on the snout, eyes or gills.
8. Avoid using your bare hands if possible – the shark's rough skin will rip them and the bleeding will compound problems by exciting it.
9. Powerheads (explosive charges fitted to a shaft or spear and usually only used by spear-fishermen diving in shark-rich waters) can be effective in the right situation. They require expertise and accuracy, as the powerhead is only effective against a single shark. Using it in a school can easily precipitate a frenzy.

FEATURES OF A SHARK BITE

Depending on the size of the shark and the severity of the attack, the injury may consist of minor lacerations and skin abrasions, major lacerations, a single parabolic wound, multiple huge ragged wounds, or even limb amputations in many cases. Over 70 per cent of shark attacks involve the lower limbs only. Major shark bite injuries inevitably cause haemorrhage and shock.

MANAGEMENT OF SHARK BITES

There are only three primary things to do:
1. **Get the casualty out of the water.** This is critical for survival and must be done with the greatest speed possible. Do not waste time trying to ventilate the casualty in the water by mouth-to-mouth respiration. He or she is simply bleeding all the oxygenated blood back into the sea.
2. **Stop the bleeding.** The casualty must be placed lying on his or her back in a flat or slightly head-down position on a firm place clear of the water or on the boat. The casualty has lost blood, is shocked as a result, and may be near-drowned. Uninjured limbs should be elevated 30 degrees above the horizontal.
   (a) **Pressure bandages** are the first method to be used. Pack the wound with anything, ideally, pressure dressings from a Shark Attack Pack (see page 284), but even a towel or T-shirt will do, then apply pressure. In most cases, this will staunch the flow of blood. Finger pressure over the femoral artery, in the case of a leg, or the brachial artery, in the case of an arm, will help while the pack is being fitted.
   (b) If a big artery is spurting, it may be tied off with whatever is at hand – fishing-line, length of string or a shoe-lace.
   Do not worry about sterility at this stage.

(c) **Tourniquets** should be used on limbs if bleeding persists despite firm packing and pressure. A limb can survive for two to three hours without its blood supply. The tourniquet should be wide and flat to distribute pressure over a reasonable surface area. Tight cords or rubber tubing tend to result in pressure injuries to underlying tissues. Tourniquets are potentially dangerous and must be removed after two hours maximum. The surgeon who will be doing the definitive repair will not thank you for destroying normal tissue around the wound by cutting off its blood supply; nor will the casualty. Don't forget to inform the rescue service that a tourniquet is in place. Attach a prominent label to the casualty, clearly reading:

> **Tourniquet applied to**
> **right / left   leg / arm**
> at .... am/pm on (date) ....

3. **Control shock.** If there are a few people available, one person should control the bleeding while the others should:
   (a) Ensure a clear **airway**.
   (b) Ensure proper ventilation (**breathing**).
   (c) Ensure **circulation**.
       These first three steps are the basis of CPR (see page 230).
   (d) Administer 100 per cent oxygen by demand valve, if available.
   (e) Cover the casualty with a towel, blanket or space blanket.
   (f) Summon emergency help.
   (g) Keep the crowds at bay.

In order to alleviate shock, it is essential to replace some of the lost blood volume. Intravenous infusions of Haemaccel and Ringer's lactate should be set up simultaneously, as soon as the casualty is stable. Haemaccel is an efficient plasma expander and should be used when severe bleeding has occurred (maximum initial dose Haemaccel 1500 ml, thereafter alternate with blood 1:1). Ringer's lactate is a solution containing a mixture of salts for intravenous use. The idea is to replace lost blood volume so that the blood pressure can be improved until blood itself can be administered.

In 1998, a cell-free polymerised haemoglobin solution manufactured from cattle blood and providing virtually all of the oxygen-carrying capacity of whole human blood was introduced by the US-based company, Biopure, and marketed under the name Hemopure (HBOC-201). It can be stored at room temperature for up to three years and laboratory blood typings are not required because the haemoglobin solutions are cell free and can be administered to any blood group. In many cases, the administration of HBOC-201 has been life saving when whole blood was not an immediate option in the treatment of acute and severe blood loss. As yet, no record exists of its use following a shark attack.

Under no circumstances should a shark attack victim be moved until major bleeding is controlled, respiration and circulation are restored, an intravenous line has been established, and shock has improved. Do not rush a shocked, bleeding casualty to hospital. He or she will die.

The importance of not moving a shocked casualty until his or her blood pressure has stabilised cannot be overstressed. Do not be persuaded by anxious but untrained bystanders, or even ambulance personnel who are not paramedics, to move a shark attack victim. Most deaths from shark bites occur because of inadequate attention to stopping haemorrhage, and then moving a shocked casualty too soon.

If you are not paramedically trained, concentrate on stopping the bleeding, and ensure that the casualty is breathing and that there is circulation. Give oxygen if available and **wait** for a qualified person to give intravenous assistance. Injured limbs may be splinted for support. All dive boats must have shark attack packs on board for handling just such a problem before returning to shore.

Quick guide to immediate action:
1. Get the casualty out of the water.
2. Shout for someone to summon trained emergency help.
3. Lay the casualty flat on his or her back.
4. Stop the bleeding by applying:
    (a) digital pressure,
    (b) pressure bandage, or
    (c) tourniquet.
5. Control shock by:
    (a) ensuring a clear **airway**,
    (b) ensuring proper ventilation (**breathing**),
    (c) ensuring **circulation**,
    (d) administering 100 per cent oxygen,
    (e) elevating non-injured limbs,
    (f) splinting injured limbs,
    (g) covering the casualty (use a towel, space blanket or clothing), and
    (h) setting up intravenous lines.
6. Transfer the casualty to hospital when shock is controlled.
7. Do not forget about the tourniquet!

SHARK ATTACK PACK

All diving groups, dive operators and commercial dive boats should possess a shark attack pack – an advanced form of primary first aid that requires paramedic training or a doctor on site. Paramedic skills are a great asset when any incident occurs, such as a near-drowning or an injury caused by a marine animal. Dedicated scuba divers should consider undergoing the necessary training.

Recommended contents of shark attack pack:

1 x non-return airway
2 pairs of rubber gloves & goggles ⎫
2 pairs of protective plastic goggles ⎬ HIV protective wear for CPR operators
2 x full-length plastic aprons ⎭
2 x 1 litre Ringer's lactate solution
3 x 500 ml Haemaccel
3 only IV administration sets with blood filters and 18 gauge needles
3 only 16 gauge IV cannulae
1 only butterfly needle 21 gauge
2 only plastic syringes 10 ml
1 only plastic syringe 50 ml
5 only disposable needles 21 gauge
5 packs alcohol swabs
1 only adhesive tape reel 2.5 cm wide
4 only 25 cm x 50 cm trauma pads – sterile
4 only crepe bandages 15 cm
1 only crepe bandage 10 cm
5 only steripad dressings 12.5 cm x 10 cm
1 only Esmarch's bandage 10 cm (tourniquet)
2 only artery forceps, disposable 10 cm (used to clamp bleeders)
1 only aluminium foil blanket (space-blanket)

OTHER MARINE ANIMALS THAT BITE

Sharks are not the only creatures in the sea that can deliver a nasty bite. Divers and spear-fishermen need to be on their guard when in the presence of any of the following creatures, preferably moving slowly away and observing them from a safe distance.

BARRACUDA

There are about 20 species of barracuda worldwide, but only one species is known to bite divers, the great barracuda (*Sphyraena barracuda*). It reaches a size of about 1.5 metres, although specimens of over two metres have been described. They usually make only one strike and their bite is a straight or V-shaped wound as they have nearly parallel rows of teeth.

Management of injury is identical to that for shark bites.

MORAY EELS

These are commonly found in coral reefs, but can occur even in temperate water. Moray eels favour crevices and cracks between rocks and an attack by one is invariably due to a diver poking where he or she shouldn't. When habituated to divers,

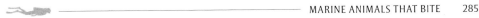

they can become 'tame', even welcoming a scratch on the head but, if threatened, startled or cornered, they are vicious and savage. They have narrow jaws with sharp pointed teeth. Once they bite, they tenaciously maintain their grip like terriers, lacerating the tissue. Their skin is extraordinarily tough so attempting to free oneself with a knife is going to be quite a performance. Treat them as you would a vigilant watchdog – approach with caution and then stay clear. Large moray eels can reach up to three metres in length.

Management of a bite follows the treatment for shark bites.

GROUPER (SEA BASS, GARRUPA)

These are large fish; the biggest can reach a size of over three metres, with a mass of 300 kg or more. Curious and non-aggressive, but bold, they cause injury through diver stupidity. When attacked or annoyed, a bite from their large mouth can cause ragged lacerations with extensive bruising, while being rammed by their huge head can cause extensive bruising and injuries to internal organs.

Management of grouper bites is as for shark bites, but remember to check for internal injuries which may have occurred as a result of being rammed.

KILLER WHALES (ORCAS)

These beautiful mammals live throughout the oceans of the world. They are the largest members of the dolphin family and probably the most intelligent. Previously described as ferocious killers, they are no longer believed to be deliberate man-eaters, but they are carnivores, hunting seals, walrus, squid, ocean-going fish and even other smaller whales with power and speed. Their massively powerful jaws can bite a seal in half, so do not let them think you are a new kind of seal in your eight-millimetre expanded neoprene wet suit. Stay well clear of killer whales.

The above are just some of the biters of the sea, but there are plenty of fish and other marine creatures with sharp teeth who are quite willing to oblige an incautious diver. For example, manta rays, seals and sea-lions, needlefish, snoek (*Thyrsites atun*), and even salt water crocodiles, can all inflict a potentially deadly wound.

38

MARINE ANIMALS THAT STING AND SHOCK

There are thousands of 'stingers' on and under the ocean. They are found in many different marine zones; corals cling to rocks, stonefish hide among the reefs, zebra fish flagrantly expose themselves, while bluebottles and sea wasps just hang around. Their shape and form also varies enormously; sea snakes are long and sinuous, for example, but stingrays are flat. Being stung by some will simply cause an itchy skin irritation, but others can kill in minutes.

Basically, as with many other creatures, the 'stingers' fall into two groups:
– animals without spinal columns (invertebrates), and
– animals with spinal columns (vertebrates).

STINGERS WITHOUT SPINAL COLUMNS

Invertebrates have no spine, so zoologists had to look for other features by which to classify them. This brings us to the first group, all of which have hollow guts. Since you can't call a whole group of creatures 'hollowguts', they are called Coelenterates which is the same thing in Greek – *coele* meaning hollow and *enteron* being the word for intestine (or gut).

1. COELENTERATES

When a hollow gut is your licence to join a club of spineless creatures, an amazing variety of members turn up. This group of stingers includes:

(a) HYDROIDS With stinging tentacles around their mouths, these hollowguts look like disguised versions of the mythical monster Hydra. Some stay put during their mature life and build a limestone shelter around themselves – these are the fire corals (which only look like coral as they are really hydroids). Others, the *Pennaria* or fire ferns, have long plume-like tentacles disguised as feathers. Some just float around – these are the bluebottles, or Portuguese men-of-war. There are thousands of hydroids but these examples illustrate the type.

(b) SCYPHOZOA This group of hollowguts is also unable to speak English and gets its name from the Latin *scyphus*, meaning a deep hollow cup, and the Greek *zoa*, meaning an animal. They have the unpleasant habit of discharging their sexual organs into their intestines. Included in this group are the inverted 'hollow cups' that are the jellyfish and the deadly sea wasp. Their stinging tentacles are grouped around the edge of an inverted bell.

(c) ANTHOZOA Once again *zoa* appears, so these are animals too. *Anthos*, from the Greek, means flower, so these are the 'flower animals'. Not surprisingly, sea anemones belong to this group. Less obviously, the stony corals and the soft corals also belong to the hollowgut flower animals.

HOW DO THESE ANIMALS STING? All of the hydroids have stinging cells, called nematocysts, which are found mostly on their tentacles. These cells are capsules filled with venom and each possesses a hollow, needle-like tube. If a diver touches the tentacles, the sharp tip of the tube is everted, penetrates the skin and injects the venom. Contact with fire coral, jellyfish, a bluebottle or an anemone results in thousands of these tiny intradermal injections. The effect depends on the organism, individual sensitivity and the area of the sting.

– The **hydroids** usually only cause skin reactions at the site of the sting – although the Portuguese man-of-war can cause great pain. Death is not usually a feature of hydroid stings.

– The **anthozoans**, such as some of the anemones, can cause severely painful stings which later break down and ulcerate.

– The effect of contact with **scyphozoans** varies from a very mild prickle, in the case of many jellyfish, to violent agony, even death, in the case of the sea wasp, probably the most venomous marine animal known (see below).

FIRE CORAL, found on many reefs around the world, presents a particular problem. Stinging may occur but, more often, it is the sharp edges of the calcified shell that lacerate the skin. These wounds almost always become infected and healing is slow. **All** coral injuries should be:

(a) thoroughly cleaned as soon as possible,

(b) washed with an antiseptic,

(c) treated with local antibiotic ointments, and

(d) kept dry, as further diving invariably results in a spreading infection or the formation of an abscess.

SEA WASP (BOX JELLYFISH)

The **sea wasp** (*Chironex fleckeri*) is patently the real problem in the whole group of coelenterates so let's look at it in more detail. A member of the class Cubozoa, it is often referred to as **the** box jellyfish, although it is only one of a number of different species, not all of which share its deadly reputation.

Box jellyfish occur in the warm tropical waters of northern Australia and the Indo-Pacific region and are most common in the summer months. They are usually found in shallow, sheltered waters, such as protected coves and bays.

The bell-shaped body can grow up to 20 cm across but, being pale blue and transparent, they are often difficult to see in the water, and can swim at a rate of up to four knots, which easily beats any diver. Tentacles are attached to the lower edge of the bell at four points and there may be as many as six tentacles at each point, each growing up to three metres in length. This results in a large 'danger area' around a sea wasp, and potential rescuers can easily become the next casualty, so great care must be taken when attempting to rescue a presumed sea wasp victim.

The venom is found in nematocysts, or stinging cells, on the tentacles, and is rapidly absorbed into the circulation. It has cardiotoxic, dermatonecrotic and neuro-toxic components and the initial pain is excruciating. The tentacles become sticky and adhere tightly to the skin. This causes the pain to rapidly worsen, and the victim may collapse and lose consciousness, which could easily lead to drowning.

Locally at the site of the sting, numerous crossing and irregular red or purple lines develop within seconds. These form large welts which break down and form ulcerating sores during the next week. Early administration of antivenom will reduce the likelihood of scarring.

General effects with absorption of the venom are threefold:
–   terrible and shocking pain,
–   depression of heart and circulatory function, and
–   depression of breathing and brain function.

Agony dominates a picture of a casualty experiencing progressive heart failure, inability to breathe, paralysis, generalised muscle cramps, rigidity of the abdomen, vomiting, frothing at the mouth, constriction of the throat, delirium and convulsions. If effective assistance is not immediately available on the dive boat or on shore, death may occur in as little as two or three minutes in healthy individuals, or even within 30 seconds in young children and people with respiratory or cardiac disease.

MANAGEMENT OF SEA WASP STINGS

(a) Get the victim out of the water as fast as possible. Assess his or her condition and begin rescue breathing or CPR if necessary (see page 230).

(b) Apply a compression immobilisation bandage, tourniquet, rope, string or any ligature **above** the sting if it is on an arm or leg to try and stop progressive or generalised envenomation.

(c) Pour **vinegar** over the stings and any pieces of tentacle. Acetic acid inactivates the venom and specifically inhibits the discharge of further nematocysts. This must be done before any attempt is made to remove the tentacles, still loaded with active nematocysts, which will worsen the condition of the diver and even poison the rescuer.

(d) Scrape off the inactivated tentacles with a knife. Drying them with talcum powder makes this easier.

(e) Apply more vinegar to the area as a poultice. This can help to break down venom in the skin.

(f) Summon medical assistance:
    – morphine given intramuscularly will help the pain,
    – sea wasp antivenin must be given if available. Trained first aiders can administer antivenin intramuscularly, but only paramedics should set up an IV line, and
    – transfer the casualty to hospital when shock is stabilised.
(g) Do not forget to release the tourniquet (maximum two hours).

The management of severe stings from other coelenterates, such as bluebottles, stony coral and jellyfish, is along similar lines, except that antivenin is not given.

2. MOLLUSCS

The second group of invertebrates are the softies – the molluscs (from Latin *moluscus* or *mollis*, meaning 'soft'). They may be soft-bodied but there is nothing soft about the venom of their poisonous members. Molluscs are named according to where their feet are situated. This group includes:

- octopuses – called *cephalopods* (feet on head), and
- cone shells – called *gastropods* (feet on stomach).

(a) Blue-ringed octopus

Your average octopus is shy and retiring and its bite, although painful, is usually uneventful. This, however, does not apply to the blue-ringed or spotted octopus (*Octopus maculosis*), which lives in shallow tropical waters and tidal pools from Japan to Australia. It is small, about 20 cm across, and yellowish or orange brown in colour until it is disturbed, when its rings change to bright blue.

Despite its size, the blue-ringed octopus can kill. It bites with a parrot-like beak and its saliva contains **tetrodotoxin**, a paralysing poison that attacks the nervous system (see also Fugu, page 303). Death can result from respiratory failure, but victims may be saved if artificial respiration is begun before cyanosis and hypotension develop. As paralysis sets in, the victim may retain his or her senses and awareness, but is unable to respond.

Pressure immobilisation is a recommended first aid treatment and prolonged artificial respiration, including mechanical ventilation, may be required until the effects of the envenomation disappear. No antivenom is available.

Other cephalopods are cuttlefish, squid and nautilus, but these are not poisonous.

(b) Cone shells

Cone shells, also known as cone snails or marine snails, occur in warm, tropical seas worldwide, although some are adapted to more temperate environments. They are cousins of land snails and, like them, have a single spirally coiled shell, a distinct head with two or four tentacles, two eyes, and a fleshy foot (they are called gastropods because they 'walk' on their bellies). Their conically shaped shells are often very decorative and are sought-after by shell collectors. All of the ±500 species of cone shell are venomous, with the composition of the venom varying from one species to another. However, a few larger species have venom that also contains tetrodotoxin.

The cone shell's stinging system is ingenious. Venom is stored in a venom bulb within the body. Before stinging, the venom passes along a duct to a tapering set of spiral teeth much like the drilling end of a borehole drill. These teeth lie inside the shell. To sting, they are moved out (like grandpa's teeth), grasped by a trunk-like 'nose' (proboscis) and rammed into the victim.

Locally, the sting of some small cone shells may be no worse than a bee sting but, generally, symptoms include numbness, swelling, burning or pain. Numbness and tingling start at the site of the wound and spread over the whole body – sometimes immediately, although onset can be delayed for days. The lips and mouth are particularly numb. Muscle paralysis may occur, ranging from mild weakness to total body paralysis. Speech and swallowing can become difficult. In severe cases, paralysis of the breathing muscles causes death. If the victim lives six hours, survival is probable. After 24 hours the victim will be better.

MANAGEMENT There are no antivenoms for cone shell stings. In severe cases, the emphasis is on artificial respiration to keep the victim alive over the first few hours, while the venom metabolises. This may mean rescue breathing for extended periods if in a remote area, or until the victim can be placed on a hospital respirator. In milder cases, apply pressure immobilisation and administer tetanus toxoid. Broad-spectrum antibiotics may be needed to reduce the risk of infection.

PREVENTION Although colourful, patterned cone shells are highly collectible, don't pick up ANY sea shells unless you are sure they are not occupied!

> Keep in mind that virtually all the poisoners of the sea, irrespective of whether they are invertebrates or fishes, use nerve poison as their weapon of choice. Anticipate paralysis and respiratory failure in any stung diver, irrespective of the stinger.

3. ECHINODERMS

The third group of invertebrates that sting divers are the prickly-skins or *echinoderms*. They get their name from the Greek *echino*, meaning a hedgehog or sea urchin, and *derm* meaning skin. They are a neat group in that they are radially symmetrical. Included in this clan are starfish, sea urchins and sea cucumbers. Sea cucumbers are fine; it is the starfish and sea urchins that have stingers among them.

(a) Starfish

Usually, only one starfish is problematic to divers – the crown of thorns (*Acanthaster planci*). It has caused massive overgrowth and destruction of the Indo-Pacific coral reefs, something it apparently does from time to time as a cyclical event. The crown of thorns starfish measures over 60 cm in diameter, has about 16 arms and is covered with sharp, thick, 6-cm-long venomous spines that are covered in slime. These may break off after penetrating the skin.

(b) Sea urchins

There are many different sea urchins, some with spines over 30 cm long, others with short spines. Some are very venomous, others less so but, aside from their spines, sea urchins have another, more venomous, stinging system. Delicate, long, stalk-like appendages, called pedicellariae, project between the spines. Each of these has a swollen end equipped with a set of jaws and a poison bag. Contact causes these pedicellarial jaws to close and venom to be injected. And these jaws do not let go as long as the prey moves. A diver is far too powerful for them to overcome, so they break off and continue to inject their poison. Pedicellarial venom is more potent than that of the spines. A Japanese species, *Toxopneustes elegans*, has long floral pedicellariae that waft beyond the spines. Contact with this urchin can kill.

PRESENTATION OF STARFISH AND SEA URCHIN STINGS The presentation of a sting from the crown of thorns starfish and most sea urchin spines is similar and is usually local only.

Local effects are immediate severe burning pain and the area around the wound becomes numb. Spines may be seen in the skin. Infection is common, with spreading inflammation occurring around the site, with pain and aching.

General effects involve a nerve poison. In the case of sea urchins, it is the delicate pedicellariae that work this effect with their exotic venom. Severe local burning pain is followed by weakness, faintness, numbness and progressive muscular paralysis. The pain usually disappears after about an hour, but paralysis may last for over six hours. Speech and swallowing may become difficult, and progression to respiratory paralysis may lead to death. Note that this sequence of events is very similar to the effects from the sea wasp, blue-ringed octopus and cone shell stings.

MANAGEMENT First aid is directed at the local injury and its generalised problems.
(a) It is difficult to remove sea urchin spines. They break off easily and, being composed largely of calcium carbonate, usually will be absorbed spontaneously by the body within a few weeks. If the spines penetrate a joint or an eye, surgical removal becomes necessary. Sometimes the site of penetration becomes infected, and medical help and antibiotics will then be needed.
(b) The venom of these spines and pedicellariae is **heat-sensitive**, so application of heat to the area will inactivate the poison. Treat the sting with water at 50°C,

taking care not to scald the victim, who is already in pain. Heat is the most effective way of destroying the venom.

(c) If available, unripe pawpaw sap is useful in alleviating pain. Cut into a green fruit and allow the milk-like sap to drip on to the wound.

(d) Medicinal alcohol may now be applied. It is antiseptic and inactivates pedicellariae, which can now be removed if visible.

(e) Oral antihistamines may provide some relief and painkillers, such as paracetamol, taken by mouth can assist pain.

(f) Any signs of paralysis or respiratory difficulty may mean that rescue breathing will be needed, so **keep a watchful lookout**. Don't put a stung diver to bed to suffocate in solitude while everyone else parties into the night.

4. ANNELIDS

The fourth group of stingers is the segmented worms or *annelids*. (Familiar non-marine varieties are earthworms and leeches.) Within most marine environments, tubeworms on the seabed are the usual annelids that scuba divers may encounter. They have long, segmented bodies and work their mischief in two ways:

— the bite is inflicted using biting jaws, and
— the sting is inflicted by brushing against the bristles on each segment with bare limbs.

The bite or sting causes a painful local reaction. First aid treatment involves immersing the affected limb in hot water, applying topical antiseptics and the administration of painkillers. Bristles can be removed using sellotape or adhesive tape.

5. PORIFERA

These are the sponges, and there are literally thousands of species of these simple animals occurring throughout the world. Some sponges cause painful skin irritations after contact with the surface of their fibrous outer skeletons. Management is along general first aid lines.

GENERAL APPROACH TO SEA STINGERS

The average diver will not remember the technicalities of scientific nomenclature nor the stinging methods used by the multifarious invertebrates. It is also seldom that a victim can identify the exact species of stinger involved. Unfortunately, the stingers couldn't care less about identification either, and will continue to injure careless or unsuspecting divers, whose dive buddies will then be presented with the potentially lethal problem of what treatment to apply.

Therefore, a practical, simple, easy-to-remember approach is necessary.

— **If the stinger has spines (starfish, urchin or fish), there will be a puncture wound: use hot water.**
— **If the stinger has no spines (but usually tentacles), there will be welts or a rash: use vinegar.**

Example

> Pete Muckitt was diving with Charlie Crumpet at the sunken temple near Trincomalee in Sri Lanka. As the water was warm Pete had decided not to bother with his wet suit. Clad only in swim shorts, he explored the shattered temple, squeezing between broken columns and peering under fallen plinths. Suddenly, excruciating pain lashed at his bare back. Yowling in agony into his regulator, he crawled from under the ruins and made for the surface. Charlie, seeing Pete kicking frantically above him, followed. At the surface, he helped the screaming Pete aboard the boat. Pete was thrashing in pain, with no idea as to what had happened, but a purpling welt on his bare back told Charlie that Pete had been stung. But by what? And what to do?

This is the type of problem that may occur when a diver is injured underwater. The absence of a major wound excludes a large biting animal, but the presence of intolerable pain indicates a stinger. At this point, what did Charlie know? He knew that stingers use nerve poisons and that paralysis and respiratory arrest were possibly on the way. He knew that heat, vinegar and alcohol are treatments for stings. He also knew that antihistamines and oral painkillers might help.

So Charlie tried the lot. While waiting for water to heat on the boat's stove, he poured vinegar over the welt. He followed this with hot water compresses (45–50°C) to Pete's back for 30 minutes. He gave Pete an antihistamine and two painkillers and watched for any sign of weakness or paralysis. As the boat returned home, he radioed ahead for medical assistance.

This would be a reasonable approach to any sting. Without knowing anything about the cause, it is possible to render effective assistance. It would even help with vertebrate stings, because stinging fish also utilise spines to sting and their venoms are destroyed by heat too.

STINGERS WITH SPINAL COLUMNS – THE VERTEBRATES

Up to now we have examined some aspects of stingers without spinal columns, but when a spinal column becomes the ticket of admission into the stingers' club, a whole host of horrible members enrol. Stingrays, scorpionfish, ratfish, catfish, toadfish, rabbitfish, weevers and stargazers make up only a portion of the prickly pack waiting for an unsuspecting diver.

The interesting thing about this gang is that the more venomous and spiky the fish, the more indolent and less aggressive it becomes. Who needs to attack when your first defence is a knockout? When it comes to the stinging vertebrates, in most cases, the effect of the venom can be lethal, and specific treatment is largely unknown.

Like sea urchins, stinging fish use spines to sting. These spines form part of the dorsal, pelvic or anal fins, or are situated just in front of the dorsal or pectoral fins. In the case of the stingray, the sting is on the tail.

In general, the venom glands of stinging fish are commonly placed on either side of the base of the stinging spine, or around the spine. The spines may be either sharp and needle-like, or have backward-facing barbs, which cause extensive laceration of tissue on withdrawal of the spine. The spine is covered by a sheath which is pushed back when the spine enters the victim. This sheath compresses the venom gland and causes it to inject the poison.

Stinging fish are generally reclusive and hide by burying themselves in sand, or use camouflage, so contact with them occurs inadvertently. The lionfish is the exception; hidden within its beautiful, lacy dorsal and pectoral fins are venomous spines. Contact can also occur when stinging fish are netted or caught. These fish must never be handled!

The two most important stinging fish are the stingrays and the scorpionfish.

STINGRAYS

There are many different species of stingray, all of which are characterised by their long, whip-like tail, which bears a venomous spine. They are commonly found in shallow coastal water where they lie partially buried in the sand, making it easy for an incautious bather or diver to step on them.

Although stingrays (also known as whip-tailed rays) are generally docile, they will act in self-defence, flipping their tail upwards to strike. In some species, the sting is situated very close to the body, but in others the sting is placed further down the tail, enabling them to lash out and sting very viciously. The 'sting' comprises a long, barbed spine with a venom gland at its base and a protective, membrane-like sheath that covers the entire sting mechanism. The barbs are serrated, with a sharp tip. When the sting enters a person's body, the pressure causes the protective sheath to tear, releasing the venom into the wound.

Most stingray injuries are to the legs and ankles and, while these are not fatal, they are very painful, as enzymes contained in the venom cause intense spasm in the smooth muscle, with localised pain and swelling, and even tissue and cell death. Significant tissue damage can also result from the removal of the barb, with subsequent infection at the site.

If the sting penetrates the abdomen or chest cavity, the resultant injuries to major body organs, accompanied by severe lacerations, massive blood loss and the fact that the venom affects the cardiovascular system, can prove fatal (see page 296).

This was the case when Australia's famed 'crocodile hunter', Steve Irwin, died in September 2006, after being accidentally pierced in the heart by a stingray barb, while filming a wildlife programme for television.

MANAGEMENT OF STINGRAY INJURIES

- Get the diver out of the water and monitor the vital signs. Look out for nausea, vomiting, muscle cramps and chills, as these could indicate imminent anaphylaxis (allergic shock) or developing venom effects.
- Stop any bleeding, but take care to ensure that further damage is not done to the casualty or rescuer if the sting is still embedded in flesh.
- Manage the pain. Stingray venom is protein-based and causes extreme pain that is maximal 30–90 minutes after envenomation but will continue to fluctuate in intensity for several hours. The venom is heat-labile (broken down by heat), so the most effective treatment is to immerse the injured area in water as hot as the casualty can stand (up to 45°C) for 30–90 minutes.
- Additional intramuscular or intravenous pain-relieving medication can be administered, as well as injection of a local anaesthetic, such as 2% lignocaine, into the injured area.
- Vinegar and other liquids are NOT effective for stingray injuries.
- The wound will need to be properly cleaned and sutures may be required.
- Antibiotics and tetanus toxoid should be given to prevent infection. Surgical debridement (the removal of dead tissue) may be necessary.
- **If the abdomen or chest cavity has been penetrated,** or there is severe tissue injury, seek emergency medical help. The venom can affect the cardiovascular system, causing peripheral vasoconstriction (blanched white extremities), dilation (beefy red extremities), arrhythmia (irregular heartbeats) or even asystole (the heart may stop beating altogether). It can also act on the brain centres causing respiratory failure and convulsions.

SCORPIONFISH FAMILY

Members of this family, among the most poisonous fish known, can be divided into three groups, using their venomous spines as a distinguishing character:

(a) **Zebra fish** (*Pterois*), also called lionfish or turkeyfish, have long, delicate venomous spines. They are showy and indifferent to visitors, but are a hazard in coral reefs.

(b) **Scorpionfish** (*Scorpaena*) have fairly thick spines. They rely on camouflage, blending their colouring to match the crevices and seaweed in which they lurk.

(c) **Stonefish** (*Synanceja*) have very heavy venomous spines covered in warty, thick sheaths. They are well camouflaged, lie quietly in sheltered rocky niches and are very difficult to see. Their poison is the most dangerous of all.

The known venoms of all stinging fish are heat-labile, that is, destroyed by heat. On contact, the venom causes intense pain, which may be so severe that the victim screams, thrashes around and even loses consciousness. The venom is toxic to muscle, causing paralysis. In severe cases, the respiratory muscles can be affected, leading to respiratory failure, while paralysis of the heart muscle may cause cardiac failure.

The result is a diver who may be screaming, writhing, vomiting in pain, losing consciousness and possibly drowning, while developing a progressive paralysis which involves breathing and stops heart action. Survivors are likely to suffer infection, even gangrene, of the affected area.

MANAGEMENT OF STINGING FISH INJURIES

First aid treatment of venomous fish stings has three dimensions – initial control of pain, reducing the effects of the venom and treating potential sites of infection.

1. Rescue the casualty from the water and lay him or her flat on the ground.
2. Irrigate the wound to rinse out some of the poison (use saline solution if available, otherwise fresh cold water or even sea water). Remember that some of the venom-producing sheath may remain in the wound, continuing to poison the diver.
3. While the wound is being cleaned, heat fresh water as quickly as possible.
4. Immerse the limb in water at 50°C (as hot as bearable without scalding) for 30–60 minutes. The addition of Epsom salts to the water has been reported to be useful. If done quickly, heating the infected area rapidly destroys the venom and provides dramatic relief from pain. Treat wounds on the head and torso with hot water compresses.
5. Tourniquets have been used to try to stop generalised absorption of the venom, but their use is questionably effective and some formal emergency training is needed.
6. Injecting local anaesthetic (2% lignocaine or xylocaine) into the area around the wound may help the pain. Again, some emergency training is needed.
7. Once the above has been done, keep a watch for respiratory and/or cardiac failure. If necessary, begin EAR and/or CPR (see page 230).
8. Call for medical help. The wound must be properly cleaned and dressed. Lacerated wounds may need suturing, antibiotics may be needed and, in severe cases, hospitalisation may be indicated.
9. Remember that the casualty is frightened, and in great pain and distress. Be calm and reassuring.
10. If specific stonefish antivenin is available, it should be given in all cases of stonefish stings.

SEA SNAKES

Sea snakes occur in the warm tropical waters of the Indian and western Pacific oceans, particularly around Singapore and Borneo. There are about 50 species in total, more than 20 of which have been recorded in Australia's coastal waters.

One pelagic species, *Pelamis platurus*, the yellow-bellied sea snake, has an exceptionally wide range and has been found from the Pacific across the Indian Ocean to eastern and southern Africa and even on the western coast of the Americas.

Sea snakes are marine reptiles – they have lungs and breathe air. They have no fins, and swim by using their flattened tails as paddles, along with undulating sideways body movements. Although they are generally regarded as docile, they can become aggressive during the mating season, if stepped on, or when caught on a line or netted. In general, they are far more venomous than land snakes. Their venom is neurotoxic, myotoxic and haemotoxic, causing:

- nerve poisoning with paralysis,
- muscle-tissue breakdown, and
- blood cell destruction.

The good thing is that sea snake fangs are short and are easily torn out, so that not everyone who gets bitten is poisoned. As the sea snake can control the amount of envenomation, just a small proportion of sea snake bites are fatal to man.

Sea snakes are most commonly found in shallow water near river mouths where the water is turbid. A wader stepping on a sea snake may not even know that he or she has been bitten, as the bite is usually painless. This can be very awkward, because serious illness is on the way. Depending on the site, the species of sea snake, the amount of venom injected and the victim's characteristics, there is a time period ranging from 10 minutes to a few hours before anything is noted.

The first signs are that the victim becomes restless and a little excitable. As the muscle-toxin component works, the tongue becomes 'thick', and generalised body aches and stiffness appear. Drooping of the eyelids is an early sign and spasm of the jaw muscles or lockjaw occurs. The nerve-toxin then causes an ascending paralysis, starting in the legs and working up to the neck. Speech becomes difficult, swallowing is an effort, and vomiting may occur.

The blood-toxin causes a breakdown of red blood cells with progressive shock. The destruction of muscle cells and red blood cells causes the urine to become red-pink and kidney failure can occur. Finally, convulsions, coma, cardiac failure and respiratory failure can lead to death.

MANAGEMENT OF SEA SNAKE INJURIES

1. The victim must lie down and remain absolutely quiet. No walking, effort or any physical exertion must be allowed. Splint the afflicted limb.
2. Apply a tourniquet above the site of the puncture wound. It must be released after two hours.
3. Obtain medical help urgently.
4. Provide rescue breathing (EAR) or CPR as needed.
5. If trained to do so, give sea snake antivenin if available, otherwise use polyvalent serum with Krait (Elapidae) fraction.
6. If possible, the snake should be kept for identification.

MARINE ANIMALS THAT SHOCK

A number of fish, including catfish and electric eels in fresh water, and stargazers and electric rays in sea water, possess voltage-generating electric organs.

The **electric ray** (family Torpedinidae) has a typically flattened disc-shaped body but, unlike other rays, the tail is fish-shaped rather than whip-like. The electric organs are situated on either side of the front of the disc, the lower surface of the fish being electrically negative and the upper surface positive. Depending on the species, a voltage of 8–220 volts can be generated. Contact with a diver may result in short-lived incapacity, but rapid recovery invariably occurs.

The **electric eel** (*Electrophorus electricus*) is the most advanced battery known. This South American river fish is an air breather, having to surface from time to time to breathe. Measuring about 1.2 metres long, it can generate a voltage of 370–550 volts at 40 watts, which can easily knock a man out. The output lasts 0.002 seconds at a frequency of 400 cycles per second and the eel can maintain a steady output at this rate for about 20 minutes. After a five-minute break, the output can be repeated. Eat your heart out, Duracell!

A POINT OF IMPORTANCE FOR MEDICAL RESCUERS

Many invertebrates and vertebrates inflict a sting that can cause temporary paralysis. When administering first aid, always remember that the casualty may be able to both hear and see, even if he or she cannot move, talk, or even breathe. If a casualty is conscious, he or she is probably aware of what is going on. It is absolutely imperative that you continually give reassurance and explain what you are doing.

If the rescuers are in a state of uncontrolled excitement or loudly discuss what is happening, the temporarily paralysed casualty could be overhearing everything being said around him or her. While you are performing mouth-to-mouth resuscitation and ignorant onlookers are proclaiming 'it's too late' or 'he's gone!', the afflicted diver may be conscious, terrified and desperately praying that you do not listen to the bystanders and stop your possibly life-saving efforts.

39

MARINE ANIMALS THAT ARE POISONOUS TO EAT

Most divers love a good seafood meal, whether it be grilled linefish, seafood potjie or tuna sashimi. Under the wrong circumstances, however, almost any fish or seafood can be toxic, even lethal. Fortunately, genuine seafood poisonings are relatively rare, although a lot of people are allergic to various types of seafood, particularly shellfish such as mussels and oysters, often only discovering this in the most unpleasant way.

Some seafood poisonings are important, either because they are common or because they can affect whole communities. These are:
- shellfish,
- ciguatera,
- tetrodotoxin, and
- scombroid.

SHELLFISH POISONING
If you do not obtain your shellfish in a responsible manner, you may poison your guests in any number of ways with a fine seafood platter.

1. Gastroenteritis
Gastroenteritis follows the eating of 'off' shellfish (particularly fresh mussels or oysters) that have been contaminated by bacteria. Nausea, vomiting, diarrhoea and cramps occur, lasting a day or two. Treatment is dietary restriction, lots of fluids, antiemetics and anti-diarrhoeals.

2. Allergic reactions
People who have previously eaten shellfish without any problems may develop acute allergic reactions on their second or subsequent meal. This can present as a violently itchy and spreading red rash with large welts; an acute episode of asthma; or as a sudden collapse due to circulatory shock. The last two can kill, so this is a potentially serious problem.

MANAGEMENT OF ALLERGIC REACTIONS

1. Itching and rashes can generally be controlled by the use of antihistamines.
2. Acute breathing difficulties – due to sudden severe asthma, or sudden circulatory collapse and shock – are medical emergencies. **Summon a doctor or emergency paramedic service without delay.**
3. If the casualty is in a remote place with no recourse to any medical help:
   (a) Inject adrenalin 1:1000 **subcutaneously** at a dose of 0.01 ml/kg body mass, **very slowly over five minutes**. Draw back on the syringe before injecting to ensure that a blood vessel has not been entered by the needle. Do not inject adrenaline into a blood vessel! Automatic adrenalin injectors with a concealed spring-activated needle are now available (e.g. EpiPen, Ana-Guard).
   (b) Monitor the pulse continuously. It will become forceful and accelerate as the injection is given. If it rises above 120 beats per minute, stop injecting and wait until the pulse settles.
   (c) Watch the casualty's face. It will become extremely pale due to the vasoconstriction effect of adrenaline.
   (d) Monitor respiration continuously. Be prepared for CPR.
   (e) Inject 100–200 mg of hydrocortisone intramuscularly into the upper outer quadrant of the buttock muscle.
   Adrenaline and hydrocortisone are emergency life-saving drugs and may only be considered when it is impossible to get any trained help. These medications are then being given without expert opinion or training and offer only a hope of success in extreme circumstances.
   (f) Administer CPR if breathing and heart function fail.

3. Paralytic shellfish poisoning (PSP)

This is a potentially lethal condition that occurs during 'red tides', which are caused by the sudden and massive proliferation of a tiny plankton organism called a dinoflagellate. In 1936, the dinoflagellates causing this sudden bloom were first described as a species of the genus *Gonyaulax*. In 1990, the particular toxin-producing species were confirmed as *Alexandrium catanella* and *A. tamarense*.

Fish that eat these organisms may die en masse. However, molluscs (mussels, clams, oysters, scallops and perlemoen/abelone) simply store the contaminating *Alexandrium* and pass it on to the person who eats them. This can cause an epidemic of PSP at the time of the red tide and for some time afterwards, as the molluscs may retain the poison for several months after a flush of red tide.

The poison is a nerve toxin (saxitoxin) that blocks movement of sodium through nerve cell membranes. Without sodium transmission, nerve cells cannot function. This results in the symptoms of PSP – numbness, paralysis, respiratory failure and coma. There is no specific antidote for PSP toxicity.

PRESENTATION OF PARALYTIC SHELLFISH POISONING

Symptoms begin within one hour after eating contaminated molluscs. Numbness around the mouth, nausea and vomiting occur, followed by headache, difficulty in talking, swallowing, and walking. Within the next hour, difficulty in breathing, respiratory arrest and cardiac failure may follow.

MANAGEMENT OF PSP

1. Using emetics to induce vomiting will reduce the amount of toxin absorbed.
2. Other management is purely supportive and involves very prolonged EAR (Mouth-to-mouth, see page 233). In a hospital environment, the patient must be intubated and placed on mechanical ventilation. Although neurological examination after the onset of respiratory arrest may even suggest that the patient is brain dead, supportive therapy must be continued. In the majority of cases, consciousness will be regained within the next six to ten hours and, within 24 hours, complete symptom resolution should occur.
3. Monitor the pulse and heart beat continuously. Be ready to administer CPR (see page 235).
4. Remember that a paralysed victim who is conscious may be aware of what you are doing. It is **extremely** important to give constant reassurance.
5. Following vigorous resuscitative treatment, death due to PSP is uncommon.

CIGUATERA POISONING

Like PSP, this is transmitted to man by eating tainted fish products. With PSP, eating shellfish contaminated with the dinoflagellate *Alexandrium* caused the problem. With ciguatera, another dinoflagellate, *Gambierdiscus toxicus*, is believed to be the culprit. *Gambierdiscus* lives on brown seaweed.

Fish that eat the seaweed become contaminated and, if they are caught and eaten by man, the toxin can be passed on, as the heat-stable ciguatoxin is not destroyed by cooking or frozen storage. Alternatively, the herbivorous fish may be eaten by a carnivorous fish which becomes contaminated in turn. If it is caught and eaten, the carnivorous fish will cause the disease to manifest in man, although the fish itself is unaffected. The disease is mainly confined to tropical waters.

Many common reef fish, including file-fish, grouper, parrot-fish, surgeon-fish, trigger-fish, trunk-fish and wrasse are carriers, and moray eels are particularly poisonous when affected. However, these are seldom eaten. The real problem arises when popular eating fish, such as anchovies, herrings, barracuda and shad (elf), suddenly become poisonous. The difficulty is compounded by the fact that there is no way of knowing what their status is, so determinations for ciguatera are usually limited to diagnosis based on symptoms.

PRESENTATION OF CIGUATERA POISONING

Symptoms of ciguatoxic fish poisoning can begin within less than six hours. Initial symptoms are gastrointestinal, including nausea, cramping and vomiting. Early neurological signs are headache, flushing, muscle aching and weakness, followed by a tingling and numbing sensation of the lips, tongue and mouth, dizziness and joint pains. Skin symptoms are typical: cold feels hot and hot feels cold, and redness, itching, burning and blistering of the skin may occur. The muscle pains progress to severe weakness, tremors and paralysis.

Convulsions, coma and death occur in up to 10 per cent of ciguatera cases. Victims usually recover within a few days, but severe neurological disorders may persist for months, sometimes for years. Symptoms may recur following alcohol consumption.

MANAGEMENT OF CIGUATERA POISONING

The same treatment principles as outlined for PSP apply. From the point of view of prevention, the safest solution is not to eat reef fish, and especially to avoid their gonads and guts.

TETRODOTOXIN (PUFFER FISH) POISONING

Worldwide, there are more than 120 representatives of Tetraodontidae, a family of tropical and subtropical fish that includes puffer fish (*blassops*) and tobies. Most species are small, with round bodies embellished with spiky scales on the back, flanks and belly. They can inflate themselves to many times their size, hence the name.

The skin, liver, gonads and gut (viscera) of puffer fish, porcupine-fish and ocean-going sun-fish contains tetrodotoxin – a potent nerve poison (the same as used by both the blue-ringed octopus and venomous cone shells).

Although it is widely accepted that puffer fish flesh is also toxic, it is regarded as something of a delicacy in Japan, where it is called *fugu*. Only very highly trained and esteemed chefs are permitted to prepare the fish for their gourmet clientele. The intention is to cause slight numbness of the lips without any further problems but, unfortunately, accidents do happen, and every year a few risk-taking Japanese diners don't make it home.

Tetrodotoxin poisoning commences with numbness around the mouth, after which the tongue and whole body become numb. Twitching, progressive paralysis, difficulty with speech and swallowing, and convulsions occur, with the victim remaining conscious all the while. This can be followed by severe respiratory distress with a hypoxic blue colour and bleeding into the skin. Recovery is possible, but about 60 per cent of poisoned victims die.

MANAGEMENT OF TETRODOTOXIN POISONING

This is purely supportive, as for PSP and ciguatera.

SCOMBROID POISONING

The scombroid family includes mackerel, tuna, albacore, swordfish and bonito. The firm muscle flesh of all these fish is rich in the amino acid histidine. Improper preservation or canning procedures allow bacteria to enter the flesh of the fish, where they break down the histidine into a poisonous amine called saurine, which has many of the properties of histamine – the basic cause of allergic reactions in humans. From time to time, one hears of a mass recall of canned tuna for this reason.

The affected fish has a sharp peppery taste and should only be given to your neighbour's pesky cat! In humans, the reactions are a mixture of nausea, vomiting, diarrhoea, abdominal pain and gut irritation, along with migraine or an intense headache, an intensely itchy spreading rash or urticaria, asthma, tightness of the chest with wheezing, and palpitations. In extreme cases, circulatory shock can occur.

Scombroid poisoning can be avoided by prompt freezing, or by cooking these fish soon after catching. Do **not** allow your mackerel catch to stand in the sun all day. Deep-sea fishermen who catch tuna and other big-game fish in open water must have adequate fridges or blocks of ice on board to chill their catch.

MANAGEMENT OF SCOMBROID POISONING

1. Induce vomiting as soon as possible, unless the victim has already vomited or is very agitated by severe breathing difficulty.
2. Give antihistamines, preferably by injection.
3. Obtain medical help.
4. **If medical help is absolutely unavailable**, administer adrenalin and hydrocortisone as detailed above under management of allergic reactions (see page 301).

40

UNDERWATER EXPLOSIONS

An explosion under water is far more vicious than an equivalent blast on the surface and can be extremely dangerous for any diver in the vicinity. A diver may be exposed to an underwater explosion for several reasons, among them:
- underwater mining or salvage work,
- accidental exposure to unexploded ordnance on a sunken wreck, or
- deliberate acts of sabotage or war.

When an underwater explosion is triggered, the following occurs:
1. A large gas bubble suddenly forms; this is under very great pressure and is very hot.
2. Pressure and heat cause the gas bubble to expand immediately, increasing its size. A very rapidly moving pressure wave is forced through the water. This first pressure wave (primary wave) is called the **short pulse**.
3. All liquids are incompressible and water is no exception. The surrounding water opposes the expanding bubble, tending to recompress it. A series of oscillating increases and decreases commences, each increase causing another, but progressively weaker, pressure wave.
4. The pressure waves move very rapidly near the centre of the explosion, then slow down as distance increases. Eventually they reach the speed of sound and behave like sound in water, losing energy inversely to the square of the distance travelled.

    In simple terms, this means that a series of high-speed pressure waves follow one another from a central high-pressure source of expanding gas. As distance increases, energy decreases but, because water is denser than air, pressure waves move further in water than they do in air. They are also reflected from the surface and from the bottom if it is solid (i.e. rocky). A soft, sandy seabed will absorb some of the force. Reflected waves then add their force to other pressure waves, increasing their power and effect. At the surface, some of the reflected waves may move in the opposite direction to oncoming waves and reduce their effect.
5. Depending on the force and depth of the explosion, a well-described series of events takes place at the surface.

(a) If the detonation is large or shallow enough, the surface water is torn or shreds and then bulges up. This bulge is called the **dome**.

(b) Next comes a rapidly widening ring of dark water due to the advancing pressure waves. This is termed the **slick**.

(c) Finally, the ascending gas reaches the surface and breaks through, causing a spout of water to spray into the air. This is the **plume**.

If the explosion is deep or small, the above may not occur.

What happens to a diver in range of these pressure waves?

If a diver is in the water at the time of an underwater explosion, he or she will be unaware of any increased pressure on the arms and legs. As these are technically fluid systems, without any gas spaces, pressure is transmitted directly through them from the water. What the diver may be aware of are the reactions that occur in the body's air spaces:

- ears and sinuses,
- lungs and airways, and
- the abdomen.

When the pressure wave reaches the diver, the pressure is transmitted through tissues with little or no effect, being a fluid-to-fluid transmission. But, as the pressure wave reaches the lining of the air spaces, destruction commences. Shredding and pluming occur, as at a water surface. The membranes and tissues of the ears, sinuses, airways, lungs and gut are simply torn to pieces.

This is very different from an explosion on land, where most of the damage is caused by flying bits of bomb casing, shrapnel and other debris hitting the victim. In water, movement of solid objects is greatly impeded by water resistance and they do not travel far. The pressure wave does the killing.

MANAGEMENT OF UNDERWATER BLAST INJURIES

Obviously, the best way to avoid being injured by an underwater blast is not to dive in areas where explosions are likely to occur. However, commercial and naval divers often work with explosives underwater and are therefore exposed to risk.

PREVENTION

1. If you are required to work with explosives, it is imperative that you wear protective clothing, such as explosive blast body-shields or air-containing suits. Blast shields consist of a jacket with an impervious outer layer and a perforated inner section open at the lower end to absorb an explosive blast of water and gas. The air in air-containing suits reflects the pressure waves, causing shredding of the first water–air interface, which happens to be the suit and not a lung.

2. If a diver is at the surface at the moment of an explosion, he should try to get his body's air spaces – the head, chest and abdomen – out of the water. At best, the diver should lie on some floating material, and at worst he should float on his back to try and minimise the injury. Remember though, that near the surface, and at the bottom, reflection may augment the force of oncoming pressure waves – neither of these are good places in which to be.

TREATMENT

1. Externally, the diver may appear intact and any injuries may initially seem to be relatively minor. Serious injuries, such as a ruptured bowel or torn lung, may only manifest later. All victims of an underwater blast must be hospitalised as a precaution, even if only for observation until it is clear that there are no life-threatening consequences.
2. Do not give any fluids or food by mouth in case the gut has been penetrated. A thorough examination in hospital is needed to rule this out.
3. In the case of a critical injury, CPR and oxygen may be required.
4. If a lung injury has occurred, administer 100 per cent oxygen by mask.

41

MANAGEMENT OF AN UNCONSCIOUS DIVER

When one is presented with an unconscious diver above or below water, there may be no immediate way of knowing the cause. The diver could have experienced equipment problems, the gas mix may be incorrect, he or she might have suffered a non-diving-related incident such as a heart attack, diabetic coma or stroke, or been exposed to hypothermia, dangerous sea creatures, electricity or an underwater explosion. But, whatever the primary cause for loss of consciousness, there is a very real possibility that a submerged, unconscious diver will suffer bends and a burst lung with arterial gas embolism during the rescue ascent.

QUICK ACTION – THE 'SEVEN Bs'

Going through check lists of causes takes time and a cool head. In an emergency, time is a luxury and a cool head is a rarity. A quick aid is to memorise the inverted triangle of the 'seven Bs'. Whatever the primary or secondary causes of unconsciousness, effectively handling the 'Bs' can save the victim. Is the diver:

Below water?

Breathing?

Bleeding?

Beating?

Burst?

Bent?

Bit?

1. Below water

The first step is instinctive: return the diver to the surface using a controlled emergency swimming ascent (CESA, see page 170). However, getting the diver there requires understanding. The danger is inducing pulmonary barotrauma of ascent (see page 161). If the diver is convulsing, wait for the convulsion to pass, as returning to the surface may be lethal if exhalation is inadequate. Dump the casualty's weight belt, then commence a controlled **deep diver rescue ascent**, ensuring that the diver's head is extended well back to allow expanding air to be exhaled (see page 216).

Remain calm! Do not perform an uncontrolled, fast ascent – the result will probably be a dead diver and a bent rescuer.

2, 3, 4. Breathing, bleeding and (heart) beating

Once the diver is at the surface, breathing, bleeding and heartbeat are managed as a group, because controlling them restores vital functions. This means stopping major blood loss, and then providing rescue breathing and/or external cardiac massage – the latter two comprising CPR (see page 230).

Control bleeding first. Don't perform CPR if arterial blood is spurting from a gaping wound. **Pack the wound and apply pressure** (AIDS caution!) before you begin **rescue breathing or CPR**. If bleeding is absent, start rescue breathing on the surface of the water if necessary. If there is no pulse, start **chest compressions** as soon as the diver is on a firm place in the boat or on land.

If there are two or more rescuers, one should start CPR while the other attempts to control bleeding. If you are alone, control massive bleeding as quickly as possible, then start rescue breathing or CPR.

Before commmencing resuscitation, take a moment to study the casualty's skin colour, as it can provide valuable clues as to the possible cause of the unconsciousness. Is he or she:

– a blue unconscious diver (hypoxic),
– a white unconscious diver (oxygen toxic, in shock or hypothermic), or
– a red unconscious diver (carbon dioxide, carbon monoxide toxic, or hyperthermic).

5. Burst

If unconsciousness occurred during ascent or very soon after surfacing, the diver **must** be considered to have AGE (arterial gas embolism, see page 164), which will require urgent transportation to a recompression facility (see page 166).

6. Bent

If unconsciousness is due to DCI (decompression illness, see page 178), the diver will very rarely be in the water. Bends occur later after ascent, unless the dive was so prolonged or so deep that instant acute cerebral decompression illness developed. In nearly all cases of bends, though, the diver will be at the surface and several minutes will have passed. Urgent transport to a recompression facility is needed.

7. Bit (or stung)

A major bite, such as from a shark or barracuda, will be obvious, but a sting may be less so. Check for the mark of the poisoner – look for welts, discoloured streaks and tentacles on exposed areas, urchin spines in any area (spines penetrate suits and fins), and the puncture wounds of scorpionfish. Apply vinegar to welts and hot water to puncture stings (see page 293).

In all the above instances, contact a diving physician urgently. Administer basic first aid until professional assistance is available.

DO THE PAPERWORK

Having controlled breathing, bleeding, beating, bursting, bending or bites, and got the casualty safely off for the appropriate treatment, the dive leader, or an appointed person, must now try to establish the causes that led to unconsciousness. Speak to the victim's dive buddy, the dive master, fellow divers and the dive-boat operator. Get **exact** details of the dive profile for this and any recent dives (check the diver's wrist computer, if he was wearing one) and his behaviour during the dive. Establish when the diver had his last medical and whether he had any known ailments, injuries or was taking any medication. Determine whether there was any potential for contact with marine life, explosives or electricity during the dive.

Next, do a thorough check of the casualty's equipment and list any anomalies. Keep this equipment aside for possible further analysis. Measure the air pressure remaining in the scuba cylinder. Could the diver have run out of air, or was the air supply contaminated with carbon monoxide as a result of careless or inadequate filtration? Was he using pure oxygen or a gas mix? Did he use a contents gauge and a depth gauge? Did he have a buoyancy device and, if so, had it inflated prematurely, causing an uncontrolled ascent? Was the weight belt too heavy for the diver?

Ask questions about whether the diver was familiar with the equipment used. For example, if the gear was hired, did the diver borrow a weight belt with an unfamiliar buckle release or a buoyancy jacket with a differently-positioned dump valve?

Write a full accident report for the attending DMO to assess (see page 352).

CAUSES OF UNCONSCIOUSNESS

Before preparing the accident report, it is vital to have a systematic approach in determining why unconsciousness occurred. Be methodical. A perfect performance of CPR may save a diver but, if he missed his decompression stops, he may not be out of trouble yet. To establish the cause of unconsciousness, you need to consider the following:

1. What has the diver inhaled?
Water – this could cause near-drowning (see page 229).
Oxygen – this could cause hypoxia (see page 195) or oxygen toxicity (see page 197).
Nitrogen – this could lead to nitrogen narcosis (see page 202).
Carbon dioxide – a build-up could result in carbon dioxide toxicity (see page 204).
Carbon monoxide – this could cause carbon monoxide poisoning (see page 213).
Foreign material – such as dentures or vomit.

2. What equipment was the diver using?
Scuba – what gas mixture was being used?
Rebreather – was the diver experienced in its use, or a novice?
Surface air supply or standard diving suit – what gas mixture was being supplied?

3. Is the diver injured?

Is there a visible injury to the head or body or a visible bite or sting? If hypothermia can be ruled out, remove the diver's wet suit, gloves and booties to check for penetrating stings or spines. Injuries resulting from electrical contact will involve burns.

4. Can you determine when the diver lost consciousness?

If anyone in the dive group witnessed the diver losing consciousness, it may help you to determine the cause.

On descent:
>   Chest or helmet squeeze
>   As a result of any of the causes in 1 and 3 above

At the bottom:
>   Any of the causes in 1 and 3 above

On ascent:
>   Acute decompression illness including arterial gas embolism
>   Blackout of ascent (in breathhold divers)
>   Any of the causes in 1 and 3 above

Immediately on return to the surface:
>   Arterial gas embolism
>   Bubble formation with acute decompression illness
>   Any of the causes in 1 and 3 above, except narcosis

Later after surfacing:
>   Acute decompression illness
>   Arterial gas embolism
>   Any of the causes in 3 above.

5. What is the diver's temperature?

When the diver was first recovered, was there evidence of hypothermia (diver's body too cold or a low body temperature) or hyperthermia (diver's body too hot or an elevated temperature)?

6. Any known medical problems?

Try to establish whether the diver has experienced any of the following:
– previous heart attack or stroke,
– diabetes or low blood sugar (hypoglycaemia), or
– epilepsy.

The final presentation may be multiple, for example, a marine animal sting that causing near-drowning, followed by a missed decompression stop, leading to bends as a result of a hasty rescue attempt, plus lung damage and arterial gas embolism as a consequence of inadequate regard for exhalation during the rapid emergency ascent performed to save the diver's life.

The following table depicts the common possible causes of unconsciousness, based on where unconsciousness first occurred:

ONSET OF UNCONSCIOUSNESS					
	DESCENT	BOTTOM	ON ASCENT	AT SURFACE	AFTER DIVE
N_2 narcosis	X	X			
Hypoxia	X	X	X		
O_2 toxicity	X	X	X		
CO_2 toxicity	X	X	X		
CO poisoning	X	X	X	X	
Water inhaled	X	X	X	X	
Foreign matter	X	X	X	X	X
Pulmonary barotrauma			X	X	X
Decompression illness			X	X	X
Squeeze	X				
Marine sting				X	X
Marine bite	X	X	X	X	X
Sea snake					X
Seafood					X
Hypothermia		X	X	X	
Head injury		X	X	X	X
Electrocution		X			
Explosion		X	X	X	
Other medical	X	X	X	X	X

If unconsciousness commenced during the dive descent, the following are the usual reasons and their causes:

UNCONSCIOUSNESS ON DESCENT USING SCUBA	
N_2 narcosis	Deep air dive, wrong nitrox mix
Hypoxia	Cylinder empty, faulty regulator, wrong mix
O_2 toxicity	Pure oxygen, Nitrox, Heliox, Trimix
CO_2 toxicity	Air contamination, tight gear, dense nitrox
CO poisoning	Air contamination
Water inhaled	Panic, alcohol, equipment problem, coughing
Foreign matter	Dentures, vomit
Squeeze	Rapid negative descent with regulator failure
Marine bite	Shark, barracuda, grouper; etc.
Other medical	Epilepsy, diabetes, heart attack, stroke

If unconsciousness commenced at the bottom, the following are the usual reasons and their causes:

UNCONSCIOUSNESS AT BOTTOM USING SCUBA	
N_2 narcosis	Deep air dive, wrong nitrox mix
Hypoxia	Cylinder empty, faulty regulator, wrong mix
O_2 toxicity	Pure oxygen; nitrox; heliox; trimix
CO_2 toxicity	Air contamination, tight gear, dense nitrox mix, strenuous exercise, skip breathing
CO poisoning	Air contamination
Water inhaled	Panic, alcohol, equipment problem, coughing
Foreign matter	Dentures, vomit
Marine bite	Shark, barracuda, grouper etc.
Other medical	Epilepsy, diabetes, heart attack, stroke
Head injury	Wreck, cave diving
Hypothermia	Alcohol, inadequate insulation, ice diving
Electrocution	Contact with underwater cables, welding
Explosion	Explosives in wrecks, setting explosives

If unconsciousness commenced during ascent, the following are the usual reasons and their causes:

UNCONSCIOUSNESS ON ASCENT USING SCUBA	
Arterial gas embolism	Inadequate exhalation, tight gear, rapid ascent, asthma, respiratory infection, patent foramen ovale
Tension pneumothorax	Inadequate exhalation, tight gear, rapid ascent; asthma, respiratory infection
Acute decompression illness	Rapid ascent with substantial gas load and missed decompression stops
Hypoxia	Cylinder empty, faulty regulator, wrong mix
O_2 toxicity	Pure oxygen, nitrox, heliox, trimix
CO_2 toxicity	Air contamination, tight gear, dense nitrox mix, strenuous exercise, skip breathing
CO poisoning	Air contamination
Water inhaled	Panic, alcohol, equipment problem, coughing
Foreign matter	Dentures, vomit
Marine bite	Shark, barracuda, grouper etc.
Other medical	Epilepsy, diabetes, heart attack, stroke
Head injury	Wreck or cave diving
Hypothermia	Alcohol, inadequate insulation, ice diving
Explosion	Too short fuse after setting explosives

If unconsciousness commenced on surfacing after the dive, the following are the usual reasons and their causes:

UNCONSCIOUSNESS AT THE SURFACE USING SCUBA	
Arterial gas embolism	Inadequate exhalation, tight gear, rapid ascent, asthma, respiratory infection, patent foramen ovale
Tension pneumothorax	Inadequate exhalation, tight gear, rapid ascent, asthma, respiratory infection
Acute decompression illness	Rapid ascent with substantial gas load and missed decompression stops
CO poisoning	Air contamination – persisting effect
Water inhaled	Panic, alcohol, strong currents, coughing
Foreign matter	Dentures, vomit
Marine bite	Shark, barracuda, grouper etc.
Marine sting	Following vertebrate or invertebrate stings
Other medical	Epilepsy, diabetes, heart attack, stroke
Hypothermia	Alcohol, inadequate insulation, ice diving
Head injury	Collision with boat, rocks
Explosion	Too short fuse after setting explosives

If unconsciousness commenced after the dive, the following are the usual reasons and their causes:

UNCONSCIOUSNESS FOLLOWING SCUBA DIVING	
Arterial gas embolism	Occurs immediately or very soon after diving
Tension pneumothorax	Occurs very soon after diving
Mediastinal emphysema	Compression of heart and lung function, occurs soon after diving
Acute decompression illness	Majority of cases occur within 30 minutes after diving
Marine bite	Shark, barracuda, grouper etc.
Marine sting	Following vertebrate or invertebrate stings
Snake bite	Occurs soon after diving, bite may be painless
Other medical	Epilepsy, diabetes, heart attack, stroke
Head injury	May be delayed after head injury underwater
Seafood	Ingestion of poisonous or contaminated seafood

Emergency management of an unconscious diver

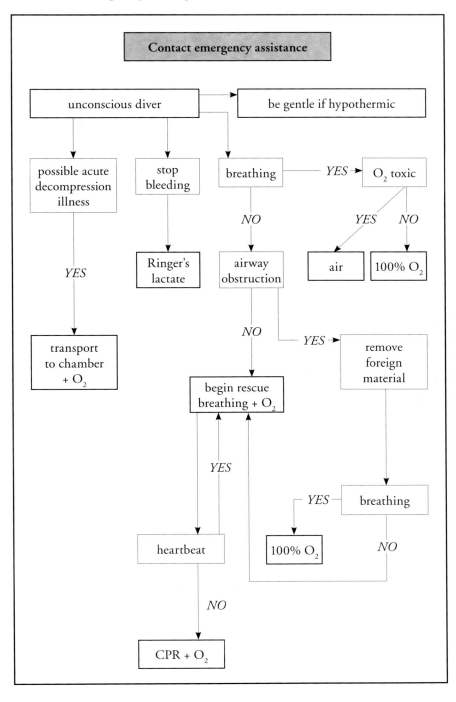

 **42**

EMERGENCY PROTOCOL
FOR DIVER RESCUE

In an emergency situation, someone needs to take control. Amidst the chaos and panic that tends to accompany any crisis, there has to be one person keeping a clear head, monitoring what is happening and able to relay accurate and relevant information to the next link in the rescue chain. While a 'simple' rescue might involve no more than the diver, his buddy and the boat operator, a complicated emergency at sea may require teams of specialists from a variety of disciplines – technical divers, EMTs, helicopter pilots, traffic officials, hyperbaric chamber staff and medical personnel. Then there are the bystanders, sometimes just gawking, often willing to help, but always needing to be prevented from interfering with the rescue.

What role each individual plays will depend on his or her skills and competence, the moment at which one arrives on the scene and the extent of involvement in the incident. If it is just you and your buddy, you have to step up, no matter what, but if an emergency occurs in a large group, you may have to make a quick decision about where you can be most effective, taking into account the situation as well as your own abilities and the abilities of other people present.

If an emergency involves someone you are close to, it is often best to let a neutral person take control, as emotion may prevent you from acting rationally.

Trained rescue divers spend hours going through drills and preparing for the day when they have to do it for real. Recreational divers can do their bit by paying attention during safety briefings, making sure they check and double-check their equipment and that of their dive buddy, and by diligently sticking to the agreed dive plan.

But accidents can, and do, happen. When you are faced with a diving emergency you may have to rely on those hours spent in training to get you through. So, even if you skip some of the other chapters in this book, make sure that you read this one thoroughly, and often!

Do not become part of the emergency!
Willingness to help is all very well, but if you are not competent to cope
with the situation, you could find yourself needing to be rescued as well.
Many tragedies have occurred when one rescue incident has turned into two.
Don't let it be you!

NOTE: The information in this chapter is not set out in 'sequence'. In an emergency, there are many variables, and it is almost impossible for a book to describe precisely what has to be done, at what moment and by whom. Familiarise yourself with all the information given here. You never know what function you may have to fulfil when an emergency occurs; the best you can do is to be prepared for all eventualities.

TAKE CONTROL OF THE SITUATION

(a) Ensure that the casualty and the rescuers are in a safe place. Divers should be out of the water and beyond any wave or tidal action of the sea, or on the deck of the dive boat. Check for the presence of any other hazards, such as traffic.

(b) Determine whether anyone at the site is CPR-trained.

(c) **Check the casualty's airway, breathing and circulation** (ABC).

(d) **Check for signs of external injuries.**

(e) If there is visible bleeding, apply pressure and pack any wounds to control the bleeding.

(f) Commence rescue breathing and/or CPR if required.

(g) Appoint someone to act as a contact person to summon trained help.

(h) Appoint an assistant (preferably two people if available) to assist you with hands-on resuscitation.

(i) Try to determine whether the casualty belongs to a diver rescue service and obtain the local contact number.

ESSENTIAL INFORMATION TO BE CONVEYED BY THE CONTACT PERSON

In the course of the rescue operation, essential information about the casualty may be required by a large number of people: the emergency call centre operator, diver rescue service, hospital admissions desk, diving medical officer (DMO), hyperbaric chamber operator, medical aid call centre etc.

Before you make any calls, **write down the details** (see next page); don't hope that you will remember them when you are on the phone.

EMERGENCY TELEPHONE NUMBERS

Space is provided on page 368 for a personal list of emergency numbers.
Ensure that you have the applicable numbers programmed into your
cell phone and easily accessible near your phone at home.
Keep a written copy of all your emergency contact information in a waterproof (zip-lock) bag in your dive bag, first-aid kit, vehicle cubby-hole etc.

The first call you make will be to summon emergency services. Take a deep breath before you dial. It is essential that you keep calm and relay all the relevant information clearly and accurately.

(a) Name and telephone number (with area code) of the contact person.

(b) Name, age, gender and telephone/cell number of the casualty.

(c) Approximate nature and severity of the emergency:
  – whether the emergency is life-threatening and whether resuscitation (CPR and/or emergency oxygen) is required,
  – number of people requiring assistance,
  – ability of those on hand to render interim assistance, and
  – whether a hyperbaric chamber is likely to be required (state that it is a scuba diving emergency).

(d) Location of casualty or incident:
  – If you are at sea, state where you intend to come ashore (harbour, launch site, etc.).
  – If in an urban environment, give the full street address or, failing that, the suburb and nearest cross streets or prominent landmarks.
  – If in a remote location, give the nearest town or village, or identify prominent landmarks. Try to indicate the direction and/or distance (e.g. south of the river mouth; turn-off is three kilometres after the general store, etc.).

(e) Details of the casualty's membership particulars with a diver rescue service and/or medical aid or emergency medical insurance cover (have membership details on hand if possible).

(g) Names and details of casualty's next of kin or other emergency contacts. If the casualty is a member of DAN or any other diver rescue service, you should be able to obtain their personal particulars from its call centre or central register, as well as determine whether they have any known illnesses or are on any medication or treatment.

Once you have made the initial call, ensure that someone reliable remains at the telephone in case the emergency service needs to call back to locate you. Regardless of whether you are using a landline or mobile phone, **do not** tie up that line with non-essential calls. If your only access is by a landline some distance away, or you have to travel to get a mobile signal, you may need a to appoint a 'runner' to relay information between the primary rescuer/s and the contact person.

If your location is not easy to find, you may need to appoint helpers to direct the rescue personnel to the scene. They should wait at an agreed landmark or crossroad and must make themselves clear to any rescue services who are rushing to assist.

ON-SITE MANAGEMENT IF NO PARAMEDIC IS AVAILABLE

If you have to take control of the situation until trained emergency personnel arrive, it is important to act systematically, and endeavour to provide treatment that is appropriate for the casualty's condition.

(a) Casualty fully conscious:
   - Reassure the casualty.
   - Lie the casualty flat (take great care not to aggravate any neck or spinal injury).
   - Encourage consumption of oral fluids (150 ml of water per hour). Do not give fluids orally if abdominal or chest trauma has occurred.
   - Give 100 per cent oxygen by regulator or face mask if available.

(b) Casualty unconscious, but breathing:
   - Lie flat in left lateral position (see page 232) to avoid the risk of inhaling any vomit.
   - Ensure airways are clear and chin is supported (see page 231).
   - Give 100 per cent oxygen by regulator or face mask.
   - Monitor pulse and breathing.
   - Be ready to perform CPR (see page 235) if no heartbeat is detected. (AIDS warning!)

(c) Casualty receiving CPR (i.e. unconscious/not breathing and no evidence of a pulse):
   - Continue CPR until trained help arrives.
   - Use 100 per cent oxygen if available.
   - Use a ventilation bag if available. Otherwise, the person administering rescue breathing should inhale oxygen from a face mask before each mouth-to-mouth breath to the casualty. An assistant can hold the mask for the person in charge of airway and breathing.

(d) Definite victim of marine animal sting:
   - Injury caused by stinging spines: immerse limb in hot water or apply hot packs (as hot as helpers can reasonably bear), taking care that you do not scald the casualty.
   - Sting not caused by spines: pour vinegar onto the wound and apply a hot vinegar poultice.
   - Watch the casualty carefully and be prepared to commence prolonged rescue breathing at any time.

(e) Definite victim of sea snake bite:
- Immobilise affected limb and keep limb below level of heart.
- Casualty must lie absolutely still. **No walking about.**
- Apply a tourniquet above the wound on limb bites. Note the time. The contact person must inform the paramedics, diving medical officer or hospital that a tourniquet has been applied, notify them of the time and request advice on how long to maintain it. It **must** be removed after two hours maximum in any event.
- Keep casualty warm and give fluids. No alcohol.
- If possible, keep the sea snake for identification.

ON-SITE ACTION IF PARAMEDICALLY TRAINED

(a) Ensure access and safety of the site.
(b) Control **Airway, Breathing, Circulation** and **Bleeding**.
(c) **Administer 100 per cent oxygen** by demand valve/breathing bag.
(d) Once the casualty is stable, perform field neurological assessment.
(e) Unless the cause of the incident is clear, assess possibilities:
- Hyperbaric disease
    acute decompression illness (see page 178)
    pulmonary barotrauma (see page 160)
    AGE (see page 164)
- Non-hyperbaric disease
    near-drowning (see page 229)
    marine animal bite (page 278) or sting (see page 287)
    hypoxia (see page 195)
    oxygen toxicity (see page 197)
    carbon dioxide (see page 204) or monoxide toxicity (see page 212)
    hypothermia (see page 258)
    heat exhaustion and/or heat stroke (see pages 256–257)
    electrical injuries or explosives (see page 305)
    undetermined diver injury.
(f) **Obtain medical history:** heart disease, hypertension, hypoglycaemia or diabetes (assess using finger-prick Dextrostix), epilepsy, current medications, recent use of drugs or alcohol, date of last diving medical.
(g) **Establish IV line:**
- For trauma: use Ringer's lactate and Haemaccel (maximum dose Haemaccel 1500 ml, thereafter alternate with blood 1:1). Rate to depend on degree of blood loss and shock.
- For acute decompression illness and AGE: use Ringer's lactate. Request advice from a diving physician re possible use of Dextran 40 (Rheomacrodex) – 500 ml in first half-hour then 1000 ml over an 8-hour period (maximum total dose 2 g/kg bm).

- In non-diving, non-trauma cases: use 5% glucose. With hypoglycaemia confirmed with glucose stick on finger-prick blood, infuse 50 ml of 50% glucose into the IV line.

(h) **Administer medication:**
- Do not give sedatives (e.g. Valium), without permission from diving medical officer (DMO).
- No aspirin or anticoagulants (heparin) with spinal or vestibular bends or pulmonary barotrauma. These may precipitate bleeding and worsen the victim's condition.
- No steroids (e.g. Decadron, Dexamethasone) without permission from the DMO. These can worsen acute spinal and cerebral decompression illness.
- Ascorbic acid (Vitamin C) 1000 mg may be given orally.
- With non-hyperbaric disease, administer drugs as per EMA protocol.

(i) **Monitor urine output:** note volume; if trained, insert a urinary catheter if the casualty is unconscious or if urinary retention is present.

EVACUATING A CASUALTY

Ideally, decisions about the mode of evacuation will be made by the emergency rescue service. Depending on the type of injury or ailment, the severity of the case, geographical location, cost limitations, membership of DAN or other medical cover, the rescue service will tell the contact person what has to be done to ensure the evacuation. They will also inform the contact person of the availability of DMOs, hyperbaric chambers, hospital facilities, etc.

If this information is not forthcoming, any decisions regarding evacuation should be made by the dive leader, following evacuation plans prepared in advance, and in accordance with standard dive training protocol.

TRANSPORT OPTIONS FOR EVACUATION

Road transport Travel time may be long and, depending on the state of the roads, the journey could be bumpy, but the costs are low. If a one-man decompression chamber is anticipated, there must be enough room in the vehicle for the chamber plus the operator.

Helicopter Travel time is short. Costs are high. Low flying is possible without pressurisation. If a decompression chamber is needed, it must fit inside the helicopter. A suitable landing site must be available.

Fixed-wing aircraft Travel time is short. Costs are high. If a chamber is required, the aircraft must either be pressurised or be able to fly at a low altitude. A suitable airstrip or landing field is necessary, and the state of any roads leading to it must be taken into account.

When contemplating the evacuation of a casualty, the following procedures apply:

(a) Consider the location of the incident in relation to how easy it is to access the site by road, as well as the distance by road to the nearest medical facility. Estimate the amount of time it will take to get there by road.

Consider the suitability of the site for helicopter landing, and/or the proximity of the site to the nearest landing strip for fixed-wing aircraft. Remember also to take account of the distance the casualty may have to travel by road from the arrival site (e.g. an airport) to the hospital or intended destination.

If you are diving inland, the flight controller or pilot may need to know the physical altitude of your location.

(b) Choose the most practical transport mode according to the accessibility of the site, estimated distance and travelling time to the medical facility, and extent of the medical urgency (see previous page).

(c) Obtain the street address and telephone number of the nearest suitably equipped hospital, ambulance service and police station.

(d) Notify a DMO. Ask whether the doctor wishes to travel to the casualty or will meet the casualty at the hospital or other agreed location.

(e) Notify the nearest decompression facility.

(f) Ensure that **all** the equipment used by the diver has been collected for expert assessment and analysis. This must be delivered to the responsible authority, hospital, decompression facility or, in the event of death, to the police.

(g) Prepare a detailed report for the DMO or other attending physician. Obtain exact details from the casualty and/or his or her dive buddies regarding the circumstances of the dive on which the incident occurred, recent dives, all equipment used, hazards encountered and rescue techniques used.

DECOMPRESSION USING A ONE-MAN CHAMBER

A one-man decompression chamber should be used with extreme caution, and only after discussion with DMO.

Indications:

(a) Acute skin or limb decompression illness.

(b) Acute severe decompression illness (use chamber only if DMO advises). The therapeutic schedule will have to be aborted if the victim vomits with inhalation of vomit, becomes confused or loses consciousness during pressurisation.

(c) Carbon monoxide poisoning.

Contraindications:

(a) Unconscious or confused hyperbaric casualty.

(b) Pneumothorax.

Check the following before the casualty enters the chamber:

(a) Chamber fully functional, and all hoses clean and grease-free.
(b) Adequate HP air for blowdown and flushing at 18 msw.
(c) Adequate oxygen for at least three hours under pressure.
(d) Couplings to inlets:
  - Chamber pressure using air inlet coupling, and
  - Face mask oxygen inlet coupling.
(e) Couplings to outlets:
  - chamber exhaust,
  - overboard oxygen dump, and
  - pneumofathometer.
(f) Communications functional.

Once all the pre-checks have been completed: remove all IV lines from the casualty. At this stage, reconsider the need for a one-man chamber pressurisation schedule versus rapid transportation to a hyperbaric facility using oxygen at surface pressure.

- Place the casualty in the chamber after removing his or her shoes and all metal objects (including watch, jewellery and coins). Explain what you are doing and reassure the casualty. Instruct the casualty on the need for middle ear equalisation during repressurisation.
- Open the oxygen supply and fit the oxygen demand mask to the casualty's face. Ensure that the head straps are properly positioned and that the inlet and overboard dumps are functional – ask the casualty to breathe.
- Close the hatch. Inform the casualty that pressurisation will commence and request acknowledgement. **Note the time.**
- Begin slow pressurisation to 18 msw using **air**. Ensure that the hatch has a good seal. Watch the casualty constantly to ensure that he or she is equalising adequately. If the casualty cannot equalise, **stop** pressurisation and open the exhaust valve until the casualty signals relief. If the casualty is still unable to equalise on recommencing pressurisation, exhaust the chamber, remove the casualty, replace the IV lines and give 100 per cent oxygen by demand valve.
- With successful pressurisation to 18 msw:
  - Note the time and start the stopwatch.
  - Inform the casualty that pressurisation was successful and that decompression will now begin. Give reassurance.
- Use the therapeutic decompression schedule as outlined in US Navy Table 5 (see page 343) or Royal Navy Table 61 (see page 333). Observe all air breaks carefully.
- Observe the casualty constantly for any deterioration and request him or her to report any worsening or improvement.

- Keep communications short and clear and avoid unnecessary chatter. Keep coms **from** the chamber open constantly. Ensure coms **to** the casualty is off except when the chamber operator is giving instructions. The casualty must not hear idle chatter or unguarded comments about his or her condition.
- Keep a close watch on the chamber pressure. As the casualty's body heat warms the chamber, the chamber pressure will begin rising (Amontons' Law). Use the exhaust valve to maintain 18 msw depth.
- Flush the chamber smoothly every 10 minutes by simultaneous slow partial opening of both air inlet and exhaust valves for 15 seconds. Ensure that the chamber pressure stays at 18 msw. **Do not violently pressurise or vent the chamber.**
- Maintain a close watch for possible oxygen toxicity.
- Instruct the casualty to hyperventilate chamber air if oxygen toxicity is suspected. **Do not bring a convulsing casualty to surface pressure.** Wait for the convulsion to pass before commencing ascent.
- Evacuation must commence when the casualty is stable at 18 msw. Transport the casualty to the appropriate facility (such as a decompression unit or suitably equipped hospital). Notify the facility of your ETA, the casualty's condition, treatment given and anticipated requirements. En route to the facility, monitor the casualty continuously.
- At the decompression facility, the DMO will decide whether to:
  - continue with the 18 msw table, or
  - transfer the casualty under pressure into a therapeutic chamber for further hyperbaric treatment.
- Prepare a full written report about the event (see Diving Accident Report Form on page 352).

43

NEUROLOGICAL ASSESSMENT

The following protocol can be used as a guideline for on-site neurological assessment, which may be required following a head injury, suspected stroke, marine animal sting, inhaled gas problem, near-drowning, hypothermia, exposure to electricity or explosives, coma or acute decompression illness. If physical trauma is suspected, immobilise the neck and spine and take great care when moving the casualty.

The requirement for a neurological assessment arises whenever an abnormality occurs in any of the three major aspects required for normal brain function, i.e.:

- highest brain faculties: self-awareness, thought, speech, reading and writing,
- motor system: movement, muscle power and co-ordination, and
- sensory system: sight, sound, taste, smell, fine and coarse touch, pressure, hot and cold appreciation, body position awareness, vibration sense and pain sensitivity.

In the event of any abnormality being detected in a diving-related case, the casualty must be treated as if he or she is a case of acute decompression illness, including pulmonary barotrauma (see page 160).

Neurological assessments of an unconscious diver should be repeated every 15 minutes and assessments of a conscious diver at one-hour intervals. These assessments should be performed by the person most qualified to do so under the prevailing circumstances. This might be a dive buddy, dive leader, a paramedic or a non-hyperbaric doctor.

In all cases, an official Diving Medical Officer (DMO) must be contacted as soon as possible in order to obtain specialised on-site guidance and ensure that the case is properly managed.

Any neurological deficit will necessitate urgent hospitalisation. The decision on whether the casualty requires a hyperbaric or non-hyperbaric facility will depend on the quality of the information that is conveyed to the DMO, who has the final responsibility of deciding the future management of the case. All the neurological assessment reports should be handed to the doctor in charge at the hospital.

Depending on whether or not the casualty is conscious, there are different ways in which to make a neurological assessment.

ASSESSMENT OF AN UNCONSCIOUS DIVER

The **Glasgow coma scale** is widely used to assess an individual's level or depth of unconsciousness. Points are given as shown below. A fully conscious person will score 15 points, while a deeply unconscious person will score just three points.

To assess response to pain in a comatose person, a normally painful stimulus must be given. Firmly squeezing the Achilles tendon between thumb and forefinger for two seconds will suffice. Any painful stimulus normally causes limb withdrawal from the source of pain, i.e. the knee and hip joints flex. This is called a flexion response. If the limb thrusts straight out following a painful stimulus, this is an abnormal 'extension to pain' response. Any response must be noted as indicated below.

Glasgow Coma Scale

Eye opening	Score
Spontaneous	4
Responds to speech	3
Responds to pain	2
None	1
Verbal response	
Oriented	5
Confused	4
Inappropriate words	3
Incomprehensible sounds	2
None	1
Motor response	
Obeys commands	6
Localises to pain	5
Flexion to pain	4
Abnormal flexion	3
Extension to pain	2
None	1
	Score 3–15

In addition to the casualty's responses to the Glasgow coma scale tests, the following must be checked and monitored in an unconscious casualty:

1. Pupillary responses

Comparing the pupils with a nearby person's eyes, are they:

(a) Normal in size?

(b) Equal in size?

(c) Do the pupils:

   (d) Contract when a light is shone into them?

   (e) Contract together, and equally, when a light is shone into each of them?

2. Pulse rate

Monitor the pulse rate. A very rapid but weak pulse indicates circulatory shock. A very slow pulse may indicate increased pressure on the brain within the skull.

3. Blood pressure

Monitor this if possible. Increasing or decreasing blood pressure must be noted.

4. Respiratory rate

Monitor the number of breaths per minute. Note any increase or decrease in the casualty's respiratory rate.

5. Temperature

Monitor rectally if possible. Increasing or decreasing temperature must be noted.

Repeat and record all these observations every 15 minutes while consciousness is reduced, or confusion and disorientation are present. When the casualty is fully conscious, repeat these observations at hourly intervals.

Pinpoint or unequal pupil size, slowing of the pulse and respiratory rate, and an increase in blood pressure indicate increased intracranial pressure on the brain.

ASSESSMENT OF A CONSCIOUS DIVER

If the diver is conscious, proceed with the neurological evaluation as indicated in the neurological assessment form on the following pages. Tick the appropriate block in each section.

NEUROLOGICAL ASSESSMENT FORM

1. C.O.M.A. (Consciousness, Orientation, Memory, Arithmetic)

CONSCIOUSNESS	YES	NO		Is the diver experiencing seizures?
ORIENTATION Time	YES	NO		Ask the diver: 'what is the time?' 'what day is it?'
Place	YES	NO		Ask the diver: 'where are you?'
Person	YES	NO		Ask the diver: 'what is your name?'
MEMORY Immediate	YES	NO		Ask diver to repeat: 11, 3, 79, 8.
Recent	YES	NO		Ask the diver: 'where do you stay?', 'what did you last eat?'
Remote	YES	NO		Ask the diver: 'what is you phone number?', 'where do you work?'
ARITHMETIC	YES	NO		Ask diver to subtract serial 7s from 100.

2. EYES

SIGHT NORMAL IN BOTH EYES	YES	NO		Can he count 2–4 fingers, one eye at a time? Can he read this page?
PUPIL LIGHT REFLEX NORMAL	YES	NO		Are the pupils equal in size? Do they contract in a bright light?
ACCOMMODATION NORMAL	YES	NO		Are the pupils larger on looking far, smaller on looking close?
EYE MOVEMENTS NORMAL	YES	NO		Can both eyes follow a moving finger up, down, L and R? Check for any rapid abnormal jerking movements, up, down or sideways (nystagmus).

3. FACE

FACIAL MOVEMENTS NORMAL ON BOTH SIDES	YES	NO		Can he or she close/open eyes, wrinkle forehead, smile, clench teeth tightly (feel that the jaw muscles do tighten).
FACIAL SENSATION NORMAL ON BOTH SIDES	YES	NO		Can he or she feel a light touch on both sides of chin, cheeks, nose and forehead?

4. HEARING AND SPEECH

HEARING NORMAL IN BOTH EARS	YES	NO		Can he hear two fingers rubbed 5 cm from each ear in a quiet place?
SPEECH INTACT	YES	NO		Is there any huskiness? Are there any misplaced words or slurring?

5. TONGUE					
TONGUE MOVEMENT NORMAL	YES		NO		Can he or she put out the tongue and move it L and R. Check for deviation to one side?

6. TASTE AND SMELL					
TASTE NORMAL	YES		NO		Can he or she taste sweet (sugar), salty (salt) and sour (lemon)?
SMELL NORMAL	YES		NO		Can he or she smell coffee, garlic, vinegar with each nostril?

7. SWALLOWING REFLEX					
SWALLOWING NORMAL	YES		NO		Watch the larynx move up and down as the diver swallows.

8. MUSCLE POWER					
SHOULDER MOVEMENTS EQUAL AND NORMAL	YES		NO		Press down on the diver's shoulders and ask the diver to shrug. Look for equal power on both sides.
GRIP	YES		NO		Can he or she firmly grasp two of your fingers? Check that R and L grip are more or less similar.
ARMS	YES		NO		Can he or she pull and push against resistance with both arms and with similar power?
LEGS	YES		NO		Can he or she lift, part and push legs together against resistance?

9. RANGE OF MOVEMENTS

Check that the diver can move all limbs equally and easily in all directions – up, down, outwards and inwards. Check that each joint can be fully flexed and extended.

SHOULDERS	YES		NO	
ELBOWS	YES		NO	
WRISTS	YES		NO	
HIPS	YES		NO	
KNEES	YES		NO	
ANKLES	YES		NO	
SPINE	YES		NO	

10. MUSCLE TONE				
SPASTIC	YES	NO		Are one or more limbs very stiff or fixed in flexion or extension?
FLACCID	YES	NO		Are one or more limbs very floppy when lifted and allowed to drop?

11. SENSORY FUNCTION

Use a cotton wool ball for light sensation; the point of pin or injection needle for sharp sensation; the back of pin or injection needle for dull sensation; tuning fork (middle C) for vibration sense.
Are all modalities of sensation intact in:

HANDS	YES	NO		Back of hands; base of thumbs; base of 5th fingers.
ARMS	YES	NO		Back of arms; front of arms.
TORSO	YES	NO		Back of torso; front of torso.
LEGS	YES	NO		Front of legs; back of legs.
FEET	YES	NO		Tops of feet; soles of feet.

12. COORDINATION (cerebellar function)

POINT ORIENTATION *(Test both hands)*	YES	NO		Using an index finger, can the diver touch an object in front of him or her.
FINGER-NOSE TEST *(Test both hands)*	YES	NO		Can the diver rapidly touch his or her nose, then your finger held in front of him/her?
GAIT NORMAL	YES	NO		Check for wobbly legs, stagger, unsteadiness, walking heel-to-toe.
BALANCE (RHOMBERG) *(Normal answer is NO)*	YES	NO		Does the diver sway when standing with eyes shut, arms crossed and feet together?

13. LIMB REFLEXES

Use a patellar hammer or a blunt object. Test both sides.

KNEES	YES	NO		With the knee flexed and relaxed, tap the tendon below the kneecap. The lower leg should jerk up.
ANKLES	YES	NO		Pull the foot upward and tap the Achilles tendon. The foot should jerk down.

BICEPS	YES		NO		Rest the diver's arm on his or her lap. Place your free thumb in front of the diver's elbow and tap your thumb. The lower arm should jerk up.
TRICEPS	YES		NO		Rest the diver's arm on his or her lap. Tap the tendon just above the elbow. The lower arm should jerk down.

14. BABINSKI RESPONSE

This is an abnormal reflex. It indicates brain damage. Run a blunt object up the soles of the feet. A normal response is curling down of the toes. A Babinski response is an upward movement of the big toe with the other toes fanning out.

BABINSKI RESPONSE	YES		NO		

FINAL ASESSMENT

Note all abnormal findings here:

44

THERAPEUTIC OXYGEN TABLES

Therapeutic oxygen tables are used to recompress and then decompress divers suffering from acute decompression illness, including arterial gas embolism, as well as to treat divers with carbon monoxide poisoning.

Worldwide, the most commonly used therapeutic oxygen tables are those supplied by the Royal Navy (RN) or US Navy (USN). The decompression times of their equivalent tables are identical. In South Africa, USN tables are often used. (Note that the US tables are calibrated in feet, not metres.)

The choice of which table to use traditionally depends upon the circumstances of the specific case:
- With mild skin-only or pain-only DCI – Table 5 (USN) or Table 61 (RN).
- With more severe or neurological DCI – Table 6 (USN) or Table 62 (RN).
- With definite arterial gas embolism – Table 6A (USN) or Table 63 (RN); however, many dive doctors prefer to use Table 6 or Table 62 in the management of arterial gas embolism (see page 164).

CLASSIC OXYGEN THERAPEUTIC TABLES

US NAVY	ROYAL NAVY	DECOMPRESSION TIME
Table 5	Table 61	2 hrs and 15 mins
Table 6	Table 62	4 hrs and 45 minutes
Table 6A	Table 63	5 hrs and 19 minutes

Signs and symptoms traditionally determine the choice of treatment protocols. For example, USN Table 5 is used for mild or pain-only decompression illness (DCI) when complete resolution occurs within 10 minutes at 18 msw. When more serious decompression illness occurs, or when mild decompression illness fails to resolve within 10 minutes at 18 msw, USN Table 6 is the traditional default.

The current trend is the use of the longer Table 6 in the treatment of milder cases of decompression illness. The rationale is that any neurological signs associated with apparently mild decompression illness may be vague and escape initial diagnosis by the attending dive medical officer (DMO).

Because of the largely non-invasive nature of recompression therapy, it is safest to assume that even mild symptoms may precede more serious and progressive decompression illness. The current therapeutic trend advocates the use of USN Table 6 for both initial and follow-up treatments, as well as arterial gas embolism.

USN Table 6 or RN Table 62 are preferred over USN Table 6A or RN Table 63, neither of which is currently in popular use, for the following reasons:

- Nitrogen narcosis may seriously compromise the efficiency of the attendant and the DMO at the initial chamber depth of 50 msw (165 fsw).
- A substantial inert gas burden is delivered to both casualty and attendant, which may result in extreme decompression difficulties in the event of an incomplete recovery at 50 msw.
- Table 6A has received the reputation of being a 'tender bender', as the likelihood of the attendant developing decompression illness is high unless he or she also breathes oxygen from 9 msw (30 fsw) during the ascent to the surface.
- As the duration of gas bubbles in the cerebral circulation is likely to be short, due to the powerful vasodilatation reflex which they stimulate, there is probably little need to use the pressure provided at 50 msw to reduce bubble size and allow them to pass into the venous circulation.
- The use of Table 6A is now reserved for those casualties who present with rapid onset of severe symptoms following dives with minimal inert gas uptake and who show no significant improvement, or are continuing to deteriorate after compression to 18 msw breathing oxygen.
- This means that Table 6A will rarely be used, except following submarine escape-training ascents or when 50/50 heliox is unavailable.

In addition to the three groups of tables named above, the need may occasionally arise for more complex management. These much longer tables require the use of air, nitrox or heliox and have been included for completeness.

ROYAL NAVY THERAPEUTIC TABLES

A number of tables are in current use, depending on circumstances, for the treatment of acute decompression illness. The initial options are usually the Royal Navy Tables 61, 62 and 63. For more complex cases, Tables 64, 66 and 67 are provided. These tables are acknowledged as in use with the Royal Navy and this information is offered without prejudice.

SHORT OXYGEN RECOMPRESSION THERAPY
(TABLE 61)

This table may be used for the management of missed decompression and should be considered for the treatment of acute decompression illness with limb pain, cutaneous or lymphatic manifestations ONLY.

In cases of decompression illness (DCI), the casualty should be given a careful neurological examination so that involvement of the nervous system, in particular, can be excluded.

PROCEDURE FOR TABLE 61:

1. The casualty starts breathing oxygen on the surface.
2. Descend to 18 msw over one or two minutes, stopping only if the casualty or attendant have difficulty in clearing their ears.
3. The time of the treatment starts on reaching 18 msw.
4. If the symptoms of decompression illness are completely relieved within 10 minutes, decompression may proceed in accordance with Table 61. Otherwise use Table 62. In practical terms, this will mean that only a minority of cases will complete Table 61.
5. The attendant should breathe oxygen during the oxygen period at 9 msw and during the ascent to the surface.

Table 61: Short oxygen recompression therapy

Gauge depth (msw)	Stops/ascent (minutes)	Elapsed time (hours and mins)	Rate of ascent (msw/minute)
18	20 (O$_2$)	00:00 – 00:20	–
18	5 (Air)	00:20 – 00:25	–
18	20 (O$_2$)	00:25 – 00:45	–
18–9	30 (O$_2$)	00:45 – 01:15	3 m in 10 min
9	5 (Air)	01:15 – 01:20	–
9	20 (O$_2$)	01:20 – 01:40	–
9	5 (Air)	01:40 – 01:45	–
9–0	30 (O$_2$)	01:45 – 02:15	3 m in 10 min
Surface		02:15	

STANDARD OXYGEN RECOMPRESSION THERAPY (TABLE 62)

This table is used for the great majority of cases of decompression illness which do not meet the criteria required for short oxygen recompression therapy.

PROCEDURE FOR TABLE 62:

1. The casualty starts breathing oxygen on the surface.
2. Descend to 18 msw over one or two minutes, stopping only if the casualty or attendant have difficulty in clearing their ears.
3. Timing of the treatment starts on reaching 18 msw.
4. Upon reaching 18 msw, the casualty must be re-assessed. This assessment should take no more than two to three minutes and, in most cases, will reveal the casualty's condition to have stabilised or be starting to improve. However, very occasionally, casualties who have presented with serious symptoms arising shortly after surfacing, especially after very deep dives, rapid uncontrolled

ascents or submarine escape may fail to improve or continue to deteriorate at 18 msw. In all such cases, other than those following submarine escape-training ascents, the chamber should be compressed to 30 msw on air with the casualty breathing 50/50 heliox. Decompression will then normally be completed using Table 67.

Submarine escape trainees (and divers in cases where 50/50 heliox is not available) who continue to deteriorate after initial compression to 18 msw on oxygen should be compressed to 50 msw on air breathing 32.5:67.5 $O_2:N_2$. Decompression will then normally be completed using Table 63.

In ALL such cases it is essential to contact a Diving Medical Specialist. In very rare cases, continued deterioration may require transfer to Table 64 or 65.

5. If the symptoms have remained static or improved incompletely after three 20-minute periods on 100 per cent oxygen at 18 msw, Table 62 may be extended. One, two or three further oxygen breathing periods, separated by a five-minute air break, may be added on the advice of a diving medicine specialist. If the symptoms or signs have not resolved after two extensions at 18 msw, seek further advice from the diving medicine specialist.

Depending upon the nature and severity of the symptoms or signs, it may be necessary to transfer the casualty to Table 64.

Table 62: Standard oxygen recompression therapy

Gauge depth (msw)	Stops/ascent (minutes)	Elapsed time (hours and mins)	Rate of ascent (msw/minute)
18	20 (O_2)	00:00 – 00:20	–
18	5 (Air)	00:20 – 00:25	–
18	20 (O_2)	00:25 – 00:45	–
18	5 (Air)	00:45 – 00:50	–
18	20 (O_2)	00:50 – 01:10	–
18	5 (Air)	01:10 – 01:15	–
18–9	30 (O_2)	01:15 – 01:45	3 m in 10 min
9	15 (Air)	01:45 – 02:00	–
9	60 (O_2)	02:00 – 03:00	–
9	15 (Air)	03:00 – 03:15	–
9	60 (O_2)	03:15 – 04:15	–
9–0	30 (O_2)	04:15 – 04:45	3 m in 10 min
Surface		04:45	

Symptoms may recur during decompression to 9 msw. **Halt the ascent.** Recompress slowly (1 msw/min), to no deeper than 18 msw or until resolution of symptoms or signs occurs. Oxygen should be breathed throughout. Consult a diving medicine specialist.

If symptoms recur at 9 msw, consult a diving medicine specialist. Depending on the nature and severity of the symptoms, it may be necessary to return to 18 msw or extend the table at 9 msw. Table 62 may be extended for one or two one-hour oxygen breathing periods at 9 msw, separated by 15-minute air breaks.

For an unmodified Table 62, or a Table 62 with a single extension at 9 msw or 18 msw, the attendant must breathe oxygen for the last 30 minutes at 9 msw and during the ascent from 9 msw to the surface (60 minutes in total). However, if Table 62 is extended more than once, then the attendant should breathe oxygen for the whole of the final oxygen period at 9 msw and the ascent to the surface (90 minutes in total). If the attendant has undergone a hyperbaric exposure in the preceding 24 hours, he or she should undertake an additional 60 minute period breathing oxygen at 9 msw (150 minutes in total).

DEEP AIR–OXYGEN RECOMPRESSION THERAPY (TABLE 63)

The philosophy behind Table 63 is to provide an oxygen table after a brief period spent at 50 msw during which any bubbles present in the circulation, particularly of the brain, are minimised in volume through the effects of Boyle's Law (see page 21). However, there are disadvantages to employing this approach, not least of which is the difficulty of attending casualties compressed to 50 msw on air, where inert gas narcosis may severely compromise the performance of the attendant and examining physician. Furthermore, the consequence of the deep phase of the table is to deliver a substantial inert gas burden to both casualty and attendant which may impose unattractive decompression options in the event of an incomplete recovery at 50 msw.

Recent research has shown that the residence time for gas bubbles in the cerebral circulation is likely to be brief, due to the powerful vasodilatation reflex which they stimulate. Consequently, there may be little requirement to use pressure to encourage bubbles to pass into the venous circulation.

This table was developed specifically for the treatment of arterial gas embolism (see page 164). Given the difficulties in making such a diagnosis and the potential disadvantages associated with an initial compression to 50 msw, use of this table is reserved for casualties who present with a rapid onset of severe symptoms following dives with minimal inert gas uptake and who show no significant improvement, or are continuing to deteriorate, when assessed following compression to 18 msw breathing oxygen (see Table 62, Procedure 4). In practice, this means that Table 63 is seldom used, except when 50/50 heliox is unavailable .

PROCEDURE FOR TABLE 63:

1. Pressurise the chamber, without delay, with air to 50 msw at the fastest rate that can be tolerated by the casualty and attendant – up to 30 msw per minute. If a gas mixture of 32.5:67.5 O_2:N_2 is available, this should be breathed by the casualty via Built-in Breathing System (BIBS) masks.

2. If the casualty is free of symptoms and signs after 25 minutes and oxygen is available, then decompression may be commenced using Table 63. If oxygen is not available, Table 64 should be used, omitting the oxygen.

3. If there are persisting symptoms and signs after 30 minutes at 50 msw, no matter how minor, Table 64 should be used.

4. If the casualty is deteriorating at 50 msw, contact a Diving Medicine Specialist as a matter of urgency. It may be necessary to compress the casualty further and continue treatment using Table 65. This should not be contemplated unless:
   (a) a Diving Medicine Specialist is consulted, and
   (b) the chamber is capable of supporting a prolonged treatment.

5. Decompression from 50 msw to 18 msw should take four minutes, after which Table 63 proceeds as for Table 62, except that the attendant must always breathe oxygen during the final 60 minutes at 9 msw and subsequent ascent (90 minutes in total). If the attendant has had a previous hyperbaric exposure within 24 hours, then oxygen should be breathed for both 60 minute periods at 9 msw and during the ascent (total 150 minutes).

Table 63: Deep air–oxygen recompression therapy

Gauge depth (msw)	Stops/ascent (minutes)	Elapsed time (hours and mins)	Rate of ascent (msw/minute)
50	30	00:00 – 00:30	–
50–18	4 (Air)	00:30 – 00:34	8 m in 1 min
18	20 (O_2)	00:34 – 00:54	–
18	5 (Air)	00:54 – 00:59	–
18	20 (O_2)	00:59 – 01:19	–
18	5 (Air)	01:19 – 01:24	–
18	20 (O_2)	01:24 – 01:44	–
18	5 (Air)	01:44 – 01:49	–
18–9	30 (O_2)	01:49 – 02:19	3 m in 10 min
9	15 (Air)	02:19 – 02:34	–
9	60 (O_2)	02:34 – 03:34	–
9	15 (Air)	03:34 – 03:49	–
9	60 (O_2)	03:49 – 04:49	–
9–0	30 (O_2)	04:49 – 05:19	3 m in 10 min
Surface	-	05:19	

DEEP AIR–OXYGEN RECOMPRESSION THERAPY
(TABLE 64)

This table is used for casualties who make an incomplete recovery while undergoing treatment according to USN tables 62, 63 or 67, or for the treatment of DCI in the absence of oxygen.

PROCEDURE FOR TABLE 64:

1. The table may be entered at any depth up to 50 msw from treatment tables 62, 63 or 67. Timing of the table should include any time previously spent at the depth of entry.

2. When employed *de novo* (in the absence of oxygen), the rate of descent should be as fast as can be tolerated by the casualty and attendant. This is normally of the order of 30 msw/minute. Timing of the table commences upon arrival at 50 msw.

3. Ascent between stoppages is to take five minutes. This is not included in the stoppage times, but has been allowed for in the elapsed times.

4. When used to treat a diver following a heliox dive, upon arrival at 50 msw, 40:60 O_2:He should be administered for periods of 20 minutes followed by five minutes breathing 20:80 O_2:He. During the ascent from 50 to 18 msw the casualty should breathe 20:80 O_2:He. If 20:80 O_2:He is not available, then air may be used during the breaks from breathing therapeutic gas at depths between 50 and 18 msw. Upon arrival at 18 msw, 100 per cent oxygen should be administered, with oxygen breathing periods of 25 minutes duration followed by five minutes breathing chamber air. The casualty, who must be closely monitored for evidence of pulmonary oxygen toxicity, should be given a minimum of four oxygen breathing periods (for a total time of two hours) and thereafter to suit the casualty's needs, as advised by a Diving Medicine Specialist. The attendant should begin breathing 100 per cent oxygen two hours before leaving 9 msw, and both the casualty and the attendant should breathe 100 per cent oxygen at 6 and 3 msw as shown in the table.

5. Table 64 may be entered at 30 msw (see Table 67) or 18 msw (see Table 62, Procedure 5), if advised by the Diving Medical Specialist who will also give instructions on the oxygen breathing periods required. This guidance will take into account oxygen breathing before Table 64 was prescribed.

6. Table 64 may be used while breathing air if oxygen is not available. In the absence of heliox, nitrox mixes of up to 40 per cent oxygen may be administered at 50 msw at the discretion of the Diving Medicine Specialist (the casualty must be monitored closely for evidence of pulmonary oxygen toxicity).

NOTE: this is a long Table which should not be entered into without careful consideration. Prior to committing to Table 64, the hyperbaric chamber supervisor must ensure that all life support considerations can be met.

Table 64: Deep air–oxygen recompression therapy

Gauge depth (msw)	Stops/ascent (minutes)	Elapsed time (hours and mins)	Rate of ascent (msw/minute)
50	2 hours	00:00 – 02:00	–
42	30 minutes	02:05 – 02:35	–
36	30 minutes	02:40 – 03:10	–
30	30 minutes	03:15 – 03:45	–
24	30 minutes	03:50 – 04:20	5 minutes between stops throughout
18	6 hours (*Note 1*)	04:25 – 10:25	–
15	6 hours	10:30 – 16:30	–
12	6 hours (*Notes 1, 2*)	16:35 – 22:35	–
9	12 hours	22:40 – 34:40	–
6	1 hour (O_2)	34:45 – 35:45	–
–	1 hour	35:45 – 36:45	–
3	1 hour (O_2)	36:50 – 37:50	–
–	1 hour ($O_2$2)	37:50 – 38:50	–
Surface	–	38:55	

NOTES:
1. Oxygen breathing in accordance with Table 64, Procedure 4.
2. The attendant should breathe oxygen for two hours before leaving 9 msw.

REPEAT HYPERBARIC OXYGEN THERAPY
(TABLE 66)

This table was developed specifically for the treatment of casualties who require hyperbaric oxygen therapy. By limiting the depth to 14 msw, Table 66 reduces the probability of oxygen toxicity occurring amongst casualties who may require a large number of therapies over the course of a number of weeks.

Table 66 is **not** to be used as a primary treatment for acute decompression illness or carbon monoxide poisoning. However, it may be used to re-treat cases of decompression illness and carbon monoxide poisoning in which there has been incomplete recovery or a recurrence of symptoms. (See next page for Table 66.)

PROCEDURE FOR TABLE 66:

1. The casualty should start breathing oxygen on the surface. Casualties who have difficulty clearing their ears while wearing a mask may breathe chamber air until the treatment depth has been reached. Upon reaching the treatment depth, the casualty must immediately commence breathing oxygen.

2. Descend to 14 msw slowly, allowing sufficient time for the casualty to clear his or her ears. The descent will probably be achieved in between five and ten minutes but may take up to 30 minutes.
3. Timing of the treatment commences on reaching 14 msw.
4. The casualty breathes 100 per cent oxygen for three periods of 30 minutes, with a five-minute air break between the oxygen breathing periods.
5. Ascent from 14 msw commences after 20 minutes of the third oxygen period has been completed and is at a continuous bleed rate of 1.4 msw per minute.
6. The attendant must breathe oxygen for the last 20 minutes of the table, including the 10-minute ascent from 14 msw to the surface.
7. Serious cases may require several treatments per day. Where possible, an interval of four hours should be left between treatments.

Table 66: Repeat hyperbaric oxygen therapy

Gauge depth (msw)	Stops/ascent (minutes)	Elapsed time (hours and mins)	Rate of ascent (msw/minute)
14	30 (O_2)	00:00 – 00:30	–
14	5 (Air)	00:30 – 00:35	–
14	30 (O_2)	00:35 – 01:05	–
14	5 (Air)	01:05 – 01:10	–
14	20 (O_2)	01:10 – 01:30	–
14 -0	10 (O_2)	01:30 – 01:40	1.4 m in 1 min
Surface	–	01:40	–

HELIOX/OXYGEN RECOMPRESSION THERAPY (TABLE 67)

This table, a combination of the COMEX 30 Table and RN Table 62, is to be used for treatment in cases of decompression illness with serious symptoms or signs that do not improve, or which continue to deteriorate following an initial compression to 18 msw on 100 per cent oxygen.

It should also be used in all cases of omitted decompression, whether the diver is symptomatic or not, when the diver has completed fewer than 15 minutes of stops and the stops missed were at depths in excess of 18 msw. When contemplated for the treatment of DCI which fails to respond to treatment with standard oxygen recompression tables, the advice of a Diving Medicine Specialist should be sought.

PROCEDURE FOR TABLE 67:

1. The casualty starts breathing 50:50 O_2:He on the surface (or from 18 msw when transferring from RN Table 62). Descend to 30 msw over three to four minutes, stopping only if the casualty or attendant has difficulty in clearing their ears.

Table 67: Heliox–oxygen recompression therapy

NOTE: If 20:80 O_2:He is not available, air may be used.

Gauge depth (msw)	Stops/ascent (minutes)	Elapsed time (hours and mins)	Rate of ascent (msw/minute)
30	20 (50:50 O_2:He)	00:00 – 00:20	–
30	5 (20:80 O_2:He)	00:20 – 00:25	–
30	20 (50:50 O_2:He)	00:25 – 00:45	–
30	5 (20:80 O_2:He)	00:45 – 00:50	–
30	10 (50:50 O_2:He)	00:50 – 01:00	–
30–24	30 (50:50 O_2:He)	01:00 – 01:30	1 m in 5 min
24	5 (20:80 O_2:He)	01:30 – 01:35	–
24	25 (50:50 O_2:He)	01:35 – 02:00	–
24–18	30 (50:50 O_2:He)	02:00 – 02:30	1 m in 5 min
18	5 (Air)	02:30 – 02:35	–
18	20 (O_2)	02:35 – 02:55	–
18	5 (Air)	02:55 – 03:00	–
18	20 (O_2)	03:00 – 03:20	–
18	5 (Air)	03:20 – 03:25	–
18	20 (O_2)	03:25 – 03:45	–
18	5 (Air)	03:45 – 03:50	–
18–9	30 (O_2)	03:50 – 04:20	3 m in 10 min
9	15 (Air)	04:20 – 04:35	–
9	60 (O_2)	04:35 – 05:35	–
9	15 (Air)	05:35 – 05:50	–
9	60 (O_2)	05:50 – 06:50	–
9–0	30 (O_2)	06:50 – 07:20	3 m in 10 min
Surface	–	07:20	

2. Timing of the treatment starts on reaching 30 msw.

3. Upon reaching 30 msw, the casualty must be re-assessed. This assessment should take no more than two to three minutes and, in most cases, will reveal the casualty's condition to have stabilised or be starting to improve. Occasionally, casualties who have presented with serious symptoms arising shortly after surfacing may continue to deteriorate at 30 msw. In such cases, the chamber should be compressed to 50 msw on air with the casualty breathing heliox, 40:60 O_2:He. Decompression will then normally be completed using Table 64. In ALL such cases it is essential to contact a Diving Medical Specialist. In very rare cases, continued deterioration may require transfer to Table 65.

4. If the casualty is free of symptoms and signs after 55 minutes at 30 msw, then decompression may be commenced using Table 67. If the symptoms

have remained static or improved incompletely after 55 minutes at 30 msw, up to five additional 20-minute periods breathing 50:50 O_2:He, separated by five-minute breaks breathing 20:80 O_2:He, may be added on the advice of a Diving Medicine Specialist. On completion of such extensions, decompression should be by Table 64 with 50:50 O_2:He breathed during the ascent from 30–24 msw. A five-minute break breathing 20:80 O_2:He should be taken on arrival at 24 msw with 50:50 O_2:He breathed during the remaining 25 minutes of the 24-metre stop and the ascent from 24–18 msw. Table 64 should then be completed from 18 msw to the surface.

5. If 20:80 O_2:He is not available, then air may be used during the breaks from breathing therapeutic gas at depths between 30 and 18 msw.

   On the advice of a Diving Medical Specialist, Table 67 may be extended by one or two 20-minute oxygen periods, separated by five-minute air breaks, at 18 msw and/or one or two 60-minute oxygen periods, separated by 15-minute air breaks at 9 msw.

6. For an unmodified Table 67, the attendant must breathe oxygen during both 60-minute oxygen periods at 9 msw and during the ascent from 9 msw to the surface (total 150 minutes). If Table 67 is extended at 18 msw, by either one or two additional oxygen periods, it must also be extended by an additional 60-minute oxygen period at 9 msw, during which time the attendant is to breathe oxygen (total 210 minutes).

   If Table 67 is extended at 9 msw, the attendant must breathe oxygen for an additional 60-minute period (total 210 minutes). If the attendant has undergone a hyperbaric exposure in the preceding 24 hours, then Table 67 should be extended at 9 msw to permit the attendant to breathe oxygen for an additional 60-minute period (total 210 minutes).

   In cases where Table 67 is extended at 30 msw, and decompression is by Table 64, the attendant should breathe oxygen as described in the instructions for Table 64 (see page 338).

US NAVY OXYGEN THERAPEUTIC TABLES

The discussion as presented above for the RN tables applies to USN Tables 5, 6 and 6A as well as the deep extended Table 4. The older term, decompression sickness, is still used in the USN tables, which are calibrated in Imperial units (ft and ft/min).

OXYGEN TREATMENT OF PAIN-ONLY DECOMPRESSION SICKNESS (TABLE 5)

This table is used for the treatment of pain-only decompression sickness when the symptoms are relieved within 10 minutes at 60 ft.

PROCEDURE FOR USN TABLE 5:

1. Descent rate: 25 ft/min.
2. Ascent rate: 1 ft/min. Do not compensate for slower ascent rates. Compensate for faster rates by halting the ascent.
3. Time at 60 ft begins on arrival at 60 ft.
4. If oxygen breathing must be interrupted, allow 15 minutes after any reaction has entirely subsided and resume the schedule at the point of interruption.
5. If oxygen breathing must be interrupted at 60 ft, switch to Table 6 upon arrival at the 30 ft stop.
6. Attendant breathes air throughout. If treatment is a repetitive dive for the attendant or tables are lengthened, the attendant should breathe oxygen during the last 30 minutes of ascent to the surface.

USN Table 5: Oxygen treatment of pain-only decompression sickness

Depth (ft)	Time (minutes)	Breathing media	Total elapsed time (hrs:min)
60	20	Oxygen	0:20
60	5	Air	0:25
60	20	Oxygen	0:45
60–30	30	Oxygen	1:15
30	5	Air	1:20
30	20	Oxygen	1:40
30	5	Air	1:45
30–0	30	Oxygen	2:15

OXYGEN TREATMENT OF SERIOUS
DECOMPRESSION SICKNESS (TABLE 6)

This table is used to treat serious or pain-only decompression sickness when the symptoms are **not** relieved within 10 minutes at 60 ft.

PROCEDURE FOR USN TABLE 6:

1. Descent rate: 25 ft/min.
2. Ascent rate: 1 ft/min. Do not compensate for slower ascent rates. Compensate for faster rates by halting the ascent.
3. Time at 60 ft begins on arrival at 60 ft.
4. If oxygen breathing must be interrupted, allow 15 minutes after the reaction has entirely subsided and resume the schedule at the point of interruption.
5. Attendant breathes air throughout. If treatment is a repetitive dive for the attendant or tables are lengthened, attendant should breathe oxygen during the last 30 minutes of ascent to the surface.
6. Table 6 can be lengthened by an additional 25 minutes at 60 ft (20 minutes on oxygen and 5 minutes on air) or an additional 75 minutes at 30 ft (15 minutes on air and 60 minutes on oxygen), or both.

USN Table 6: Oxygen treatment of serious decompression sickness

Depth (ft)	Time (minutes)	Breathing media	Total elapsed time (hrs:min)
60	20	Oxygen	0:20
60	5	Air	0:25
60	20	Oxygen	0:45
60	5	Air	0:50
60	20	Oxygen	1:10
60	5	Air	1:15
60–30	30	Oxygen	1:45
30	15	Air	2:00
30	60	Oxygen	3:00
30	15	Air	3:15
30	60	Oxygen	4:15
30–0	30	Oxygen	4:45

AIR AND OXYGEN TREATMENT OF GAS EMBOLISM
(TABLE 6A)

This table was designed specifically for the treatment of arterial gas embolism. The same considerations as provided for Table 63 RN (see page 336) apply to the use of this table. (See opposite for USN Table 6A.)

USN Table 6A: Air and oxygen treatment of gas embolism

Depth (ft)	Time (minutes)	Breathing media	Total elapsed time (hrs:min)
165	30	Air	0:30
165–60	4	Air	0:34
60	20	Oxygen	0:54
60	5	Air	0:59
60	20	Oxygen	1:19
60	5	Air	1:29
60	20	Oxygen	1:44
60	5	Air	1:49
60–30	30	Oxygen	2:19
30	15	Air	2:34
30	60	Oxygen	3:34
30	15	Air	3:49
30	60	Oxygen	4:49
30–0	30	Oxygen	5:19

PROCEDURE FOR USN TABLE 6A:

1. Descent rate: 20ft/min.
2. Ascent rate: 165–60 fsw not to exceed 3 ft/min, 60 fsw and shallower, not to exceed 1 ft/min. Do not compensate for slower ascent rates. Compensate for faster rates by halting the ascent.
3. Time at treatment depth does not include compression time.
4. Table begins with initial compression to depth of 60 fsw. If initial treatment was at 60 ft, up to 20 minutes may be spent at 60 ft before compression to 165 fsw. Contact a Diving Medical Officer.
5. If a chamber is equipped with high-O_2 treatment gas, it may be administered at 165 fsw and shallower, not to exceed 2.8 ATA oxygen. Treatment gas is administered for 25 minutes interrupted by five minutes of air. Treatment gas is breathed during ascent from the treatment depth to 60 fsw.
6. Deeper than 60 ft, if treatment gas must be interrupted because of CNS oxygen toxicity, allow 15 minutes after the reaction has entirely subsided before resuming treatment gas. The time of treatment gas is counted as part of the time at treatment depth. If at 60 ft or shallower and oxygen breathing must be interrupted because of CNS oxygen toxicity, allow 15 minutes after the reaction has entirely subsided and resume schedule at point of interruption.
7. Table 6A can be lengthened up to two additional 25-minute periods at 60 ft (20 minutes on oxygen and five minutes on air), or up to two additional 75-minute periods at 30 ft (60 minutes on oxygen, 15 minutes on air), or both.

8. Attendant breathes 100 per cent oxygen during the last 60 minutes at 30 fsw and during ascent to the surface for an unmodified table or where there has been only a single extension at 30 or 60 fsw. If there has been more than one extension, the oxygen breathing at 30 fsw is increased to 90 minutes.
    If the attendant has had a hyperbaric exposure within the past 12 hours, an additional 60-minute oxygen breathing period is taken at 30 fsw.
9. If significant improvement is not obtained within 30 minutes at 165 ft, consult a Diving Medical Officer before switching to treatment Table 4.

AIR OR AIR & OXYGEN TREATMENT OF SEVERE DECOMPRESSION SICKNESS OR ARTERIAL GAS EMBOLISM (TABLE 4)

This table is used to treat worsening symptoms during the first 20-minute oxygen breathing period at 60 ft on Table 6 or 6A.

PROCEDURE FOR USN TABLE 4:
1. Descent rate: as rapidly as possible.
2. Ascent rate: 1 minute between stops.
3. Time at 165 ft; this includes time from the surface.
4. If only air is available, then decompress on air. If oxygen is available, casualty begins oxygen breathing upon arrival at 60 ft with appropriate air breaks. Both attendant and casualty breathe oxygen beginning two hours before leaving 30 ft.

USN Table 4: Air or air and oxygen treatment of severe DCS or AGE

Depth (ft)	Time	Breathing media	Total elapsed time (hrs:min)
165	½ to 2 hr	Air	2:00
140	½ hr	Air	2:31
120	½ hr	Air	3:02
100	½ hr	Air	3:33
80	½ hr	Air	4:04
60	6 hr	Air or oxygen/air	10:05
50	6 hr	Air or oxygen/air	16:06
40	6 hr	Air or oxygen/air	22:07
30	12 hr	Air or oxygen/air	34:08
20	2 hr	Air or oxygen/air	36:09
10	2 hr	Air or oxygen/air	38:10
0	1 min	Oxygen	38:11

UNDERWATER AIR RECOMPRESSION THERAPY
(TABLE 1A)

As this table was originally intended for use in a chamber in the management of pain-only decompression sickness when oxygen is unavailable and pain is relieved at a depth of less than 66 feet, using Table 1A in underwater air recompression therapy is dangerous (see Disadvantages, page 189). The ascent is timed by surface tenders, using a signal line.

USN Table 1A: Air recompression therapy

Depth (feet)	Time (mins)	Breathing media	Total elapsed time (hrs:mins)
100	30	Air	0:30
80	12	Air	0:43
60	30	Air	1:14
50	30	Air	1:45
40	30	Air	2:16
30	60	Air	3:17
20	60	Air	4:18
10	120	Air	6:19
0	1	Air	6:20

PROCEDURE FOR USN TABLE 1A UNDER WATER:

1. The diver must be fully dressed and negatively weighted, so that there is no difficulty in maintaining depth under water. A tendency to drift upward is contraindicated.
2. The diver and the attendant will breathe air using conventional scuba. Adequate full spare cylinders plus attached demand valves, sufficient for two people for seven hours each, must be available on the shot line.
3. A shot line clearly marked in 10-feet lengths to 100 feet and adequately weighted is suspended from a buoy large enough to support the two divers easily.
4. If the recompression cannot be done in a sheltered, quiet area, the buoy must be tethered close to the boat.
5. Hand and foot loops, and a seating system, must be fitted to the shot line to assist both the diver and the attendant.
6. The diver and the attendant descend to 100 feet at a rate of 25 feet per minute.
7. The ascent rate is 1 minute between stops.
8. Time at 100 feet includes time from the surface.

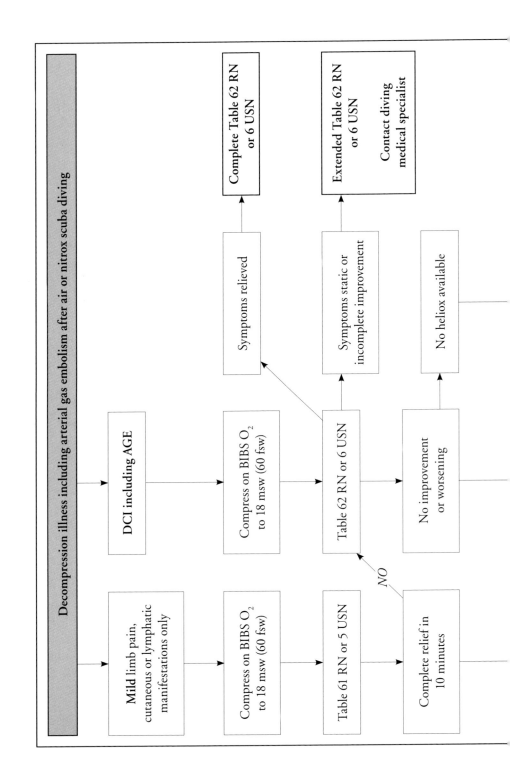

Decompression illness including arterial gas embolism after air or nitrox scuba diving

Mild limb pain, cutaneous or lymphatic manifestations only → Compress on BIBS O$_2$ to 18 msw (60 fsw) → Table 61 RN or 5 USN → Complete relief in 10 minutes

DCI including AGE → Compress on BIBS O$_2$ to 18 msw (60 fsw) → Table 62 RN or 6 USN → Symptoms relieved → **Complete Table 62 RN or 6 USN**

Table 62 RN or 6 USN → Symptoms static or incomplete improvement → **Extended Table 62 RN or 6 USN** / **Contact diving medical specialist**

NO

No improvement or worsening → No heliox available

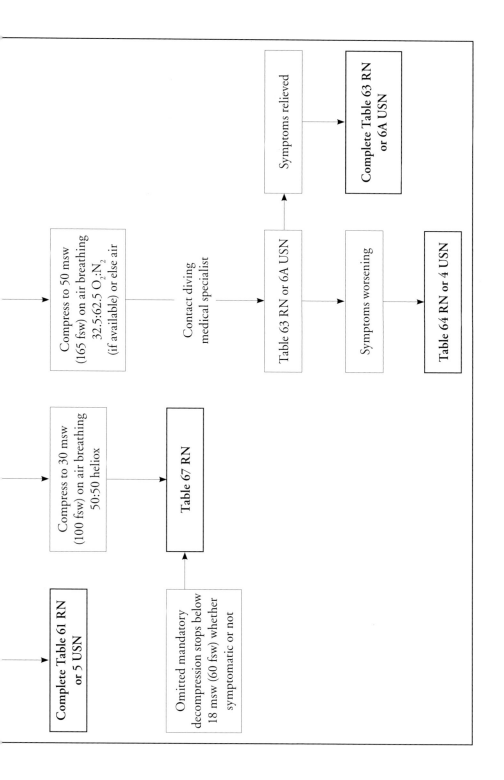

Compress to 50 msw (165 fsw) on air breathing 32.5:62.5 O_2:N_2 (if available) or else air

Compress to 30 msw (100 fsw) on air breathing 50:50 heliox

Complete Table 61 RN or 5 USN

Omitted mandatory decompression stops below 18 msw (60 fsw) whether symptomatic or not

Table 67 RN

Contact diving medical specialist

Table 63 RN or 6A USN

Symptoms relieved

Complete Table 63 RN or 6A USN

Symptoms worsening

Table 64 RN or 4 USN

45. APPENDIX

DIVERS ALERT NETWORK

The Divers Alert Network (DAN) is an internationally-operative service offering free medical and rescue facilities to its member divers, and their families, whatever their home DAN base. It is strongly recommended that all divers join DAN, because a diving emergency can occur anywhere, at any time. Contact and emergency numbers are listed below.

DAN Southern Africa
South Africa; regional responsibility for southern, east Africa; Indian Ocean islands.
Private Bag X 197, Halfway House 1685, South Africa
Tel: 0860 242-242 or +27 (0)11-312-0512; Fax: +27 (0)11-312-0054
Email: mail@dansa.org
Website: www.dansa.org

Diving emergencies:
Toll free: 0800-020-111 (within South Africa)
Emergency hotline: +27-10-209-8112 (for calls from outside SA, accepts collect calls)

DAN USA (International headquarters)
United States and Canada; regional IDAN responsibility for Central and South America, the Caribbean, Polynesia, Micronesia, Melanesia, and areas not designated below.
6 West Colony Place, Durham, NC 27705-5588. USA
Website: www.diversalertnetwork.org
Tel: 1-800-446-2671 (toll-free in the USA)
Tel: +1-919-684-2948 (general enquiries)
Fax: +1-919-490-6630
Medical fax: +1-919-493-3040

Diving emergencies:
DAN America: Tel: +1-919-684-4DAN or +1-919-684-4326 (accepts collect calls)
DAN Latin America: Tel: +1-919-684-9111 (accepts collect calls)

Non-diving emergencies/Travel Assist:
Toll-free: 1-800-326-3822 (1-800-DAN-EVAC)
Collect: +1-919-684-3483 (Use if outside USA, Canada, Puerto Rico, Bahamas, British or U.S. Virgin Islands)

DAN Europe

Continental Europe; regional responsibility for Mediterranean basin, shores of the Red Sea, Middle East (inc. Persian Gulf), Indian Ocean north of the Equator, plus overseas territories, districts and protectorates.
P.O. Box DAN, 64026 Roseto (Te), ITALY
Tel: +39-085-893-0333
Fax: +39-085-893-0050
Email: mail@daneurope.org
Website: www.daneurope.org

Diving emergencies: Tel: +39-06-4211-8685

DAN Japan

Japanese mainland and islands; regional responsibility for northeast Asia-Pacific.
Japan Marine Recreation Association
Kowa-Ota-Machi Bldg, 2F, 47 Ota-Machi 4-Chome, Nakaku, Yokohama City, Kagawa 231-0011 Japan
Tel: +81-45-228-3066
Fax: +81-45-228-3063
Email: dan@danjapan.gr.jp
Website: www.danjapan.gr.jp

Diving emergencies: Tel: +81-3-3812-4999

DAN Asia-Pacific

Australia, New Zealand; regional responsibility for southern Asia-Pacific, Indian Ocean.
DES Australia P.O. Box 384, Ashburton, VIC 3147, Australia.
Tel: +61-3-9886-9166
Fax: +61-3-9886-9155
Email: info@danasiapacific.org
Website: www.danasiapacific.org

Diving emergencies:
Toll free: 1-800-088-200 (within Australia); +61-8-8212-9242 (outside Australia)
DAN/DES New Zealand: 0800-4DES111
DAN Asia-Pacific – Philippines: (02) 632-1077
DAN Asia-Pacific –Malaysia: (05) 681-9485
DAN Asia-Pacific –Korea: (010) 4500-9113
DAN Asia-Pacific –China: +852-3611-7326
Singapore Naval Medicine & Hyperbaric Center: 6758-1733

DIVING ACCIDENT REPORT FORM

1. PERSONAL INFORMATION		
Name of casualty:		
Address:		
Telephone: Work:	Home:	
Date of Birth:	Sex:	Age:
Illnesses, injuries or operations in the past 5 years:		
Health problems in the past 3 months:		
Names and addresses of doctors consulted:		
Smoking: No. per day:	Years smoking:	
Previous smoking history:	Never:	
2. WOMEN ONLY		
At the time of the diving incident:		
Menstruating:	Pregnant:	Using oral contraceptives:

3. DIVING EXPERIENCE

Type of diving qualification: NAUI   PADI   SSI   YMCA   SAUU   Other

Date of latest qualification:	Certification No:
School at which trained:	Tel No:

Certification level:	Openwater 1	Openwater 2
Advanced diver	Dive master	Instructor
SAUU one star	SAUU two star	SAUU three star
Speciality qualifications (eg. ice, cave, wreck)		
Other:		

Total number of dives logged:	Date of most recent diving medical:
Name and address of diving physician:	

4. TYPE OF DIVE		
Sea water:	Freshwater:	Surf entry:
Boat:	Altitude:	Cave:
Night:	Wreck:	Kelp:
Ice:	Deep:	No decompression:
Decompression:	Other:	Water temp:
Was the diver experienced in this type of dive?	Yes	No
Sole dive:	Buddy system:	Trio diving:
Names of divers in group and contact tel. nos:		
Hazards: Entanglement	Entrapment	Live boating

5. TYPE OF DIVING INCIDENT	
Decompression illness:	Pulmonary barotrauma:
Arterial gas embolism:	Squeeze:
Boating:	Drowning:
Near-drowning:	Marine bite or sting:
Other:	

6. TIME AND PLACE	
Date of diving incident:	Time of incident:
Location:	
Time of first obtaining help:	Time when definitive treatment was begun:

7. DETAILS OF CONTACTS HELPING AFTER THE INCIDENT

Sea rescue: Hospital:

Physician: Diver rescue service:

Police: Ambulance Service:

Dive leader or instructor:

Other:

8. DETAILS OF DIVING INCIDENT

(a) Previous dives on the diving trip:

Number of consecutive days of diving:

Dive profiles of previous dives:

DATE AND TIME	DEPTH	BOTTOM TIME	ASCENT TIME	DECOMPRESSION (depth/minutes)

(b) Dive on which the incident occured:

Dive leader's name and address or contact telephone number:

Time dive began: Time of surfacing:

Max depth: Time at bottom: Ascent time:

First dive of day: Y/N   Repetitive dive (how many?)

Any decompression obligations?   Y/N   Stops actually done:

Decompression stops missed:

Required decompression stops (depth/mins):

Dive completed: Dive aborted:

Safety stops performed?   Y/N   Altitude correction used:

Surface interval before the dive: Residual nitrogen time at start of dive:

Ascent (state rate in metres/min where applicable):

Normal: Fast: Assisted by buddy:

Uncontrolled buoyant: Emergency:

Narcosis: Vertigo: Coughing: Vomiting:

Sneezing: Skip breathing: Buddy breathing:

Octopus rig breathing: Out of air:

Other problem:

Dive plan:

Computer (state make of computer):

Table (state table and schedule used):

Additional factors:

Flying between dives?   Y/N   After dive?   Y/N

If yes how long after?   Aircraft pressurised?   Y/N

Alcohol: None   Night before   Pre-dive

                   During dive   Postdive

Drugs or medicines used before the dive?

Exercise pre-dive   During dive   Postdive

Pre-dive fatigue or hangover:

Hot bath or shower postdive:

Other symptoms before diving:

9. EQUIPMENT USED

Suit: Wet	Thickness	Dry	Other

Cylinder size:

Date of last visual inspection of cylinder:

Date of last hydraulic testing of cylinder:

Cylinder air pressure: Pre-dive		Postdive
Cylinder contents gauge:		Depth gauge:

Compressor operator's name:

Compressor operator's registration number:

Boat skipper's name:

Boat skipper's ticket number:

Weight belt: Mass	Own	Borrowed	Dumped
Dive watch:	Own used	Buddy's used	None
Buoyancy vest:	ABLJ	BC	None
Buoyancy inflation:	CO_2 cartridge	Power	Oral
Second stage regulator:		Octopus rig	

Ropes, lines and tools used:

Dive knife	Dive torch	Cyalumes

Equipment failure?

Pre-dive equipment and signals check performed?   Y/N

Pre-dive buoyancy check performed (especially with borrowed weight belt)?   Y/N

Any equipment fault found with pre-dive check?   Y/N

Comment on any equipment fault found:

10. SYMPTOMS AND SIGNS EXPERIENCED AT THE DIVE INCIDENT

Before diving:	On descent:	At bottom:
On ascent:	Immediately after surfacing:	

Later after surfacing (state hrs/mins):

Tick below next to corresponding feature:

Confusion	Headache	Rash
Disorientation	Undue fatigue	Swelling
Dizziness	Numbness	Itching
Unconscious	Pins and needles	Chest pain
Convulsions	Weakness	Abdomen pain
Blurred vision	Difficulty standing	Arm pain R/L
Double vision	Difficulty walking	Leg pain R/L
Tunnel vision	Paralysis	Nausea
Blindness	Speech problem	Vomiting
Ringing in ears	Hoarseness	Coughing
Deafness	Skin mottling	Coughing blood
Ear pain	Squeeze	Breathless

Bleeding:	Minor	Moderate	Major	Site

Fractures:

Wounds:

Death:	At bottom	On surface	Later

Comments:

11. FIRST AID GIVEN				
Mouth to mouth:		CPR:		Oxygen:
Oral fluids:		IV fluids:		Drugs:
Position: Lying flat:		Head down:		Sitting:
Other first aid treatment:				

12. DEFINITIVE TREATMENT

    (a)   Recompression therapy: Y/N

Site of chamber:

Type of chamber: One man   Two man   Multiplace

Date recompression commenced: Time commenced:

Delay between incident and recompression (days/hrs):

Therapeutic tables used:

Chamber operator's name:

Diving physician in charge of recompression:

Result of recompression therapy: Complete relief   Partial relief   No relief

Recurrence of symptoms after recompression: Y/N

Repeat recompression therapy needed: Y/N

Residual problems of defects after treatment (describe):

Final result of therapy: Full recovery   Partial

                          Permanent disability   Death

    (b)   Other therapy:

Attending doctor's name(s):

Hospital admission:

Treatment received:

Results of treatment:

13. COMMENTS

Dated at (place):

Date (DDMMYYYY):

Full name:

Signature:

FIRST AID KITS
AND MEDICAL EQUIPMENT

Major incidents, minor injuries or medical ailments can occur at any time, so it is important that divers can render assistance to themselves and others. A basic first aid certificate should be part of all training, while an advanced first aid or diver rescue qualification is invaluable in times of need. Once trained, you need to maintain your first aid, resuscitation (CPR) and oxygen administration skills through regular practise sessions and refresher courses. Rescue divers must ensure their tetanus boosters are current (you need to get a shot every three years).

Comprehensive medical kits can be purchased from specialist suppliers, or you may elect to assemble a basic kit with the help of your local pharmacy or medical equipment supplier. Store your medical supplies in sturdy, roomy waterproof plastic boxes that are clearly marked and always accessible. When you are diving in remote areas, the contents of your first aid and medical kits should vary according to the type of injury or disease likely to occur, access to professional medical help and facilities, and the first aid skills of your party.

BASIC FIRST-AID KIT

This basic kit should be carried with you on all dive trips. Although it may seem like a long list, most of the items are small and the whole kit should fit into a medium-sized tog-bag. Don't forget to include a first aid manual, stored in a waterproof (zip-lock) bag. There is no point in having the equipment if you don't know what to do with it!

1. Bandages, wound dressings and cleansing materials
- Bandages: crepe: 3 each 50 mm and 75 mm; triangular: 2
- Dressing packs: 2 each small, medium and large
- Sterile dry gauze swabs: 1 pack
- Sterile eye pads: 2
- Paraffin-impregnated gauze squares: 1 pack
- Antiseptic ointment: 1 x 25ml tube
- Burn ointment: 1 tube
- Plasters: 1 roll adhesive tape; 1 box assorted plasters; 1 roll hypoallergenic paper tape; 1 blister kit with moleskin
- Antiseptic liquid (Dettol or Savlon): 1 small bottle
- Cotton wool balls or lint-free swabs: 1 packet
- Assorted safety pins and/or bandage clips

2. Instruments

- 1 CPR mouthpiece with non-return valve
- 2 pairs of latex gloves
- 1 pair clear plastic goggles
- 2 wooden splints
- 1 pair of bandage scissors
- 1 small forceps or tweezers
- 1 eyebath
- 1 thermometer
- 1 instant cold/hot pack
- 1 tourniquet
- 1 disposable aluminium foil blanket (space blanket)

3. Medications

- 1 pack paracetamol tablets
- 1 pack anti-seasickness pills
- 1 tube cortisone cream for sunburn (e.g. Betnovate)
- 1 tube of antihistamine cream for itches and bites
- 1 bottle calamine lotion
- 1 tube antibiotic ointment such as Bactroban or Fucidin
- 1 bottle sterile eye drops
- 1 bottle high SPF water-resistant sunscreen or total block-out cream
- 1 bottle (500 ml) spirit vinegar as a remedy for marine stings

EMERGENCY MEDICAL EQUIPMENT FOR EVERYDAY USE

In addition to a basic first-aid kit, each dive boat should carry the following items:

1. Oxygen

An adequate oxygen supply is essential on every dive trip and no dive boat should take to the water without it. DAN provides compact emergency oxygen units that should suffice for almost any emergency. Contact your local DAN office to discuss your requirements, anticipated oxygen needs and the required training in the use of these units.

2. Shark attack pack

The major trauma that follows a shark attack can prove lethal unless immediate help is available. Having a shark attack pack (see pages 284–285) available can save lives but it does need someone trained in its use, and with at least some paramedical training. The pack is intended for two CPR administrators, is HIV aware and should be assembled separately from other first-aid kits.

MEDICAL KITS FOR TRAVEL TO REMOTE AREAS

If you are travelling to remote dive sites, check beforehand whether a diving medical officer (DMO) or a suitably qualified GP is available in the area and get his/her name, telephone number/s and address. Obtain details of the nearest emergency facilities, including access to a hyperbaric chamber and/or medical oxygen.

Well before you go, make an appointment with your dive doctor or family GP to discuss the medical requirements for the trip. Many medications require a prescription, as well as professional guidance and detailed instruction in their use. Ascertain whether any members of the group have allergies to specific medications, or are taking regular medication that might react with other substances. The items in a general medical kit should be suitable for use by everyone in the group, so clearly mark anything that might cause an adverse reaction in certain members. Individuals must carry a sufficient supply of all prescription medicines they require.

About a fortnight before you leave, contact a travel medical clinic to enquire about any known problems at your destination (e.g. recent outbreaks of malaria or dysentery; the state of fresh water supplies, etc.). Check that all members of the group have been immunised against locally prevalent illnesses, such as cholera or typhoid, and begin malaria prophylaxis timeously, if indicated.

Remember to take water purification tablets and/or filtration equipment with you – do not drink unpurified, suspect water!

General medications for a 'remote areas' first aid kit

(Note: prescription medications should be dispensed with caution by a first aider; preferably with the informed consent of the person who will be taking them!)

- Antimalarial tablets *
- Mosquito repellents and insecticide sprays and coils
- Anti-inflammatories
- Broad-spectrum antibiotics
- Antiemetics, antispasmodics and antidiarrhoeals
- Cold and flu tablets, capsules or effervescents
- Pain-killers (analgesics)
- Rehydration mixtures, especially for children in the party
- Antacid suspensions and tablets
- Antibiotic ear/eye drops
- Snake bite kit if snakes are prevalent in the area
- Low-reading thermometer if any risk of hypothermia exists.
- Multivitamins can be useful on long trips to remote areas where fresh fruits and vegetables may be difficult to come by.

(* Note: Malaria tablets must be individually prescribed to each diver. See pages 248–251 for more information on malaria prophylaxis.)

REFERENCE SOURCES

Baker L. 2008. 'The where, when and who of preventing malaria in travellers'. *Continuing Medical Education*. June; 26 (6): 284–289.

Bassoe P. 1911. 'Compressed air disease'. *J Nerv Ment Dis*. 38: 368–369

Bennett P.B. & Elliot D.H., eds (1999). *The Physiology and Medicine of Diving*, 4th edition. Saunders, London, New York.

Bennett P.B, Cronje F.J, Campbell E, Marroni A, Pollock N.W. 2006. *Assessment of Diving Medical Fitness for Scuba Divers and Instructors*. Best Publishing: Flagstaff, AZ.

Bennett P.B., Marroni A., Cronje F.J., Cali-Corleo R., Germonpre P., Pieri M., Bonuccelli C., Leonardi M.G., Balestra C. 2008. 'Effect of varying deep stop times and shallow stop times on precordial bubbles after dives to 25 msw (82 fsw)'.
Erratum in: *Undersea Hyperb Med*. Jan–Feb; 35(1):6 p following table of contents.

Best C.H., Taylor N.B. 1961. *The physiological basis of medical practice*. 7th ed. Baltimore: Williams and Wilkins.

Blatteau J.E., Hugon M., Gardette B., Sainty J.M., Galland F.M. 2005. 'Bubble incidence after staged decompression from 50 or 60 msw: effect of adding deep stops'. *Aviat Space Environ Med*. May; 76(5):490–2

Blatteau J.E., Gempp E., Galland F.M., Pontier J.M., Sainty J.M., Robinet C. 2005 'Aerobic exercise two hours before a dive to 30 msw decreases bubble formation after decompression'. *Aviat Space Environ Med*. Jul; 76(7):666–9.

Blatteau J.E., Boussuges A., Gempp E., Pontier J.M., Castagna O., Robinet C., Galland F.M., Bourdon L. 2007. 'Haemodynamic changes induced by submaximal exercise before a dive and its consequences on bubble formation'. *Br J Sports Med*. Jun; 41(6):375–9.

Blumberg L. 2008. 'Management of uncomplicated malaria'. *Continuing Medical Education*. June; 26 (6): 290–292.

Boies L.R., Hilger J.A., Priest R.A. 1964. *Fundamentals of otolaryngology*. 4th ed. Philadelphia: W.B. Saunders Company.

Bove A.A. 1983. 'An approach to medical evaluation of the sport diver'. *SPUMS J*. 2: 3–17.

Bove A.A. 1992. 'If the O_2 doesn't get you the CO_2 will'. *Skin Diver*. Nov.:8–9.

Bove A.A 1992. 'Diving science in '92'. *Skin Diver*. Dec.:18–19

Bove A.A. 1996. 'Medical aspects of sport diving'. *Med Sci Sports Exerc*. 28 (5) 591–595.

Bove A.A. 2003. 'Fitness to dive'. Bennett & Elliott's *The Physiology and Medicine of Diving*, pp 700–717, 5th edition, eds Brubakk A.O., Neuman T.S. Saunders, London, New York.

Bove A.A. 2004. Bove and Davis, *Diving Medicine*. Saunders, Philadelphia, USA.

Buehlmann A.A. 1987. 'Decompression after repeated dives'. *Undersea Biomedical Research*. 14(1): 59–66.

Butler F.K. Jr., Thalmann E.D. 1986. 'Central nervous system oxygen toxicity in closed-circuit scuba divers II'. *Undersea Biomedical Research*. 13 (2): 193–223.

Butler F.K. 1995. 'Diving and hyperbaric ophthalmology'. *Survey of Ophthalmology*. 39: 347–366.

Caruso J., Bove A., Uguccioni D., Ellis J., Dovenbarger J., Bennett P. 2001. 'Recreational diving deaths associated with cardiovascular disease: Epidemiology and recommendations for pre-participation screening'. *Undersea Hyper Med*. 28 (sup): 75–6

Clark J.M., Lambertsen C.J. 1971. 'Pulmonary oxygen toxicity: a review'. *Pharmacology Review*. 23(2):37-133

Cousteau J.Y., Cousteau P. 1970. *The shark: splendid savage of the sea*. New York: Doubleday & Co., Inc.

Cross, E.R. 1992. 'Why I won't use nitrox for recreational diving'. *Skin Diver*. Nov.: 10–11.

Currents. Winter 2005–2006. 'Emergency cardiovascular care'. Vol.16; No. 4.

Daniels S., Halsey M.J., Smith E.B. 1980. 'Techniques for diving deeper than 1500 ft'. *23rd Undersea Medical Society workshop*. 19–21 Mar. 1980. Bethesda: Undersea Medical Society, Inc.

Davis B. 1983. Lecture on shark attacks at Aqua-Medic Disaster Symposium. Wild Coast SA: Personal observations.

Davis J.C. 1986. *Medical examination of sport divers*. 2nd ed. San Antonio, Texas: Medical Seminars Inc.

Davis R.H. 1955. *Deep diving and submarine operations*. London: St. Catherine's Press.

Decloedt E., Cohen K., 2008. 'Asthma pharmacotherapy – the goal is optimised control'. *Continuing Medical Education*. April; 26 (4): 206-210.

Diving Medical Advisory Committee Workshop. 1981. 'Thermal stress in relation to diving'. 19–20 Mar. 1981. Institute of Naval Medicine, Gosport: Undersea Medical Society, Inc.

Dueker C.W. 1970. *Medical aspects of sport diving*. London: A.S Barnes & Co.

Dujic Z., Duplancic D., Marinovic-Terzic I., Bakovic D., Ivancev V., Valic Z., Eterovic D., Petri N.M., Wisløff U., Brubakk A.O. 2004. 'Aerobic exercise before diving reduces venous gas bubble formation in humans'. *J Physiol*. Mar 16;555(Pt 3):588.

Dujic Z., Palada I., Obad A., Duplancic D., Bakovi D., Valic Z.. 2005. 'Exercise during a 3-min decompression stop reduces postdive venous gas bubbles'. *Med Sci Sports Exerc*. Aug;37(8):1319–23.

Dujic Z., Palada I., Valic Z., Duplancic D., Obad A., Wisløff U., Brubakk A.O. 2006. 'Exogenous nitric oxide and bubble formation in divers'. *Med Sci Sports Exerc*. Aug;38(8):1432–5.

Edge C., Lindsay D., Wilmshurst, P. 1992. '*The diving diabetic*'. Diver Feb.: 35–36.

Edge C. 'Diving and Diabetes'. UK Sports Diving Medical Committee. http://www.cru.uea.ac.uk/ukdiving/medicine/diabetes.htm

Edmonds C., Lowry C., Pennefather J. 1981. *Diving and subaquatic medicine*. 2nd ed. N.S.W. Australia: Diving Medical Centre.

Egstrom G.H., Bachrach, A. 1971. 'Diver Panic'. *Skin Diver* magazine. Nov. 1971.

Elliott D.H., ed 1994. 'Medical Assessment of Fitness to Dive'. Proceedings International Conference, Edinburgh. Best Publishing Co., Flagstaff, AZ, USA.

Encyclopaedia Britannica. 1970. 'Diving, deep-sea'. 7:507-510D. Chicago: William Benton.

European Undersea Biomedical Society. 1991. Proceedings XVIIth annual meeting on diving and hyperbaric medicine. 29 Sep– 3 Oct. 1991. Heraklion/Crete: EUBS.

Feldman C. 2008. 'Asthma: second-line therapies'. *Continuing Medical Education*. April; 26 (4): 184-186.

Francis T.J.R., Dutka A.J. 1989. 'Methyl prednisolone in the treatment of acute spinal cord decompression sickness'. *Undersea Biomedical Research*. 16(2): 165-172.

Gleason B. 1992. 'Just say no to nitrox?' *Skin Diver*. Nov: 6–7.

Graver D.K. 1993. 'Flying and diving'. *Skin Diver*. Aug: 23–24.

Greer H.D. 1994. 'Diabetes and diving'. *Pressure*. 23(4): 7.

Grimstad J. ed. 1979. 5th Annual Scientific Meeting 5–6 July 1979, Bergen/Norway: European Undersea Biomedical Society.

Halstead B.W. 1980. *Dangerous marine animals*. 2nd ed. Maryland: Cornell Maritime Press.

Hamilton R.W. 1975. 'Development of decompression procedures for depths in excess of 400 ft'. The 9th Undersea Medical Society workshop. 21–23 Feb 1975. Bethesda: Undersea Medical Society, Inc.

Hamilton,R.W. et al. 1988. 'REPEX: Development of repetitive excursions, surfacing techniques, and oxygen procedures for habitat diving'. National Undersea Research Program. Technical reports 88-1A & 88-1B. Maryland: NOAA, US Dept. Commerce.

Harrison J.L. 1992. 'Drugs and diving'. *Journal Florida Medical Assoc*. 79:165–167.

Harrison T.R. et al. 1962. *Principles of internal medicine.* 4th ed. New York: McGraw Hill

Hickey D.D. 1984. 'Outline of medical standards for divers'. *Undersea Biomedical Research.* 11(4): 407-430.

Hughes G.S., et al. 1996. 'Physiology and pharmokinetics of a novel haemoglobin-based oxygen carrier in humans'. *Crit Care Med.* 24:756–764.

Irusen E.M. 2008. 'Asthma: primary therapies'. *Continuing Medical Education.* April; 26 (4): 180–182.

Jenkins C., Anderson S.D., Wong R., Veale A. 1993. 'Compressed air diving and respiratory disease'. *The Medical Journal of Australia.* 158: 276–279.

Kent M.B. ed. 1980. 'Effects of diving on pregnancy'. The 19th Undersea Medical Society Workshop. 2–3 Nov 1978. Bethesda: Undersea Medical Society, Inc.

Kent M.B. ed. 1979. 'Emergency ascent training'. The 15th Undersea Medical Society Workshop. 10–11 Dec 1977. Bethesda: Undersea Medical Society, Inc.

Kling S., 2008. 'Exercise-induced asthma'. *Continuing Medical Education.* April; 26 (4): 202–204.

Kloeck W.G.J. 1993. 'New Recommendations for basic life support in adults, children, and infants'. *CME.* April 11(4): 763–780.

Kloeck W.G.J. 1993. 'Choking'. *South African Family Practice Manual.* Jun–Aug 6:06.

Kuehn L.A. ed. 1980. 'Thermal constraints in diving'. The 24th Undersea Medical Society Workshop. 3–4 Sep 1980. Bethesda: Undersea Medical Society, Inc.

Landsberg P.G. 1988. 'Hyperventilation: an unpredictable danger to the sports diver'. Ch18: 292–305. *South Africa's second underwater handbook.* ed. A.J. Venter. Rivonia, Johannesburg: Ashanti Press.

Lanphier E.H. ed. 1980. 'The unconscious diver: Respiratory control and other contributing factors'. 25th Undersea Medical Society Workshop. 18–20 Sep 1980. Bethesda: Undersea Medical Society.

Lee H.C., Niu K.C., Chen S.H. et al. 1991. 'Therapeutic effects of different tables on Type II decompression sickness'. *J. Hyperbaric Medicine.* 6(1): 11–17.

Lloyd's Register of Shipping. 1980. 'Rules and regulations for the construction and classification of submersibles and diving systems'. London: Lloyd's Register Printing House.

Lundgren C.E.G. ed. 1978. 'Monitoring vital signs in the diver'. 16th Undersea Medical Society Workshop. 17–18 Mar 1978. Bethesda: Undersea Medical Society, Inc.

Marroni A, Bennett P.B., Cronje F.J., Cali-Corleo R, Germonpre P, Pieri M, Bonuccelli C, Balestra C. 2005. 'A deep stop during decompression from 82 fsw (25m) significantly reduces bubbles and fast tissue gas tensions'. *Undersea Hyperb Med.* Mar–Apr;32(2):85–8; author reply 89–92.

Mebane G.Y. & McIver N.K. 1993. 'Fitness to dive'. *The Physiology and Medicine of Diving*, pp 53–76, 4th edition. Eds, Bennett P.B. & Elliott D.H. Saunders, London, New York.

Melamed Y., Shupak A., Bitterman H. 1992. 'Medical problems associated with underwater diving'. *The New England Journal of Medicine.* Jan 2 1992: 30–33.

Miller J.W. ed. et al. 1976. 'Vertical excursions breathing air from nitrogen-oxygen or air saturation exposures'. National Oceanic and Atmospheric Administration, Washington DC: US Government Printing Office.

Ministry of Defence. 1972. *Diving manual B.R. 2806.* London: Ministry of Defence (Navy).

Moon R.E., Camporesi E.M., Kisslo J.A. 1989. 'Patent foramen ovale and decompression sickness in divers'. *Lancet* 1(8637): 513–514.

Morgan W.P., 1995. 'Anxiety and panic in recreational scuba divers'. *Sports Medicine.* 20:398–421.

Murphy G. 1992. 'Nitrox ban in the Caribbean'. *Skin Diver.* Nov: 12.

Murphy G. 1992. 'Nitrox: Miracle gas or double jeopardy?' *Skin Diver.* Dec.: 30–31, 167.

O'Brien J., 2008. 'Difficult asthma'. *Continuing Medical Education.* April; 26 (4): 196–199.

Payling Wright G. 1960. *An introduction to pathology.* 3rd ed. London: Longmans.

Pollock N.W. 'Aerobic fitness and underwater diving'. 2007. *Diving Hyperbaric Medicine*. 37(3): 118-124.

Richardson D. 1993 'Current philosophy and practice for emergency ascent training for recreational divers'. *SPUMS J*. 23 (4):214–222

Richardson D. 1994. 'A training organisation perspective of emergency ascent training'. *The Undersea Journal*. 2nd Quarter: 93-99.

Shilling C.W., Story P. 1982. *Man in the cold environment. A bibliography*. Bethesda: Undersea Medical Society, Inc.

Smith D.J., Francis T.J.R. 1991. 'A descriptive approach to reclassifying decompression disorders'. *Proceedings XVIIth annual meeting on diving and hyperbaric medicine*. 29 Sep–3 Oct 1991. Heraklion, Crete: EUBS.

Smith E. 1993. 'Malaria treatment and prophylaxis'. *Modern Medicine of South Africa*. June: 53–66.

SPUMS Policy on emergency ascent training. *SPUMS J*. 1993: 23 (4):239.

Strauss R.H. ed. 1976. *Diving medicine*. New York: Grune & Stratton.

Taylor M.B. 1997. 'Women in diving'. In ed Bove A.A. *Diving Medicine*. pp 89–107.

Teichler M. ed. 1993. 'Burns'. *South African Family Practice Manual*. Jun–Aug. 6:48-49.

Tuerk G.M. ed. 1975. 'Emergency medical technician/diver workshop'. Bethesda: Undersea Medical Society, Inc.

Undersea Medical Society. 1978. 'Decompression theory'. 17th Undersea Medical Society Workshop. 6–7 Sep 1978. Bethesda: Undersea Medical Society, Inc.

US Navy Diving Manual. 1979. Washington, DC. US Govt. Printing Office.

Walker R. 2002. 'Medical standards for recreational divers'. *Diving and Subaquatic Medicine*, ch 53-61, pp 533-614, 4th ed. Eds Edmonds C, Lowry C, Pennefather J, Walker R., Arnold, London, New York.

Walsh J.M. ed. 1980. 'Interaction of drugs in the hyperbaric environment'. 21st Undersea Medical Society Workshop. 13–14 Sep 1979. Bethesda: Undersea Medical Society, Inc.

Wendling J., Ehrsam R., Knessl P., Nussberger P., Uske A. 2001 'Medical assessment of fitness to dive'. International Edition. *Hyperbaric Editions*, CH 2502 Biel. ISBN 3-95222284

Wendling J., Elliott D., Nome T. 2004. 'Medical Assessment of Working Divers'. *Hyperbaric Editions*, Biel, Switzerland.

INDEX

EMERGENCY NUMBERS